W9-CCG-085

H_1 AND H_2 HISTAMINE RECEPTORS

H_1 AND H_2 HISTAMINE RECEPTORS

Edited by

Guy A. Settipane, M.D.

Associate Clinical Professor of Medicine, Brown University and
Department of Medicine, Rhode Island Hospital

FIRST EDITION

OceanSide Publications, Inc.

Providence, Rhode Island 1988–1989

OceanSide Publications, Inc.

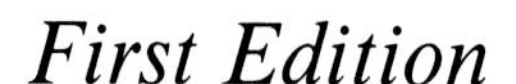
First Edition

Library of Congress Catalog Card Number 87-90733

Published by OceanSide Publications, Inc., 95 Pitman Street,
Providence, Rhode Island 02906

Copyright © 1988–1989 by OceanSide Publications, Inc.

All rights reserved. No part of this publication may be reproduced, stored in a retrieval system, or transmitted, in any form or by any means, electronic, mechanical, photocopying, recording, or otherwise, without prior written permission from the publisher.

Printed in the United States of America

ISBN 0-936587-02-4

Contributors

Robert Altman, M.D.
Clinical Instructor of Pediatrics
New York University Medical School
New York, NY

Peter J. Barnes, D.M., F.R.C.P.
Department of Clinical Pharmacology
The Cardiothoracic Institute
Brompton Hospital
London SWE, UK

Michael A. Beaven, Ph.D.
Deputy Chief
Laboratory of Chemical Pharmacology
National Heart, Lung, and Blood Institute
National Institutes of Health
Bethesda, Maryland

Dennis J. Beer, M.D.
Assistant Professor of Medicine
Pulmonary Center
Evans Memorial Department of Clinical Research
Boston University School of Medicine
Boston, MA

Sidney S. Braman, M.D.
Associate Professor
Bio-Med Medicine, Brown University
Director, Division of Pulmonary Diseases
Rhode Island Hospital
Providence, Rhode Island

C. Edward Buckley III, M.D.
Professor of Medicine and Assistant Professor of Immunology
Duke University Medical Center
Durham, North Carolina

Robert B. P. Burns, M.D.
Director of Clinical Research, Sandoz, Inc.,
East Hanover, New Jersey 07936

Thomas B. Casale, M.D.
Assistant Professor
Department of Internal Medicine
University of Iowa Hospital and Clinic
Iowa City, Iowa

John T. Connell, M.D.
Director, Nasal Diseases Study Center
Holy Name Hospital
Englewood, New Jersey

James W. Cooper, Jr., Ph.D., FCP
Associate Professor
Head, Department of Pharmacy Practice
University of Georgia School of Pharmacy
Athens, Georgia

Joel L. Cristol, M.D.
Associate Professor of Medicine
Chief, Allergy Teaching Program
Chicago Medical School
North Chicago, Illinois

Saul Feldman, M.D.
Associate Clinical Professor of Gastroenterology
Yale University Medical Center
New Haven, Connecticut

Harold M. Friedman, M.D.
Associate Professor of Clinical Medicine
Dartmouth Medical School
Hanover, New Hampshire

C. Robin Ganellin, Ph.D.
Honorary Professor of Medicinal Chemistry
University of Kent at Canterbury, England

Monique Garbarg, Dr. Sci.
Maitre de Recherches CNRS
Unite de Neurobiologie
Centre Paul Broca de l'INSERM
2 ter rue d'Alesia 75014
PARIS

Steven S. Gross, Ph.D.
Department of Pharmacology
Cornell University Medical College
New York, New York

Basil I. Hirschowitz, M.D.
Division of Gastroenterology
University of Alabama
Birmingham, Alabama

Philip N. Johnson, Ph.D.
Associate Director
Department of Pharmacy
Rhode Island Hospital, 593 Eddy Street,
Providence, Rhode Island 02906

Michael A. Kaliner, M.D.
Allergic Diseases Section
Chief, Laboratory of Clinical Investigation
National Institute of Allergy and Infectious Diseases
National Institutes of Health,
Building 10, Room 11C205
Bethesda, Maryland 20205

James P. Kemp, M.D.
Chief of the Division of Allergy
Children's Hospital & Health Center
San Diego, CA

Stephen J. Klemawesch, M.D.
Duke University Medical Center
Durham, North Carolina

Roberto Levi, M.D.
Professor of Pharmacology
Cornell University Medical College
New York, New York

Stephen K. Lucas, M.D.
Duke University Medical Center
Durham, North Carolina

Jonathan Moss, M.D., Ph.D.
Associate Professor of Anesthesiology
Harvard Medical School
Boston, Massachusetts

James L. Perhach, Ph.D.
Director, Clinical Investigation
Wallace Laboratories
Cranbury, NJ

James A. Ray, D.V.M., Ph.D.
Janssen Pharmaceutica, Inc.
40 Kingsbridge Road
Piscataway, NJ 08854

Jean-Charles Schwartz, Dr. Sci.
Professor, Universite Rene Descartes, Paris
Head, Unite de Neurobiologie
Centre Paul Broca de l'INSERM,
2 ter rue d'Alesia 75014
PARIS

Guy A. Settipane, M.D.
Clinical Associate Professor, Brown University
Director, Division of Allergy
Department of Medicine
Co-Director, Allergy Training Program
Rhode Island Hospital
Providence, Rhode Island

F. Estelle R. Simons, M.D.
Professor of Pediatrics
University of Manitoba, Canada

Sheldon L. Spector, M.D.
Professor of Medicine
University of California School of Medicine
Los Angeles, CA

Andrew A. Wolff, M.D.
Department of Pharmacology
Cornell University Medical College
New York, New York

Elizabeth WoldeMussie, Ph.D.
Laboratory of Chemical Pharmacology
National Heart, Lung and Blood Institute
National Institutes of Health
Bethesda, Maryland

FOREWORD

As an intern in 1944 by happenstance I had the good fortune to rotate through the department doing the initial clinical trials of diphenhydramine in this country (though of course other antihistamines had been in use in Europe for some time). The excitement over this drug's efficacy was pervasive. It seemed that this was THE cure for most allergic diseases—an expectation which was prophetic of the initial reaction to cortisone therapy some years later. Considering the relative lack of other therapeutic options for many allergic diseases in the 1940's, there was indeed good reason for enthusiasm. Although side effects were noted, in that era they seemed much less important than in our currently more demanding milieu.

Needless to say, widespread use of the initially available antihistamine drugs revealed not only their usefulness but also their limitations with respect both to efficacy and side effects. Thus over the following 25 years interest in these compounds waned. Investigators were inclined to regard this approach to therapy as "old hat", and more attention was directed towards mechanisms of histamine release, the possible role of other mediators in allergic and other inflammatory processes, and corticosteroid effects.

The subsequent delineation of H1 and H2 receptors in the early 1970's, however, initiated a marked renaissance of interest in antihistamines which has been productively sustained until the present. Although initially based on bioassays, increasing basic knowledge of cell membrane receptor function and structure has markedly enhanced progress in this area. Of particular importance has been the application of radioligand binding techniques to the identification of cell membrane receptors and the assessment of agonist inhibitors. Also of obvious importance has been the increasing expertise of pharmaceutical chemists in designing and synthesizing compounds which would be expected to inhibit the binding of histamine by H1 and H2 receptors. In addition to their therapeutic potential, H1 and H2 antagonists provide important probes for assessing the role of histamine in various types of inflammation (although other possible pharmacologic effects of these drugs also must be taken into consideration).

As indicated in this book, much has been learned about H1 and H2 receptors, but information on this subject still is incomplete. For example, the importance of H2 receptors in some tissues is uncertain. This has significant therapeutic implications with respect to whether H2 as well as H1 histamine antagonists should be employed in treating some diseases. Situations calling for combined H1 and H2 antihistamine therapy are described in this text, and it is very possible that there are broader indications for combined treatment. Some reassessment of the clinical use of H1 antihistamines alone also is appropriate with the recently developed very potent compounds having minimal side effects. Future work of a related type no doubt will involve the study of receptors for histamine releasing factors, and of course concomitant efforts to inhibit the release of histamine and other mediators of inflammation are ongoing.

These reflections on antihistamine therapy over the professional lifetime of an interested individual are intended to induce physicians to be more appreciative of the work and progress which the contents of this volume represent.

Kenneth P. Mathews, M.D.
March, 1987

"Man has the inherent capacity to self destruct if the neatly packaged and preformed histamine in his mast cells and basophiles are released all at one time. Indeed, the status quo may be extremely fragile in some individuals whose salvation depends on still another drop in the bottomless pit of medical knowledge. The advancement of medical science is an important means of steering our day to day fate, which is the vehicle of life. In this book, the status, knowledge, and scientific advancement of histamine receptors are pitted together to help extend and understand the bridge of life."

Guy A. Settipane, M.D.

PREFACE

The human body contains enough histamine in its tissue to destroy itself if it is released in large enough quantities at one time. Indeed, this self destructive mechanism has been activated in patients with cold induced urticaria who have dived into a frigid swimming pool or in those sensitive patients who received bee stings, injections of penicillin, or nonimmunological stimuli such as radiocontrast media and other drugs. Yet, physiological amounts of histamines are needed for mucus and gastric acid production, gastrointestinal motility, cerebral neural transmission, initiating the healing phase and cellular chemotactic responses in trauma, expulsion of foreign objects by allergic reactions, and initiating protective neural reflexes, as well as many other actions. To protect itself from an abnormal release of this toxic chemical, the human body has developed elaborate check and balance systems including neurological and chemical mediators. An important part of this check and balance as well as physiological action involve the two main histamine receptors: the H1 and H2 receptor. In this book, biochemistry, physiology, pathology, mechanism and treatment involving these receptors will be reviewed in detail in the first section followed by a discussion of current and investigative antihistamines that inhibit the actions of the H1 and H2 histamine receptors. Special emphasis is placed on H1 and H2 histamine receptor action in the nose, lungs, heart, gut, skin, and brain by devoting a chapter to each of these organs.

The antihistamine section is initiated by reviewing the proper methods of studying antihistamines and by reviewing the presently commercially available drugs. The last section reports on the exciting developments of new antihistamines that certainly will have a profound effect on future treatment of patients.

Some of the material in the book has been updated from a national symposium held at Brown University on H1 and H2-histamine receptors and publications from the New England and Regional Allergy Proceedings. Other sections have been added for completeness and cohesion resulting in a very unique, informative and indexed publication that is of interest to many specialties in medicine. Histamine crosses the interdisciplinary lines of modern medical practice.

Guy A. Settipane, M.D.

Acknowledgement: I thank my assistant **Patricia J. Nocera** and our publishing staff: Carole Fico, Virginia Loiselle, Sally Martone, Joseph M. Settipane, and Linda Twardowski for their help in publishing this book.

H_1 AND H_2 HISTAMINE RECEPTORS

Editor, Guy A. Settipane, M.D.

TABLE OF CONTENTS

GENERAL CONSIDERATIONS

Chapter I

Histamine in Body Fluids: Its Measurement in Different Clinical States

Michael A. Beaven, Ph.D., Elizabeth WoldeMussie, Ph.D.

ABSTRACT

Measurement of histamine levels in plasma and body fluids is a useful indicator of mast cell or basophil degranulation during pathological reactions. Changes in histamine levels are usually well correlated with changes in pathophysiological parameters. Examples of such correlations in diseases associated with abnormal numbers of mast cells (mastocytosis) and basophils (chronic myelogenous leukemia, polycythemia vera) or reactions associated with mast cell degranulation (asthmatic attacks, physically-induced urticarias, anaphylactic or drug reactions) are described. Procedures developed in the authors' as well as other laboratories and the precautions that should be observed in the measurement of histamine in body fluids are critically reviewed.

INTRODUCTION

This Symposium is concerned with the interaction of histamine and therapeutic agents with H_1 and H_2 histamine receptors. As will be evident from other speakers at this Symposium, the sensitivity of receptor systems to histamine and the antihistamines are readily measured *in vitro* and *in vivo*. Nevertheless, we are unable to estimate the concentrations of histamine in the vicinity of these receptors under normal and pathological conditions. We do not know the intraorgan distribution of histaminocytes, the metabolizing enzymes or the target receptors nor can we assess the factors that influence the disposition of histamine at the receptors. With the techniques available, we can measure the changes in histamine levels in various body fluids during pathological reactions and, in some cases, correlate these changes with pathophysiological parameters. Although we assume that these changes reflect the extent and time course of histamine release, they do not necessarily represent the actual levels of free histamine in tissues from which histamine is released. In this paper, we will discuss the techniques for measurement of histamine levels in body fluids, indicate what these levels are in the disorders in which histamine is clearly involved, and point out some of the factors that should be considered in planning experimental protocols.

Laboratory of Chemical Pharmacology, National Heart, Lung, and Blood Institute, Bethesda, Md. 20205

HISTAMINE ASSAY PROCEDURES

As with most biologically active substances, the discovery and early measurements of histamine in tissues and fluids was dependent on the availability of reliable biological assay systems[1-3] and indeed these were the only methods available to us for over 20 years. These methods were not sufficiently sensitive to measure histamine in normal plasma even when additional purification steps were included.[4] The first reliable chemical assay was described by Shore and co-workers in 1959. In this procedure histamine was extracted and derivatized with o-phthalaldehyde (OPT) to form a highly fluorescent product. Interference, principally from polyamines, and lack of sensitivity made the method unsuitable for assay of histamine in plasma. These difficulties were circumvented by the use of column chromatography[5-7] and

Table I

Radioenzymatic Assays For Histamine

Procedure	Reagents	Max. No Samples*	Histamine Conc. Sample/vol.
1) Double isotope	HMT, ^{14}C-SAMe β-^{3}H-Histamine	50	0.5 - 50 ng/100 μl
2) Single-step	HMT, ^{14}C-SAMe	75	0.25 - 2.5 ng/10 μl
3) Multiple-step	HMT, ^{3}H-SAMe, BSA	50	0.0025-1.0 ng/10 μl

* *Maximum number of samples (in duplicate) handled in one assay.*[13,18,24]

HPLC[8] to further purify or concentrate the extracted product. An automated fluorometric assay[9,10] has also been developed. This procedure has been adopted by several laboratories, because it is convenient and permits the assay of large numbers of samples. The most recently developed category of assays are those based on radioenzymatic procedures.[11] Plasma or tissue extracts are incubated with a partially purified preparation of histamine-N-methyltransferase (HMT) and ^{3}H- or ^{14}C-labeled S-adenosyl-L-methionine (SAMe-^{3}H or SAMe-^{14}C). The radiolabeled methyl group is transferred to histamine to form labeled N_{τ}-methylhistamine which can be readily extracted into an organic solvent from the reaction mixture. Later improvements include the use of unlabeled N_{τ}-Methylhistamine as a carrier to minimize the loss of labeled product,[12] the use of a rat kidney HMT preparation which is more active than the guinea pig brain HMT preparation used in the original assay,[13] and the inclusion of additional extraction or TLC purification steps to separate N_{τ}-methylhistamine from interfering labled products.[14-18]

THE RADIOENZYMATIC ASSAY

We have used exclusively the radioenzymatic assay and for this reason I will illustrate the present state-of-the-art by discussing these assays in particular. Our choice of the radioenzymatic assay was dictated by the need to assay histamine in plasma samples from small laboratory animals[19-21] or to monitor the time course of histamine release from mast cells or basophils in suspension or tissue culture.[22-26] The volumes required for the assay, 5 to 10μl, are ideal for this type of work.

We use 3 procedures; the double isotope assay,[12,13] a rapid single step assay, and a more sensitive multiple step assay[18] (Table I). Each has special advantages and serves different purposes.

The double isotope procedure, for example, is used where precision rather than sensitivity is required. In this procedure the sample is incubated with HMT, SAMe-^{14}C and side chain labeled ^{3}H-histamine, which is added as an internal standard. The labeled product, N_{τ}-methylhistamine, is selectively extracted into chloroform at alkaline pH from unreacted labeled reagent and histamine. The chloroform is evaporated to dryness (chloroform quenches the liquid scintillation system) and assayed for ^{3}H and ^{14}C. The extracted ^{14}C counts are corrected for recovery of ^{3}H label. The data can be plotted graphically or analyzed by computer.[27]

The single step procedure is used to assay samples that contain more than 25 ng histamine/ml. The procedure,(Fig. 1) requires the incubation (90 min 37°) of 10 μl of sample or histamine standard with 30 μl of reagent (HMT, SAMe-^{14}C in pH 7.9 buffer) in a 1.5 ml polypropylene tube. The reaction is terminated by sequential addition of a solution of unlabeled methylhistamine in perchloric acid, 10 N NaOH and a mixture of toluene/isoamyl alcohol (80+20). The tubes are capped, centrifuged (18,000 g for 1 min) and 300 μl of the organic phase transferred directly to counting vials for assay of radioactivity. The toluene/isoamyl alcohol mixture does not quench the cocktail system, yields low blank values but, unlike chloroform, does not selectively extract labeled methylhistamine from labeled histamine and is unsuitable for the double isotope assay.

The multiple step assay was devised after an extensive evaluation of all aspects of the radioenzymatic assay.[18] Since then, we have found that the addition of bovine serum albumin to the reagent containing SAMe-^{3}H and rat kidney HMT stabilizes SAMe-^{3}H and thereby reduces the reaction blank which can be troublesome when the highly labeled SAMe-^{3}H is used as the methyl donor.[24] The procedure is outlined in Figure 1 and is similar to the

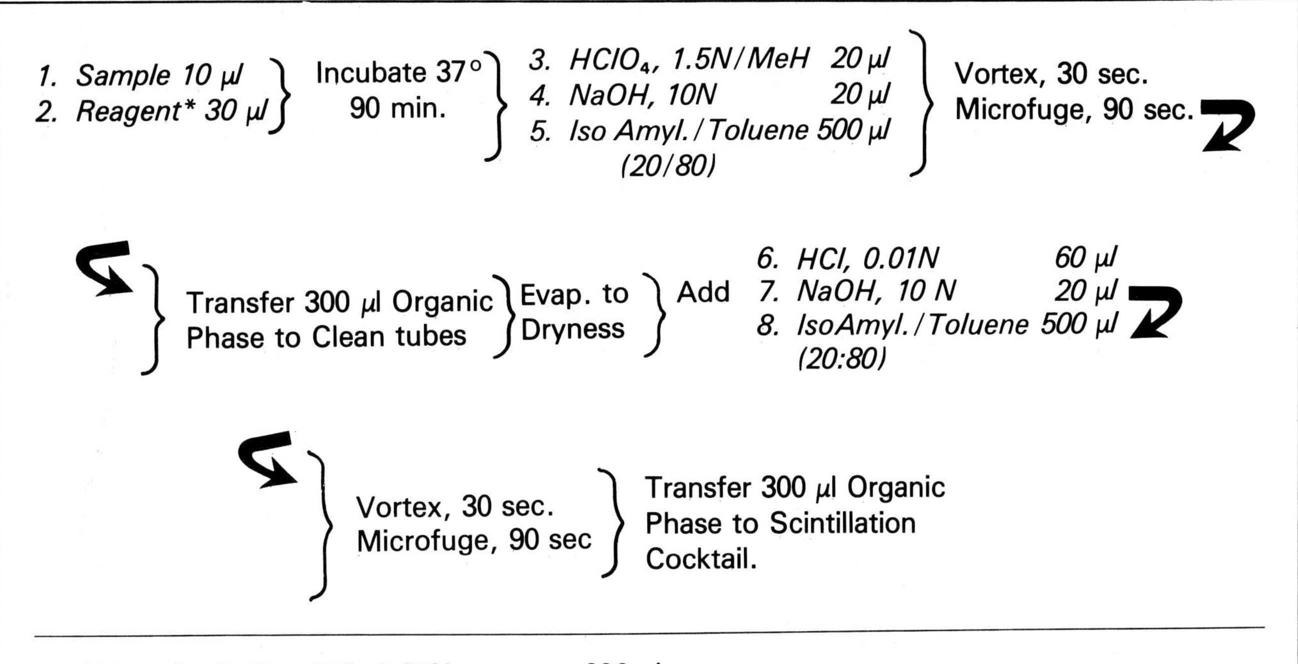

*Phosph. Buffer, 7.9, 0.05N	920 μl
Bovine Serum Albumin	33 mg
SAMe-^{3}H(10Ci/mmole:500 μCi/ml)	67 μl (33 μCi)
Rat-Kidney Enzyme	13 μl (5 μg Protein)

Figure 1. *Procedure for the single isotope assay with SAMe-^{3}H (complete scheme shown). For the single step assay, where SAMe-^{14}C is used as the methyl donor, the steps enclosed within the box are omitted and the reagent mixture consists of phosphate buffer (pH 7.9, 1000 μl), rat kidney enzyme (7* μl), and SAMe-^{14}C (0.2 μCi).[24]

single step assay except that an additional extraction step is included to reduce the reaction blank. To obtain reasonably low values for blanks, the final concentration of SAMe-^{3}H (2 x 10^{-6}M) in the incubation mixture is lower than the concentration of SAMe-^{14}C (2.5 x 10^{-5}M) used in the single step assay. The concentration of enzyme preparation is critical however. Too low a concentration will result in incomplete conversion to labeled methylhistamine when small amounts of histamine are present.[24]

SPECIFICITY AND SENSITIVITY OF THE RADIOENZYMATIC ASSAYS:ASSAY OF HISTAMINE IN SINGLE MAST CELLS

The high specificity of the enzymatic assay results from the high specificity of HMT for histamine. To date no known naturally occurring product interferes with the assay although a number of histamine agonists and antagonists drugs inhibit HMT activity and do cause problems.[28,29] With SAMe-^{3}H extraneous labeled material is extracted along with the labeled methylhistamine and additional purification steps are required to remove this material. Such steps are essential to measure histamine in plasma and fluids but are usually not required in the assay of tissue extracts.

An illustration of the sensitivity of the multiple step assay is provided by data obtained by one of us, Dr. WoldeMussie, (Figure 2). In this experiment rat peritoneal mast cells were purified by elutriation[22,24] and dilutions were made to yield 1,2 or 3 mast cells in each 10 μl aliquot. The histamine content of these different aliquots are shown. Each mast cell contained about 13 pg histamine, a value that is in reasonable agreement with previous estimates.[23] Two to five pg histamine was detectable by the assay system and 10 pg histamine gave values about twice that of blank (Fig. 2b). With this assay, it should be possible to follow histamine release from single mast cells and thereby to determine whether histamine release is a graded or "all or none" response.

APPLICATION OF THE VARIOUS HISTAMINE ASSAYS IN THE MEASUREMENT OF PLASMA HISTAMINE LEVELS

In addition to the radioenzymatic assays, the modified fluorometric assay has served equally well for plasma histamine measurements, especially, in clinical studies where sample volume is not an important constraint.

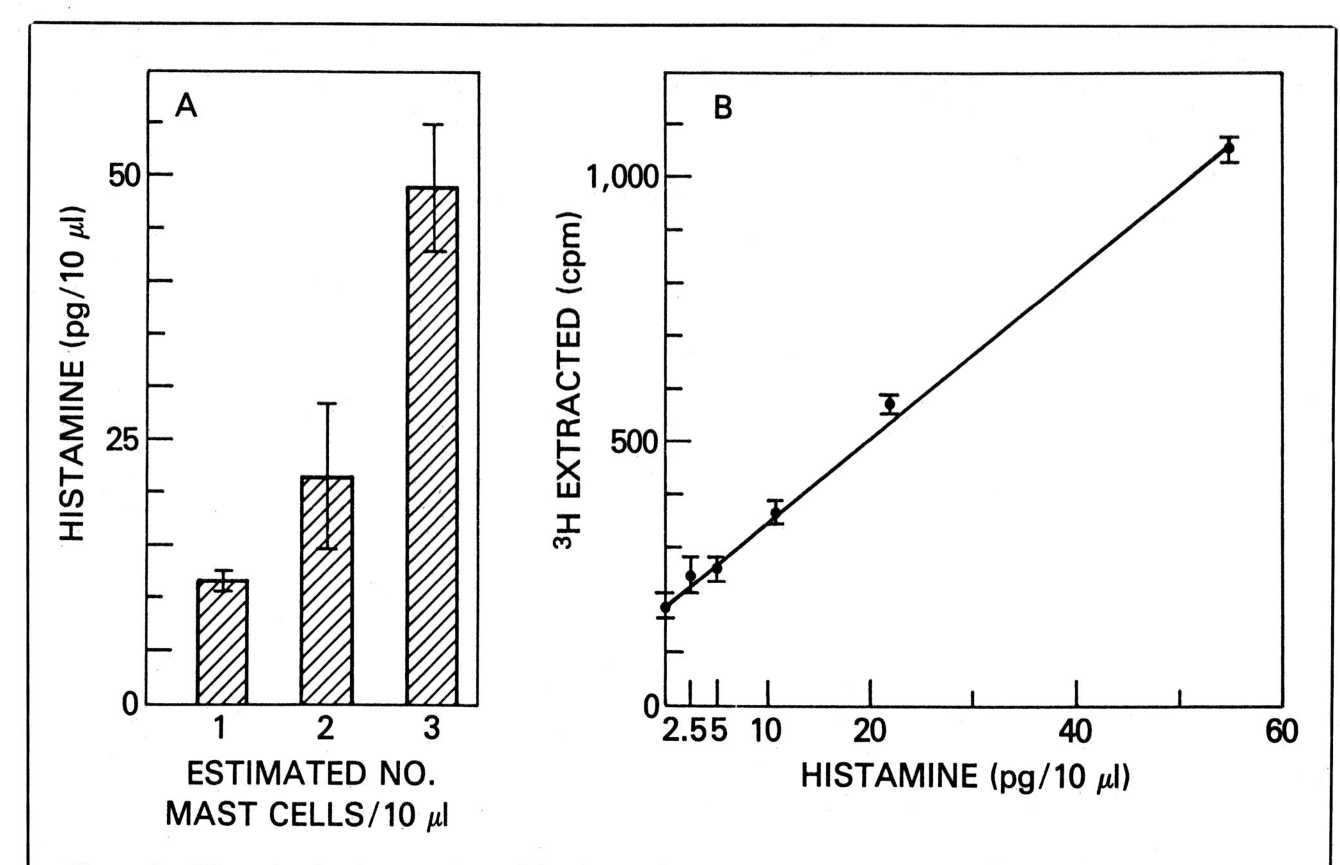

Figure 2a. *Histamine levels, as estimated by the single isotope (SAMe-³H) assay illustrated in figure 1, in cell suspensions that contain 1,2 or 3 mast cells/10 µl* aliquot. ***Figure 2b.*** *Curve for histamine standards by the same assay. See text for further details.*

Indeed over the past decade, Dr. Wilfried Lorenz has published much useful clinical data with his fluorometric histamine assays. From my perspective, these data are totally reliable and I am sure that he will touch on this subject in his talk tonight.

Although the reliability of some of the histamine measurements in plasma has been questioned,[30] the values for plasma histamine levels as reported by experienced groups are not dissimilar (Table 2). Workers from Dr. Lorenz's department report average values in the 0.3-0.4 ng/ml range as do some workers with the radioenzymatic assay. Other reports with the enzymatic assays indicate levels in the 0.6-0.8 ng/ml range and no difference between men and women (Table 2). In our laboratory, we obtain values of 0.6 ng/ml (Table 3). Estimates of blood histamine levels and urine histamine excretion (Table 3) have also remained unchanged over the past 10 years. Urinary histamine excretion in men and women are identical. Our data also indicate that serum histamine levels are 70-80% higher than those in plasma - a finding that has been noted by others and might be attributed to histamine release from basophils or platelets.[15]

Whether the true value for plasma histamine is 0.3 as opposed to 0.6 ng/ml has been of academic rather than practical interest to us, and we have not pursued the matter with as much vigor as others have in studies of atopic asthma (see later). It may well be that the lower estimates are correct, but from most studies there is consensus that well-defined, histamine-related symptoms are apparent after plasma histamine levels rise above 1 ng/ml.

HISTAMINE LEVELS IN OTHER BODY FLUIDS

Measureable histamine levels are found not only in plasma and urine but also in tears, gastric juice, blister fluid and cerebral spinal fluid (Table 4). Marked increases in histamine levels have been observed in some of these fluids in certain pathological conditions. Notably, elevated levels are observed in tears with vernal but not other forms of conjunctivitis. Histamine levels in blister fluid (produced by mild suction and heat, 48-51°, for 20-45 min) are greater when the blisters are induced over lesions produced by cold, heat, solar radiation or pressure in patients with various forms of urticaria than in blisters formed from normal skin. Cerebral spinal fluid has rather high histamine concentrations which may

Table II

Estimates of Normal Human Plasma Histamine Levels by Various Assay Procedures

Reference	Procedures	No. subjects	Histamine, ng/ml mean ± SEM	(range)
Adam *et al.*[4]	column/bioassay	7	< 1	
Porter and Mitchell[42]	" "	34	< 1	
Graham *et al.*[5]	" /fluorometric	46[c]	0.6	(0.1 - 1.4)
Lorenz et al.[6]	" "	10[b]	0.7	(0.1 - 1.4)
Lorenz and Doenicke[43]	" "	40	0.3	(0 - 0.9)
Schoning *et al.*[44]	" "	299[a]	0.35	(0 - 0.9)
Shaff and Beaven[13]	enzymatic	19	0.6 ± 0.1	(0.2 - 1.4)
Bruce *et al.*[45]	"	25	0.6 ± 0.1	
Beaven *et al.*[18]	"	57[a]	0.6	(0.2 - 1.4)
Guilloux *et al.*[46]	"	20[b]	0.79 ± 0.81	
		30[c]	0.76 ± 0.45	
Miller *et al.*[47]	ext./enzymatic	11	0.6	(0.4 - 1.0)
Dent *et al.*[14]	enzymatic/TLC	-	0.8	
Brown *et al.*[15]	" "	17[b]	0.38 ± 0.08	(0.1 - 0.5)
Moss *et al.*[16]	" "	21	1.0 ± 0.05	
Dyer *et al.*[17]	" "	51	0.32 ± 0.03	(0 - 0.9)

[a] *Includes patients with no known histamine related disorder.* [b] *Males* [c] *Females*

Table III

Histamine Levels In Normal Subjects: Summary of NHLBI Studies

Reference	Method	Plasma	Serum	Blood	Urine
			(ng/ml)		(μg/24 hr)
Beaven *et al*[18].	Double isotope (brain HMT)	---	<1 (4)	---	16 ± 14 (16)
Horakova *et al.*[48]	" " " "	<1 (11)	---	56 ± 8(11)	19 ± 3 (10)[a] 18 ± 3 (12)[b]
Shaff and Beaven[13]	" "(kidney HMT)	0.6 ± 0.1 (19)	1.0 ± 0.3 (13)	56 ± 8(7)	---
Beaven and Aiken, (unpub.)	Single isotope " " modified	0.6 ± 0.1 (6)	1.1 ± 0.1 (16) .	---	---
Range (all studies)		0.1 - 1.4	0.7 - 2.5	11 - 105	<5 - 98

Values are mean ± SEM for the number of subjects indicated in parentheses.
[a] *Male subjects* [b] *Female subjects*

Table IV

Histamine Levels in Body Fluids: Normal and Pathological Specimens

Fluid	Histamine, ng/ml Normal		Pathological		References
Blood	56 ± 5	(18)	102-27,000	(21)[a]	
Plasma	0.6 ± 0.1	(25)	<1 - 40	(42)[a]	This laboratory (see
Serum	1.1 ± 0.2	(28)	---		other tables)
Urine	14 ± 2	(38)	30-650	(33)[a]	
Saliva	<2	(3)	--		
Tears	10 ± 3	(13)	38 ± 14	(9)[b]	Abelson *et al.*[49]
	5	(23)	16	(17)[b]	Abelson *et al.*[50]
Gastric juice	11 ± 4	(9)	---		Parkin *et al.*[51]
Tissue (blister) fluid	7 ± 7	(20)	49 ± 20	(5)[c]	Kaplan *et al.*[52]
			24 - 41	(4)[d]	Kaplan *et al.*[52]
CSF	43 ± 6	(11)	---		Khandelwal *et al.*[53]

Values are mean ± SEM or range for the number of subjects indicated in parentheses.
[a] *Includes blood dyscrasias, mastocytosis, anaphylactic reaction*
[b] *Vernal conjunctivitis*
[c] *Cold induced urticarias*
[d] *Solar, heat and pressure induced urticarias*

reflect the large numbers of mast cells present in meninges. As far as I am aware, however, changes in these levels during meningeal infections have not been investigated.

FACTORS INFLUENCING HISTAMINE LEVELS IN BODY FLUIDS

Most of the histamine in humans and mammals is stored in tissue mast cells and much smaller amounts are present in basophils and neurones in the CNS. From the published data, it seems likely that average tissue histamine levels in the adult human are 5-10μg/g. Plasma histamine levels are therefore, about 1% of that in blood and less than 0.01% of that in tissues. Estimates of the excretion of histamine and its metabolites in human urine suggest that the turnover of histamine is about 3 mg/day in humans which is equivalent to about 1% of the total body pool.[18] It seems reasonable to assume that this turnover represents a combination of spontaneous release from mast cells and degradation of mast cells and basophils in the body. Basophils turnover rapidly in humans (t-½ 6 hr), but there are indications of a slow turnover of mast cells in tissues. After extensive degranulation of mast cells in rats, tissue histamine stores are slowly repleted over a period of months[31] and there is evidence that mast cells are continuously produced and degraded within body cavities and tissues.[24]

It is also becoming evident from our work that turnover of histamine in immature mast cells is more rapid than in mature cells. In the example shown in Figure 3, spontaneous histamine release was measured in different fractions of rat peritoneal mast cells which were separated according to their size by elutriation. Fractions of small cells, which contain few granules and little heparin, released as much histamine as that present in the cells within 3-4 hr, whereas, fractions of intermediate and mature cells released much smaller proportions of histamine. Mature cells, for example, released 5-8% of their total histamine pool within 3 hr. The cellular histamine content remained unchanged during this time. From this and other evidence, the appearance of histamine in the medium was due to synthesis and release of histamine rather than breakage of cells (WoldeMussie, unpublished data). Rapid turnover of histamine was also apparent in a transformed rat basophil (2H3) cell line[32] (Fig. 4). In this and other respects, the 2H3 cells resembled immature mast cells.

These findings might be relevant to certain clinical situations. In lesions with expanding populations of mast cells - for example, hypertrophic scars, keloids or urticarial lesions in young children with urticaria pigmentosa - spontaneous itching could be due to rapid histamine

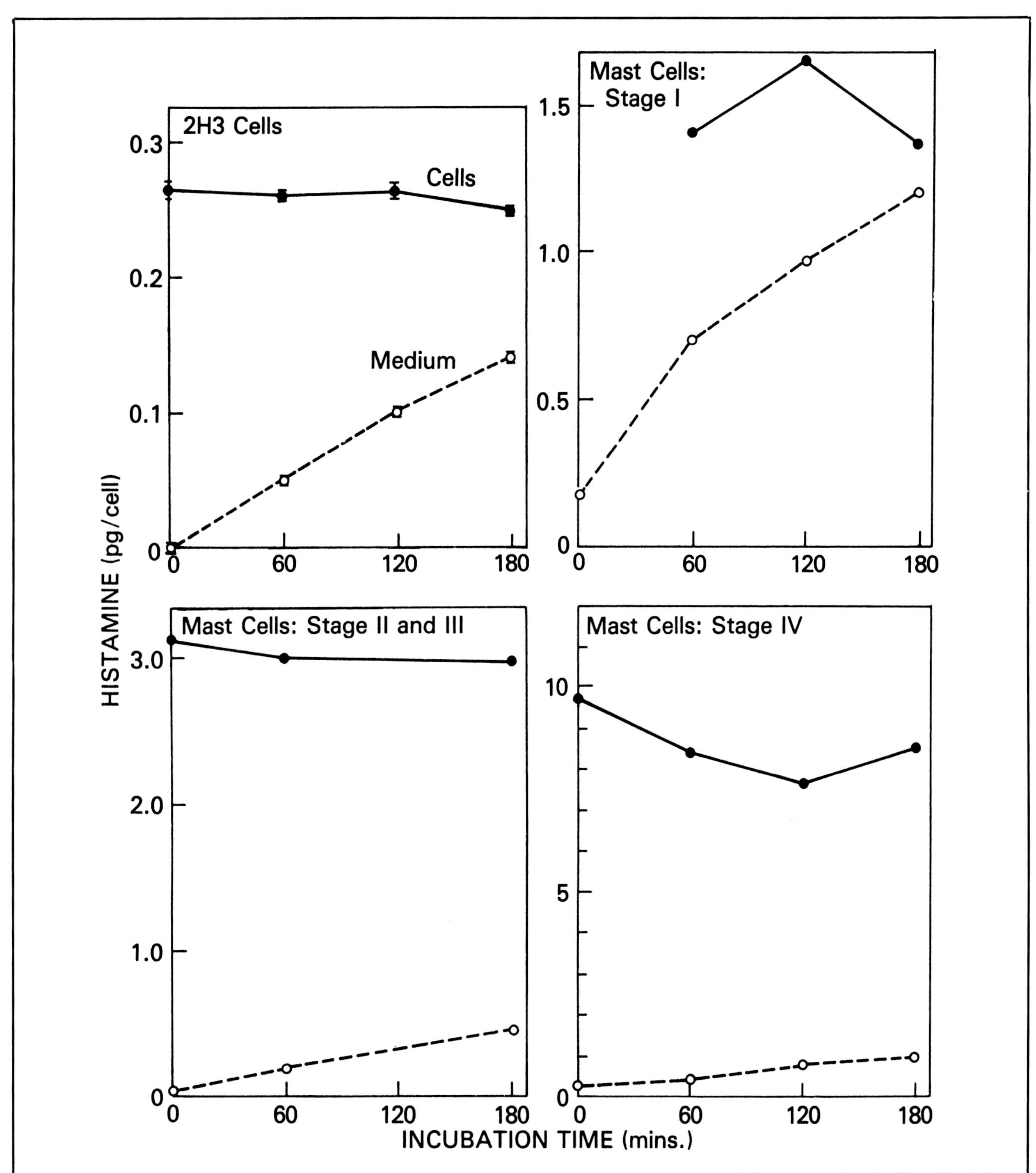

Figure 3. *Appearance of histamine in medium (o---o) in cultures of rat basophilic leukemia (2H3) cells (10^5 cells/500 μl in monolayer cultures) and suspensions of different fractions of elutriated rat peritoneal mast cells (10^5 cells/ml). Elutriated fractions 4, 6 and 11 were used in these studies.[24] Fraction 4 contains mainly (75%) immature stage I mast cells, fraction 6 stage I (65%) and stage II (25%) cells and fraction 11 more fully differentiated stage III and IV (80%) mast cells. Histamine content of cells is also indicated (●—●). The data show that histamine turnover occurs at a more rapid rate in the transformed 2H3 cell and immature mast cell than in the more mature mast cell.*

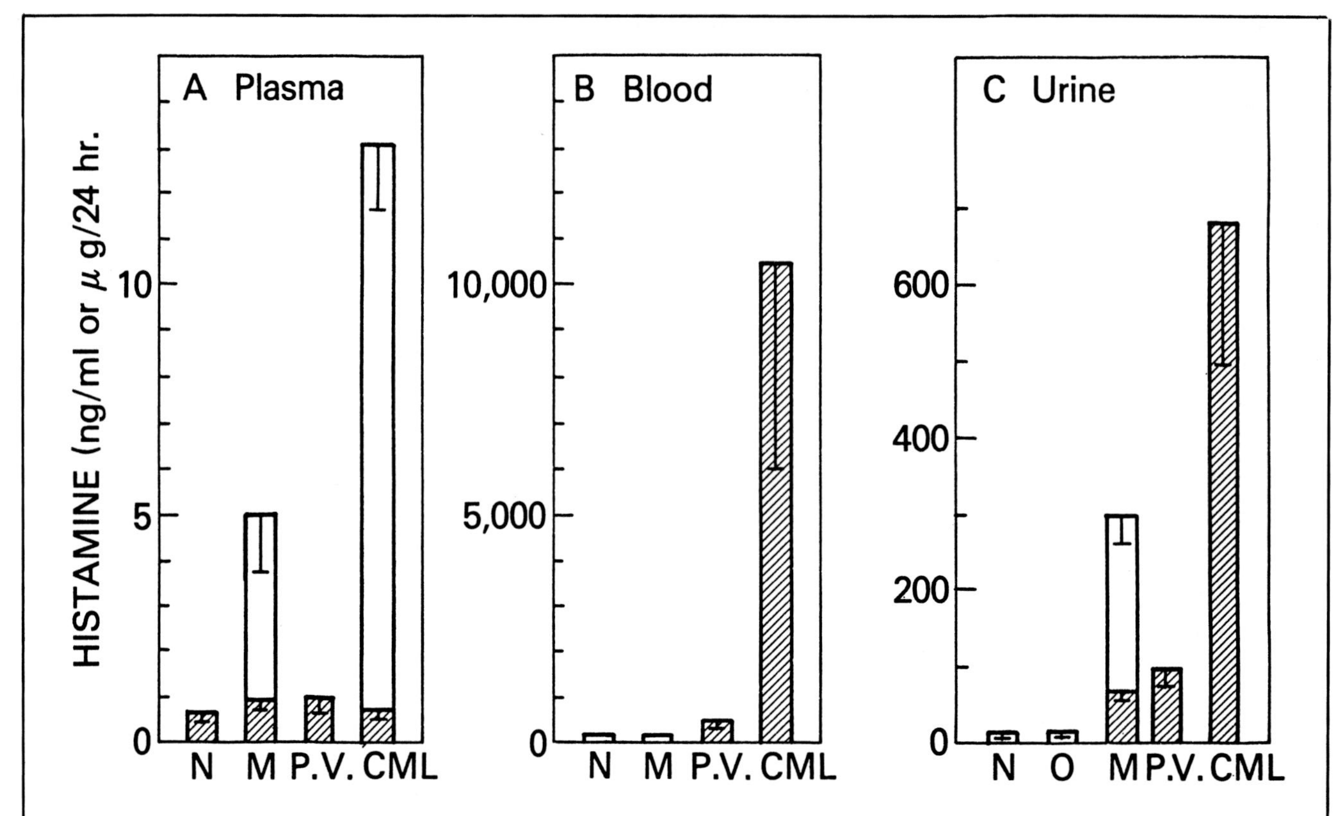

Figure 4. Histamine levels in plasma, blood and urine in 57 normal subjects (N), and 13 patients with mastocytosis (M), 10 with polycythemia vera (PV), 7 with chronic myelogenous leukemia (CML) and 10 other patients with nonhistamine related disorders (O). Mean values ± SEM are shown. Shaded portions of the bars show histamine levels in the absence of histamine related symptoms.

turnover in developing mast cells. Transformed basophils in patients with basophilic leukemias, like the transformed 2H3 cell, might have rapid histamine turnover, and there is evidence that this is so.

The basal histamine levels in plasma and urine depend not only on turnover of mast cells and basophils, the histamine pool within these cells, but also on the rate of clearance of histamine from the body. That plasma levels are low and that less than 3% of injected histamine appears unchanged in urine in man and other species,[31] means that the body possesses efficient mechanisms for degrading histamine. Histamine is, in fact, cleared rapidly from most vascular beds in experimental animals. In studies performed in collaboration with Dr. Kauffman, in which plasma samples were obtained from various vascular regions of dogs, we were able to show that 99% of the histamine given by infusion was cleared upon passage through the hind limbs, and 40-80% through other organs.[18] The differences in clearance rates do have bearing on the way experimental protocols should be designed in studies of histamine release. Ideally, blood samples should be drawn from both the arteries and the veins serving the limb or organ from which histamine release is to be studied; for example, the brachial artery and vein should be used in studies of localized reactions in the arm. The brachial vein, however, might be unsuitable for the study of changes in plasma histamine levels in more generalized reactions as we have no knowledge as to how much histamine is cleared upon passage through the arm. I realize that in clinical studies ethical considerations do not permit ideal choices in the matter, but this information should be kept in mind in interpreting one's data.

Degradation of histamine in the circulation probably occurs mainly in vascular endothelial cells. These cells contain high activities of the two enzymes involved in histamine degradation, histamine-N-methyltransferase and diamine oxidase. However, these enzymes are also present at sites of histamine action, the parietal cell and myocytes.[33]

Rapid clearance of histamine is also observed in humans. In one study, an intravenous injection of 600 ng histamine/kg resulted in maximal plasma histamine levels of 0.7 to 4.0 ng/ml (36 subjects, mean 1.5 - 2.0 ng/ml) within 1 min and a return to near normal values within 5 min in most subjects.[34] In our experience, continous infu-

Table V

Increase in Plasma Histamine Levels in Subjects with Acute Reactions

Conditions	No Subjects	Histamine, ng/ml Asymptomatic	Symptomatic	Reference
ATOPIC ASTHMA				
Normal	17	0.38 ± 0.08	---	Brown *et al.*[15]
Asthmatics	17	0.56 ± 0.11	0.84 ± 0.08	" " "
Stable asthmatics	12	0.21 ± 0.02	---	Ind *et al.*[35]
Asthmatic attack	14	---	0.64 ± 0.03	" " "
URTICARIA (COLD-INDUCED)				
Localized reaction	5	<1	10-36[a]	Kaplan *et al.*[54]
Systemic reaction (BP↓)	1	<1	240[a]	" " "
Localized reaction	1	<1	16[a]	Dyer *et al.*[17]
Localized reaction	3	<1	15-70[a]	Soter *et al.*[39]
URTICARIA (COLD-CHOLINERGIC)				
Generalized reaction	3	1	4-6	Kaplan *et al.*[55]
URTICARIA (EXERCISE/ CHOLINERGIC				
Mild	2	<1	3,4	Kaplan and Beaven[38]
Severe (gen.urticaria)	1	<1	25	" " "
Severe (BP↓, HR↑)	2	<2	8,26	Kaplan & Garofalo[56]
Severe (resp.sympt.)	7	0.6 ± 0.4	6.2 ± 2.0	Soter *et al.*[40]
URTICARIA (VIBRATION)				
Mild	2	<1	6,9	Kaplan and Beaven[38]
Severe	1	<1	53	
ANAPHYLACTIC REACTION				
Succinyl choline	1	2.1	40	Moss *et al.*[37]

[a] *Plasma from brachial vein of challenged arm.*

sion of histamine at rates greater than 200 ng/kg/min are required to produce measureable increases in plasma histamine levels and rates greater than 600 ng/kg/min are required to increase levels above 2 ng/ml (Isenberg and Beaven, unpublished data). Yet in these and another study,[35] histamine related symptoms (flushing, increased gastric secretion) were evident in all subjects once plasma histamine levels exceeded 1 ng/ml. In view of the sensitivity of humans (and most mammalian species) to histamine and the presence of potentially lethal quantities of histamine in our tissues, efficient mechanisms for histamine clearance are obviously necessary for survival. On a more practical point, it is apparent, from the data cited, that reports of plasma histamine levels much above 1 ng/ml in normal individuals without manifestation of physiological effects should be viewed with skepticism.

INCREASES IN FREE HISTAMINE LEVELS IN PATHOLOGICAL CONDITIONS

Conditions associated with abnormal numbers of mast cells (mastocytosis, urticaria pigmentosa) or basophils (chronic myelogenous leukemia, polycythemia vera) result in sustained high rates of histamine excretion in urine. In patients that we have studied, plasma histamine levels have remained below 1 ng/ml in the absence of symptoms even when histamine excretion was 2 to 20 times that in normal subjects (Fig. 4). Episodes of severe flushing or gastric discomfort were always associated with elevated (3-13 ng/ml) plasma histamine levels. In these conditions, measurements of urine histamine excretion are a more sensitive diagnostic indicator than are plasma histamine measurements. However, measurements of plasma, urine and blood levels allow us to discriminate between these different diseases.

Studies of conditions in which histamine release is induced, as opposed to those associated with abnormal numbers of histaminocytes, requires a well-controlled clinical setting and are useful only when measurements of pathophysiological parameters are made at the same time. Examples of such studies are shown in Table 5. Elevation of plasma histamine levels during asthmatic attacks has been reported by several groups[35] and data from one group is shown. This group finds small but significant increases in plasma histamine levels during acute asthmatic attacks and normal levels with asthmatic subjects in remission. These increases were inversely correlated with peak expiratory flow rates. There is, however, disagreement on the subject. Other authors report much greater increases in plasma histamine levels than those reported here, although Ind and co-workers[35] point out that leakage of histamine from basophils in blood samples drawn from asthmatic subjects may account for discrepancies in the literature.

Large increases in plasma histamine levels have been reported in urticarial conditions and anaphylactic reactions (Table 5). In patients with cold-induced urticaria pronounced increases were observed in plasma samples drawn from the arm after immersion of the arm in ice cold water. The onset and disappearance of urticarial lesions and severity of these lesions were well correlated with changes in plasma histamine levels. Generalized urticarial reactions induced experimentally in patients with other forms of physical urticaria were also associated with increases in systemic plasma histamine levels. In some of these subjects, plasma histamine levels rose from < 1 to 6-26 ng/ml and were accompanied by severe urticarial reactions, flushing, respiratory difficulties and marked changes in cardiovascular function (Table 5). Dramatic increases in plasma histamine levels have been noted during anaphylactic reactions (Table 5) or anaphylactoid reactions to drugs and adjuvants.[34,36] In some reports, whether exposure of the patient to stimulatory challenge was either deliberate or inadvertant, the reaction was sufficiently severe (cardiac arrest, collapse in blood pressure) to require resuscitative measures. Hence, my earlier comment on the need for a well-controlled clinical setting.

CONCLUSIONS

Some of the references in Table 5 provide dramatic examples of a correlation between clinical symptoms and plasma histamine levels in individual patients.[16,34,36-40] By citing these examples, I do not wish to overemphasize the importance of histamine release for it is a problem related to a group of well-defined disorders. There are examples of patients with mastocytosis in whom clinical symptoms are attributable to release of prostaglandin D_2 and histamine,[41] and in asthmatic conditions it is unlikely that histamine plays a major role. I cite them to illustrate that the techniques now available do allow us to measure small changes in plasma histamine levels and with properly designed clinical studies we are in a position to identify those reactions in which histamine plays a principal role and those where it does not.

REFERENCES

1. Barsoum GS, Gaddum JH. The pharmacological estimation of adenosine and histamine in blood. J. Physiol. Lond. 85, 1-14, 1935.
2. Barsoum GS, Smirk FH. Observations on the histamine yielding substance in the plasma and red cells of normal subjects and of patients with congestive heart failure. Clin. Sc. Lond. 2, 237-352, 1935-6.
3. Code CF. The quantitative estimation of histamine in blood. J. Physiol. Lond. 89, 257-268, 1937.
4. Adam HM, Hardwick HT, Spencer KEV. A method of estimating histamine in plasma. Br. J. Pharmacol. 12, 397-405, 1957.
5. Graham H, Scarpellini JAD, Hubka BP, Lowry OH. Measurement and normal range of free histamine in human blood plasma. Biochem. Pharmacol. 17, 2271-2280. 1968.
6. Lorenz W, Reimann H-J, Barth H, Kusche J, Meyer R, Doenicke A, Hutzel M. A sensitive and specific method for the determination of histamine in human whole blood and plasma. Hoppe-Seylers Z. Physiol. Chem. 353, 911-920, 1972.
7. Lorenz W, Doenicke A, Schöning B, Neugebaur E. The role of histamine in adverse reactions to intravenous agents. In: Thornton, JA. (ed) Adverse reactions of anesthetic drugs. Elsevier/North Holland Biomedical Press, Amsterdam, pp. 169-237, 1980.
8. Davis TP, Gehrke CW, Gehrke CW Jr, Cunningham TD, Kuo KC, Gerhardt KO, Johnson HD, Williams CH. High-performance liquid-chromatographic separation and fluorescence measurement of biogenic amines in plasma, urine, and tissue. Clin. Chem. 24, 1317-1324, 1978.
9. Siraganian RP. An automated continuous-flow system for the extraction and fluorometric analysis of histamine. Anal. Biochem. 57, 383-394, 1974.
10. Siraganian RP. Histamine release and assay methods for the study of human allergy. In: Rose, N.R. Friedman, H. (eds.) Manual of clinical immunology, American Society for Microbiology, Washington, D.C., pp. 603-625, 1976.
11. Snyder SH, Baldessarini R, Axelrod J. A Sensitive and specific enzymatic isotopic assay for tissue histamine. J. Pharmacol. Exp. Ther. 153, 544-549, 1966.
12. Beaven MA, Jacobsen S, Horáková Z. Modification of the enzmatic isotopic assay of histamine and its application to measurement of histamine in tissues, serum and urine. Clin. Chim. Acta 37, 91-103, 1972.
13. Shaff RE, Beaven MA. Increased sensitivity of the enzymatic isotopic assay of histamine: Measurement of histamine in plasma and serum. Anal. Biochem. 94:425-430, 1979.
14. Dent C, Nilam F, Smith IR. Application of thin layer chromatography to histamine radioenzymatic assay. Agents Actions 9, 34-35, 1979.
15. Brown MJ, Ind PW, Barnes PJ, Jenner DA, Dollery CT. A sensitive and specific radiometric method for the measurement of plasma histamine in normal individuals. Anal. Biochem. 109, 142-146, 1980.
16. Moss J, Rosow CE, Savarese JJ, Philbin DM, Kniffen KJ. Role

of histamine in the hypotensive action of d-tubocurarine in humans. Anesthesiology 55, 19-25, 1981.
17. Dyer J, Warren K, Merlin S, Metcalfe DD, Kaliner M. Measurement of plasma histamine: description of an improved method and normal values. J. Allergy Clin. Immunol. 70, 82-87, 1982.
18. Beaven MA, Robinson-White A, Roderick NB, Kauffman GL. The demonstration of histamine release in clinical conditions: A review of past and present assay procedures. Klin. Wochenschr. 60, 873-881, 1982.
19. Horáková Z, Beaven MA. The time-course of histamine release and edema formation in the rat paw after thermal injury. Eur. J. Pharmacol. 27, 305-312, 1974.
20. Baxter JH, Beaven MA, Horáková Z. Effects of adrenergic agents, theophylline and other drugs on dextran edema and histamine release in rats. Biochem. Pharmacol. 23, 1211-1217, 1974.
21. Almeida AP, Flye W, Deveraux D, Horáková Z, Beaven MA. Distribution of histamine and histaminase (diamine oxidase) in blood of various species. Comp. Biochem. Physiol. 67C, 187-190, 1980.
22. Soll AH, Lewin KJ, Beaven MA. Isolation of histamine-containing cells from canine fundic mucosa. Gastroenterology 77, 1283-1290, 1979.
23. Soll AH, Lewin KJ, Beaven MA. Isolation of histamine-containing cells from rat gastric mucosa: Biochemical and morphologic differences from mast cells. Gastroenterology 80: 717-727, 1981.
24. Beaven MA, Aiken DL, WoldeMussie E, Soll AH. Changes in histamine synthetic activity, histamine content and responsive to compound 48/80 with maturation of rat peritoneal mast cells. J. Pharm. Exp. Ther. 224, 620-626, 1983.
25. Beaven MA, Moore JP, Smith GA, Hesketh TR, Metcalfe JC. The calcium signal and phosphatidylinositol breakdown in 2H3 cells. J. Biol. Chem. 259, 7137-7142, 1984..
26. Beaven MA, Rogers J, Moore JP, Hesketh TR, Smith GA, Metcalfe JC. The mechanism of the calcium signal and correlation with histamine release in 2H3 cells. J. Biol. Chem. 259, 7129-7136 1984.
27. Beaven MA, Horakova Z. The enzymatic isotopic assay of histamine. In: Rocha e. Silva M. (ed.) Handbook of experimental pharmacology, vol. XVIII, part 2, Springer, Berlin, Heidelberg, New York, pp. 151-173. 1978.
28. Beaven MA, Roderick NB. Impromidine, a potent inhibitor of histamine methyltransferase (HMT) and diamine oxidase (DAO). Biochem. Pharmacol. 29, 2897-2900, 1980.
29. Bowsher RR, Verburg KM, Henry DP. Rat histamine N-methyltransferase. Quantification, tissue distribution, purification, and immunologic properties. J. Biol. Chem. 258, 12215-12220, 1983.
30. Gleich GJ, Hull WM. Measurement of histamine: a quality control study. J. Allergy Clin. Immunol. 66, 295-298, 1980.
31. Schayer RW. Catabolism of histamine *in vivo*. In: Handbook of Experimental Pharmacology, Vol. 18, part 1 (Ed. Rocha e. Silva) pp 688-725, Springer Verlag, Berlin, 1966.
32. Siraganian RP, McGivney A, Barsumian EL, Crews FT, Hirata F, Axelrod J. Variants of the rat basophilic leukemia cell line for the study of histamine release. Fed. Proc. 41, 30-34, 1982.
33. Robinson-White A, Beaven MA. Presence of histamine and histamine-metabolizing enzyme in rat and guinea pig microvascular endothelial cells. J. Pharm. Exp. Therap. 223, 440-445, 1982.
34. Lorenz W, Doenicke A, Schöning B, Ohmann C, Grote B, Neugebauer E. Definition and classification of the histamine-release response to drugs in anaesthesia and surgery: studies in the conscious human subject. Klin. Wochenschr. 60, 896-913, 1982.
35. Ind PW, Barnes PJ, Brown MJ, Causon R, Dollery CT. Measurement of plasma histamine in asthma. Clin. Allergy 13, 61-67, 1983.
36. Moss J, Philbin DM, Rosow CE, Basta SJ, Gelb C, Savarese JJ. Histamine release by neuromuscular blocking agents in man. Klin. Wochenschr. 60, 891-895, 1982.
37. Moss J, Fahmy NR, Sunder N, Beaven MA. Hormonal and hemodynamic profile of an anaphylactic reaction in man. Circulation 63, 210-213, 1981.
38. Kaplan AP, Beaven MA. *In vivo* studies of the pathogenesis of cold urticaria, cholinergic urticaria and vibration-induced swelling. J. Invest. Dermatol. 67, 327-332, 1976.
39. Soter NA, Wasserman SI, Austen KF. Cold urticaria: Release into the circulation of histamine and eosinophil chemotactic factor of anaphylaxis during cold challenge. N. Engl. J. Med. 294, 687-690, 1976.
40. Soter NA, Wasserman SI, Austen KF, McFadden ER Jr. Release of mast cell mediators and alterations in lung function in patients with cholinergic urticaria. N Engl. J. Med. 302, 604-608, 1980.
41. Roberts LJ 2nd, Sweetman BJ, Lewis RA, Austen KF, Oates JA. Increased production of prostaglandin D_2 in patients with systemic mastocytosis. N. Engl. J. Med. 303, 1400-1402, 1980.
42. Porter JF, Mitchell RG. The distribution of histamine in blood of healthy and asthmatic children. Clin. Sci. 38, 135-143, 1970.
43. Lorenz W, Doenicke A. Histamine release in clinical conditions. Mt. Sinai J. Med (NY) 45, 357-386, 1978. (78 Ref.)
44. Schöning B, Lorenz W, Doenicke A. Prophylaxis of anaphylactoid reactions to polypeptidal plasma substitute by H_1 plus H_2 receptor antagonists: Synopsis of three randomized controlled trials. Klin. Wochenschr. 60, 1048-1055, 1982.
45. Bruce C, Taylor WH, Westwood A. An improved radioenzymatic assay for histamine in human plasma, whole blood, urine and gastric juice. Ann. Clin. Biochem. 16, 259-264, 1979.
46. Guilloux L, Hartmann D, Ville G. Enzymatic isotopic assay for human plasma histamine. Clin. Chim. Acta 116, 269-275, 1981.
47. Miller RL, McCord C, Sanda M, Bourne HR, Melmon KL. Application of the enzymatic double isotopic dilution assay for the study of histamine in plasma. J. Pharmacol. Exp. Ther. 175, 228-234, 1970.
48. Horáková Z, Keiser HR, Beaven MA. Blood and urine histamine levels in normal and pathological states as measured by a radiochemical assay. Clin. Chim. Acta 79, 447-456, 1977.
49. Abelson MB, Soter NA, Simon MA, Dohlman J, Allansmith MR. Histamine in human tears. Amer J. Opthalmol 79, 417-418, 1977.
50. Abelson MB, Baird RS, Allansmith MR. Tear histamine levels in vernal conjunctivitis and other ocular inflammation. Opthalmology 87, 812-14, 1980.
51. Parkin JV, Lorenz W, Barth H, Rohde H, Ohmann C, Thon K, Weber D, Crombach M. Assay and identification of histamine in human gastric aspirate by a fluorometric-fluoroenzymatic technique. Its application in patients with chronic duodenal ulcer. Agents Actions 12, 17-25, 1982.
52. Kaplan AP,Horáková Z, Katz SI. Assessment of tissue fluid histamine levels in patients with urticaria. J. Allergy Clin. Immunol. 61, 350-354, 1978.
53. Khandelwal JK, Hough LB, Green JP. Histamine and some of its metabolites in human body fluids. Klin. Wochenschr. 60, 914-918, 1982.
54. Kaplan AP, Gray L, Shaff RE, Horakova Z, Beaven MA. *In vivo* studies of mediator release in cold urticaria and cholinergic urticaria. J. Allergy Clin. Immunol. 55: 394-402, 1975.
55. Kaplan AP, Natbony SF, Tawil AP, Fruchter L, Foster M. Exercise-induced anaphylaxis as a manifestation of cholinergic urticaria. J. Allergy Clin. Immunol. 68, 319-324, 1981.
56. Kaplan AP, Garofalo J. Identification of a new physically induced urticaria: cold-induced cholinergic urticaria. J. Allergy Clin. Immunol. 68, 438-441, 1981.
57. Lee TH, Brown MJ, Nagy L, Causon R, Walport MJ, Kay AB. Exercise-induced release of histamine and neutrophil chemotactic factor in atopic asthmatics. J. Allergy Clin. Immunol. 70, 73-81, 1982. □

Chapter II
Histamine H_1 and H_2 Receptors

Thomas B. Casale, M.D.

ABSTRACT

Histamine, one of the major mediators of immediate hypersensitivity (allergic) reactions, is capable of eliciting a variety of physiologic responses (Table 2) of major clinical importance. The mediation of histamine's actions occurs in part as a consequence of the generation of either cyclic GMP or cyclic AMP subsequent to the stimulation of specific H_1 or H_2 receptors, respectively. The development of specific histamine receptor agonists and antagonists (Table 1) and radioligand binding techniques should prove useful in the elucidation of the precise sequence of events following histamine receptor interactions. In addition, knowledge of histamine receptor subtypes and histamine-induced post-receptor events have proven beneficial in the development of treatment modalities for diseases such as anaphylaxis and the Zollinger-Ellison syndrome.

INTRODUCTION

Histamine is a β-imidazolylethylamine (molecular weight 111) of universal biologic occurrence. In man, histamine is stored predominantly in tissue mast cells and circulating basophils, and under physiologic conditions the tissue content of histamine corresponds closely to the number of mast cells[1]. Histamine is released from mast cells and basophils in response to several stimuli including antigen-IgE antibody interactions, and as such, plays a central role in allergic and inflammatory reactions.

Histamine's potent biological effects were first described by Dale and Laidlaw,[2,3] who demonstrated that histamine contributed significantly to the manifestations of anaphylaxis. However, it was not until an effective antagonist of histamine was synthesized in 1937 by Bovet and Staub[4] that the complex nature of the pathophysiologic actions of histamine began to become unraveled. The demonstration that histamine antagonists competitively inhibited histamine-induced responses suggested the presence of specific histamine receptors. It soon became evident, however, that certain effects of histamine (e.g., gastric acid secretion and rat uterus relaxation) could not be antagonized by conventional antihistamines such as mepyramine and diphenhydramine. These observations led Ash and Schild[5] to propose the existence of at least two different types of receptors, those sensitive to available antihistamines such as mepyramine (H_1 receptors) and those that were not (H_2 receptors). In 1972, Black and his colleagues[6] described a newly synthesized compound, burimamide, which competitively and specifically blocked histamine-induced gastric acid secretion and rat uterus relaxation without blocking H_1 receptors. The receptors antagonized by burimamide were designated H_2 receptors. These investigators were also able to differentiate the two different histamine receptor types by the relative agonist activities of certain histamine ana-

From the Dept. of Internal Medicine, University of Iowa Hospitals and Clinics, Iowa City, IA 52242

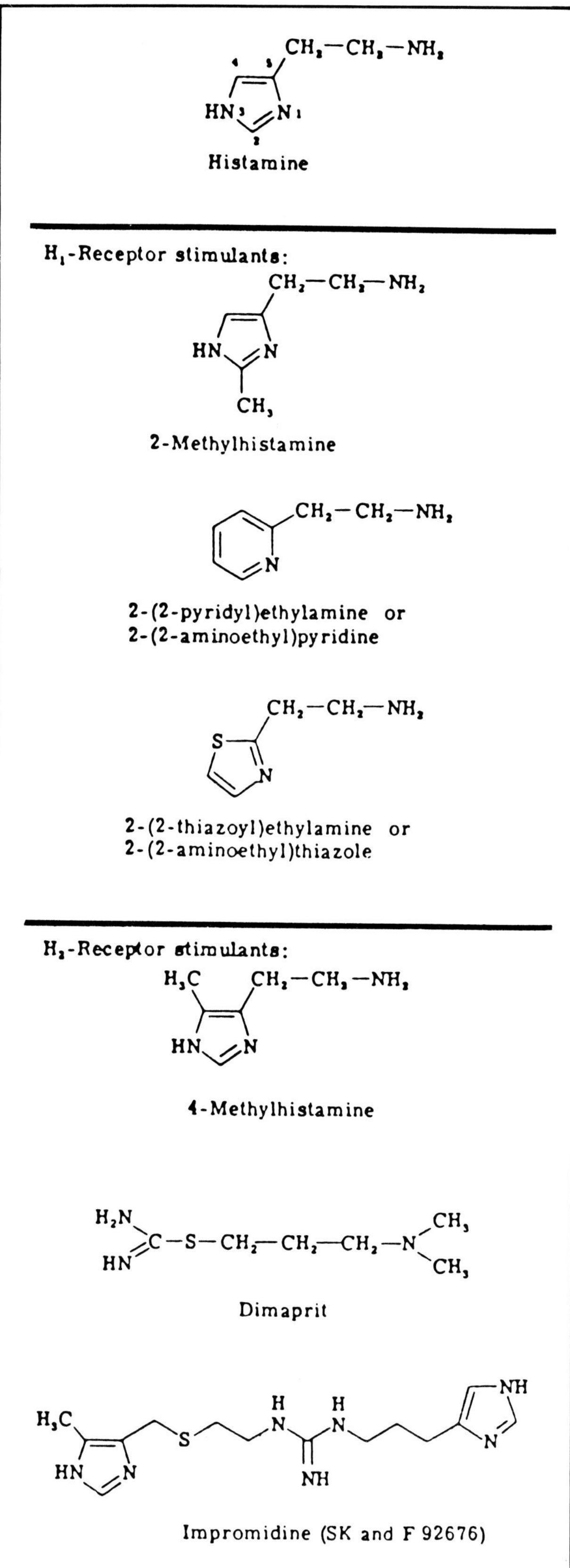

$CH_2—CH_2—NH_2$

HN N

Histamine

H_1-Receptor stimulants:

$CH_2—CH_2—NH_2$

HN N

CH_3

2-Methylhistamine

$CH_2—CH_2—NH_2$

N

2-(2-pyridyl)ethylamine or
2-(2-aminoethyl)pyridine

$CH_2—CH_2—NH_2$

S N

2-(2-thiazoyl)ethylamine or
2-(2-aminoethyl)thiazole

H_2-Receptor stimulants:

H_3C $CH_2—CH_2—NH_2$

HN N

4-Methylhistamine

H_2N, HN $C—S—CH_2—CH_2—CH_2—N(CH_3)_2$

Dimaprit

H_3C HN N S H N H N NH NH N

Impromidine (SK and F 92676)

Figure 1. *Structures of selected histamine agonists.*

logues. 2-Methylhistamine, 2-(2-pyridyl) ethylamine, and 2-(2-thiazolyl) ethylamine elicit responses mediated by H_1 receptors, whereas, 4-methylhistamine and dimaprit preferentially stimulate H_2 receptors. The different responses elicited by agonists with only minor structural variations (Fig. 1) suggest that histamine receptor subtypes are highly specialized chemical structures with well-defined specificities. Table 1 contains a list of drugs which interact with histamine receptors.

Histamine receptors, as well as all hormone receptors, perform two vital functions. First, by a process of high-affinity, very specific binding, they recognize particular biologically active structures; second, they initiate a cascade of biological reactions that culminate in physiological or biochemical responses. This second function of receptors may be the translation of a signal generated by the binding interaction with the agonist and its specific receptor. For example, the signal for stimulated histamine receptors is the generation of either cyclic adenosine monophosphate (AMP) or cyclic guanosine monophosphate (GMP), which may ultimately result in a physiologic response. Although there are exceptions, stimulation of H_1 receptors generally results in a rise in cyclic GMP, whereas stimulation of H_2 receptors results in a rise in cyclic AMP.

Studies of histamine receptors first focused on the physiologic responses induced by histamine and later on the accompanying changes in the intracellular second messengers, cyclic AMP and cyclic GMP. Most recently, investigators have directly studied these receptors by using radioligands, which are radioactively labeled drugs with high affinity for histamine receptors. Radioligand binding techniques have been used to characterize and quantitate histamine receptors and should prove useful for examining their regulation in intact tissues and cultured cells.

RADIOLIGAND BINDING STUDIES

Histamine receptors are measured by incubating the radioligand usually with a plasma membrane preparation from tissue or, occasionally, with an intact tissue preparation. The unbound radioligand activity is most commonly removed by centrifugation or filtration, and the radioactivity bound to the tissue preparation is then determined. Radioligands, however, not only bind to specific receptor sites but also to nonspecific sites. Nonspecific binding is determined by incubating the radioligand and tissue preparation with a nonradioactive drug present in a much greater concentration than the radioligand, which thereby binds to virtually all of the specific histamine receptors. Thus, since all the histamine receptors are occupied by the unlabeled drug, the radioligand should bind only to the nonspecific sites. Specific histamine receptor binding can then be calculated by subtract-

Table I

Drugs Interacting with Histamine Receptors

H_1 Antagonists	H_1 Agonists	H_2 Antagonists	H_2 Agonists
Ethanolamines	Histamine	Burimamide	Histamine
Diphenhydramine	2-Methylhistamine	Cimetidine	Ipromidine
Carbinoxamine	2-Thiazolylethylamine	Ranitidine	Dimaprit
Diphenylpyraline	2-Pyridylethylamine	Tiotidine	4-Methylhistamine
		Metiamide	4-Ethylhistamine
Alkylamines			
Chlorpheniramine			
Brompheniramine			
Ethylenediamines			
Mepyramine			
Triprolidine			
Antazoline			
Tripelennamine			
Piperazines			
Chlorcyclizine			
Cyclizine			
Meclizine			
Phenothiazines			
Promethazine			
Miscellaneous			
Hydroxyzine			

ing the radioactivity determined in the presence of the unlabeled compound from that determined in its absence. To ensure that the specific binding is actually to histamine receptors, it is necessary to check that the binding is saturable and reversible, and that unlabeled histaminergic drugs exhibit the rank order of potency predicted by pharmacologic experiments. The receptor number is determined by incubating a constant concentration of tissue receptors with increasing concentrations of radioligand that fully saturate the histamine receptors.

Identification of histamine receptor subtypes with radioligands can be achieved in two different ways. One approach involves using a radioligand that has a greater affinity for one or the other histamine receptor subtypes, such as ^{3}H-mepyramine for H_1 receptors, and ^{3}H-cimetidine for H_2 receptors. The other approach involves using a radioligand with equal affinity for both H_1 and H_2 receptors, such as ^{3}H-histamine, and then constructing competition curves for the radioligand with drugs selective for H_1 or H_2 receptor subtypes. The resulting data can then be analyzed with computer modeling techniques[7-9] that determine whether a single histamine receptor subtype or a mixture of H_1 and H_2 receptors is present and, if present, in what proportions.

HISTAMINE RECEPTORS IN ORGAN SYSTEMS

The physiologic consequences of stimulating histamine H_1 and H_2 receptors are many and diverse. A summary of the major H_1- and H_2-mediated actions is presented in Table 2. Histamine-induced responses in various organ systems are discussed below.

Cardiovascular System

The cardiovascular effects of histamine include peripheral circulatory and vascular responses as well as cardiac responses. In man, histamine predominantly causes vasodilation of the smaller vessels probably through both H_1 and H_2 receptors.[10-13] This results in cutaneous flushing and lowered peripheral resistance secondary to a drop in the diastolic blood pressure with a concomitant increase in pulse pressure. In a study by Kaliner and co-workers,[13] subjects who received intravenous histamine infusions developed flushing and hypotension which was effectively abrogated only after pretreatment with both H_1 and H_2 antagonists, but not by either antagonist alone.

Table II

Summary of the Major Histamine-Induced Responses by Receptor Subtypes

H_1	H_2	H_1 and H_2
Increased vasopermeability	Mucus production	Vasodilation (Hypotension)
Tachycardia	Cyclic AMP production	Increased pulse pressure
Triple response of Lewis	Gastric acid secretion	Neurotransmission
Bronchospasm	Inhibition of neutrophil enzyme release	
Increased pulmonary vascular resistance	Inhibition of eosinophil migration	
Cyclic GMP production	Inhibition of basophil histamine release	
Prostaglandin generation	Inhibition of delayed hypersensitivity skin reactions	
Spasmogenic contraction of stomach, gall bladder, intestine	Immunoregulation secondary to T lymphocyte effects	

Histamine also acts on postcapillary vessels causing the endothelial cells to contract, which leads to intercellular gaps and permeability. The resulting outward passage of plasma proteins and fluid into the extracellular space is accompanied by increases in lymph flow and lymph protein content and edema formation. The role of the histamine receptor subtypes in these responses will be discussed later.

The determination of the effect of histamine on the heart *in vivo* is complex because of the difficulty in distinguishing between direct cardiac effects and indirect effects of histamine such as the release of catecholamines, respiratory changes, and reflex responses to hypotension. Nonetheless, increased heart rate has been reported to be a consistent feature of histaminemia,[13,14] and in the cat and rabbit this action may be mediated through H_2 receptors.[15,16] In man, both pulse rate and pulse pressure have been reported to increase after histamine infusion, with the rise in pulse rate being effectively abrogated by H_1, but not H_2 antagonists.[13]

Cutaneous Response

Intradermal injection of histamine results in the "triple response of Lewis," which includes: 1) the formation of a small localized area of erythema caused by vasodilation; 2) a histamine-induced axonal reflex that leads to vasodilation and the characteristic "flare" that extends beyond the original area of erythema; and 3) an area of edema resulting from increased capillary permeability.[17] There have been many investigations attempting to delineate the histamine receptor subtype involved in the etiology of these responses. It appears that H_2 antagonists by themselves do not significantly inhibit histamine-induced skin responses, whereas H_1 antagonists alone or in combination with H_2 antagonists do.[18] There is only slight augmentation of the inhibitory capacity of H_1 antagonists by H_2 antagonists, indicating that histamine-induced skin responses are predominantly caused by the H_1 receptors.

Respiratory System

Stimulation of histamine receptors in the respiratory tract results in a number of physiologic responses including bronchospasm. The stimulation of H_1 receptors has been shown to induce constriction of human airways.[19-22] However, the role of H_2 receptors in airways is controversial, with both bronchodilatory[21,22] and bronchoconstrictive[19,20] effects reported. Nevertheless, it appears that the H_1 effect is the predominant one, and thus, the overall manifestation of histamine stimulation on the lower respiratory tract is bronchospasm. Histamine also dilates small radices of the pulmonary vascular tree through an H_1 receptor mechanism and increases the distance between endothelial cells of the venules, thereby increasing the potential for transudation of plasma and for extravasation of leukocytes.[23] Overall, histamine has been shown in animal models to cause an increase in pulmonary vascular resistance which is mediated by H_1 receptors.[24] Histamine has also been shown to increase mucus production through an H_2 receptor.[25]

Human peripheral lung tissue stimulated by histamine results in the production of cyclic GMP by an H_1 receptor mechanism and cyclic AMP by an H_2 receptor mechanism.[26] In addition, H_1 receptors on human peripheral lung tissue have been characterized by radioligand binding assays,[27] although the specific cell types involved are not yet identified.

Finally, stimulation by histamine has been shown to result in the production of prostaglandins from both peripheral lung tissue and airways through H_1 receptor stimulation.[26,28]

Gastrointestinal System

Histamine has been shown to stimulate gastric acid secretion through H_2 receptors linked to cyclic AMP production in oxyntic cells.[29–32] Specific H_2 antagonists competitively inhibit cyclic AMP formation in the gastric mucosa and reduce gastric acid secretion,[29–32] thus making these drugs clinicall useful in the treatment of peptic ulcer disease and the Zollinger-Ellison syndrome. Recent studies, in which guinea pigs were used, suggest that gastric cells may possess a class of binding sites for histamine that is not linked to adenylate cyclase and is unrelated to the H_2 receptor.[33] The biologic role of these sites, if any, is not yet known.

Histamine may have a relatively weak, but probably not a physiologic capacity to contract the lower esophageal sphincter through H_2 receptor stimulation.[34] Histamine has a spasmogenic effect on the stomach, intestine, and gallbladder that results from H_1 receptor stimulation. Histamine has also been reported to produce through an undefined mechanism a dose-related inhibition of the neurogenic atropine-resistant tetanic spasms in the plexus-containing longitudinal smooth muscle preparations from guinea pig ileum.[35] These histamine-induced responses are of interest clinically since subjects experiencing either an allergic or an anaphylactic reaction to food often complain of gastrointestinal cramping, pain, distension, and diarrhea which potentially could be treated with H_1 antihistamines.

Central Nervous System

Histamine's role as a neurotransmitter in brain is sub—stantiated by a variety of experimental data. [36] Although histamine itself does not cross the blood-brain barrier, its precursor, histidine, is avidly taken up.[37] It appears that histamine is stored in synaptic vesicles in the brain and is rapidly turned over, especially in the hypothalamus.[38]

Histamine in the brain has been shown to cause an increase in cyclic AMP as well as the usual increase in cyclic GMP following H_1 receptor stimulation.[39] However, using cell-free preparations from guinea pig hippocampus and cerebral cortex, only H_2 receptors were shown to be linked directly to the histamine-sensitive adenylate cyclase, whereas both H_1 and H_2 receptors are involved in the accumulation of cyclic AMP as measured in brain slices.[40] The involvement of H_1 receptors in this effect appears indirect and may occur as a result of calcium ion translocation.[40] Histamine H_1 receptors have been reported to mediate the stimulation of cyclic GMP in neuroblastoma cells and slices of cervical ganglia and to increase glycogenolysis.[41]

The presence of histamine receptors in brain have been confirmed by the use of radioligand techniques. ^{3}H-Histamine, [42] ^{3}H-mepyramine,[43,44] and 3H-cimetidine[45] have all been shown to bind to brain preparations and to selectively label histamine, H_1 and H_2 receptors, respectively.

Hematologic/Immunologic System

Histamine stimulation of H_2 receptors on neutrophils and eosinophils results in a rise in cyclic AMP levels with subsequent inhibiton of neutrophil lysosomal enzyme release and eosinophil migration, respectively.[38] In addition, histamine has been shown to inhibit phytohemagglutinin-induced proliferation of human peripheral blood lymphocytes,[46] and may be chemotactic for eosinophils.[47] H_2 Antihistamines have been reported to augment antigen-induced histamine release from human basophils *in vitro*.[48]

Through the stimulation of H_2 receptors, histamine has been shown to exert a regulatory influence on several aspects of the immune response including the diminution of delayed hypersensitivity skin test responses[49] and inhibition of *in vivo*-generated cytotoxic T lymphocytes.[50,51] Histamine and/or histamine H_2 receptor-bearing lymphocytes have been shown to interfere with the maturation of antigen-stimulated B lymphocytes,[52] antibody secretion from more mature plasma cells,[53] and immunoglobulin production by human blood mononuclear cells.[54] Finally, histamine H_1 receptors have been directly identified by radioligand binding assays on both human lymphocytes[55] and neutrophils.[56]

ACKNOWLEDGEMENTS

The author gratefully acknowledges the typing of Denise Boettcher and the editorial assistance of Karen Leighty.

REFERENCES

1. Metcalfe DD, Kaliner M, Donlon MA. The mast cell. CRC Crit Rev Immunol 3:23-74, 1981.
2. Dale HH, Laidlaw PP. The Physiological Action of β-imidazolylethylamine. J Physiol 41:318, 1910.
3. Dale HH, Laidlaw PP. Histamine Shock. J Physiol 52:355, 1919.
4. Bovet D, Staub A. Action protectrice des ethers phenoliques au cours de l'intoxication histaminique. Comp rend Soc biol 124:547-9, 1937.
5. Ash AS, Schild HO. Receptors mediating some actions of histamine. Brit. TJ Pharmacol 27:427-39, 1966.
6. Black JW, Duncan WA, Durant CJ, Ganellin CR, Parsons EM. Definition and antagonism of histamine H_2 receptors. Nature 236:385-90, 1972.
7. Hancock AA, DeLean AL, Lefkowitz RJ. Quantitative resolution of β-adrenergic receptor subtypes by selective ligand binding: application of a computerized model fitting technique. Mol Pharmacol 16:1, 1-9, 1979.
8. Feldman HA. Mathematical theory of complex ligand-binding systems of equilibrium: some methods for parameter fitting. Anal Biochem 48:317-38, 1972.
9. DeLean AL, Munson PJ, Rodbard D. Simultaneous analysis of families of sigmoidal curves: application to bioassay, radioligand assay, and physiological dose-response curves. Am J Physiol 235:E97-102, 1978.
10. Roberts LJ, Marney SR Jr, Oates JA. Blockade of the flush associated with metastatic gastric carcinoid by combined histamine H_1 and H_2 receptor antagonists. Evidence for an important role of H_2 receptors in human vasculature. N Engl JMed 300:236-8, 1979.
11. Brown R, Ingram RH Jr, Wellman JJ, McFadden ER Jr. Effects of intravenous histamine on pulmonary mechanics in nonasthmatic and asthmatic subjects. J Appl Physiol 42:221-7, 1977.
12. Hirschowitz BI. H_2 histamine receptors. Ann Rev Pharmacol Toxicol 19:203-44 1979.
13. Kaliner M, Sigler R, Summers R, Shelhamer JH. Effects of infused histamine: analysis of H_1 and H_2 histamine receptor antagonists on cardiovascular and pulmonary responses. J Allergy Clin Immunol 68:365-71, 1981.
14. Weiss S, Robb GP, Blumgart HL. The velocity of blood flow in health and disease as measured by the effect of histamine on the minute vessels. Am Heart J 4:664-91, 1928-29.
15. Albinus, M, Sewing KR. Cardiovascular effects of burimamide and metiamide. Agents Actions 4:222-26, 1974.
16. Carroll PR, Glover WE, Latt N. Cardiovascular histamine receptors in the rabbit; Aust J Exp Biol Med Sci 52:577-82, 1974.
17. Lewis T. *The Blood Vessels of the Human Skin and Their Responses.* London: Shaw and Sons, Ltd., 1927.
18. Summers R, Sigler R, Shelhamer JH, Kaliner M. Effects of infused histamine on asthmatic and normal subjects: comparison of skin test responses. J Allergy Clin Immunol 67:456-64, 1981.
19. Eiser NM, Mills J, McRae KD, Snashall PD, Guz A. Histamine receptors in normal human bronchi. Clin Sci 58:537-44, 1980.
20. Eiser NM, Mills J, Snashall PD, Guz A. The role of histamine receptors in asthma. Clin Sci 60:363-70, 1981.
21. Dunlop LS, Smith AP. Piper, PJ, The effect of histamine antagonists on antigen-induced contractions of sensitized human bronchus *in vitro.* (Proceedings) Br J Pharmacol 59:475P, 1977.
22. Nathan RA, Segall N, Glover GC, Schocket AL. The effects of H_1 and H_2 antihistamines on histamine inhalation challenges in asthmatic patients. Am Rev Respir Dis 120:1251-8, 1979.
23. Wasserman SI. The lung mast cell: Its physiology and potential relevance to defense of the lung. Environ Health Perspectives 35:153-64, 1980. (42 Ref.)
24. Ahmed T, Mirbahar KB, Oliver W Jr., Eyre P, Wanner A. Characterization of H_1 and H_2 receptor function in pulmonary and systemic circulation of sheep. J Appl Physiol: 53:175-84, 1982
25. Shelhamer JH, Marom Z, Kaliner M. Immunologic and neuropharmacologic stimulation of mucous glycoprotein release from human airways *in vitro.* J. Clin Invest 66:1400-08, 1980.
26. Platshon LF, Kaliner M. The effects of the immunologic release of histamine upon human lung cyclic nucleotide levels and prostaglandin generation. J Clin Invest 62:1113–21, 1978.
27. Casale TB, Rodbard D, Kaliner M. Characterization of histamine H-1 receptors on human peripheral lung. Biochem Pharmacol, 34:3285–3292, 1985.
28. Steel L, Platshon L, Kaliner M. Prostaglandin generation by human and guinea pig lung tissue: Comparison of parenchymal and airway responses. J Allergy Clin Immunol 64:287–93, 1979.
29. Dousa TP, Code CF. Stimulation of cyclic AMP formation in guinea pig gastric mucosa by histamine and N_x-methylhistamine and their blockade by metiamide. In *International Symposium on Histamine H_2 Receptor Antagonists.* Wood CJ and Simkins MA (Eds.). Welwyn Garden City: Smith Kline & French Laboratories Ltd., London 1973, pp. 319–330.
30. Karppanen HO, Westerman E. Increased production of cyclic AMP in gastric tissue by stimulation of histamine 2(H_2) receptors. Naunyn Schmiedebergs Arch Pharmacol, 279:83-87, 1973.
31. McNeill JH, Verma SC. Stimulation of rat gastric adenylate cyclase by histamine and histamine analogues and blockade by burimamide. Br J Pharmacol 52:104-06, 1974.
32. Sachs G, Spenney JG, Shoemaker RL, Sung CP, Jenkins BD, Wiebehaus VD. Action of H_2 antagonists on acid secretion and adenyl cyclase *in vitro.* In *International Symposium on Histamine H_2 receptor Antagonists.* Wood CJ and Simkins MA (Eds.) Welwyn Garden City: Smith Kline & French Laboratories Ltd., 1973 London, pp. 331-340.
33. Batzri S, Harmon JW, Walker MD. Identification of [^{3}H] histamine binding sites on gastric mucosal cells unrelated to histamine H_2 receptors. Biochem Biophys Res Commun 108:965-9, 1982.
34. Hirschowitz BI. H_2 histamine receptors. Annu Rev Pharmacol Toxicol 19:203-44, 1979.
35. Ambache N, Killick SW, Zar MA. Antagonism by burimamide of inhibitions induced by histamine in plexus-containing longitudinal muscle preparations from guinea-pig ileum. Br J Pharmacol 48:362P-363P, 1973.
36. Schwartz JC. Histaminergic mechanisms in brain. Annu Rev Pharmacol Toxicol 17:325-39, 1977.
37. Summers RJ, Kaliner MK. Current concepts of histamine actions through H_1 and H_2 receptors. Compr Ther 8:6-16, 1982.
38. Beaven MA. Histamine: Its role in physiological and pathological processes. Monogr Allergy 13:1-113, 1978.
39. McNeill JH. Histamine receptors and cyclic AMP. Can J. Physiol Pharmacol 58:1023-30, 1980.
40. Schwartz JC, Barbin G, Duchemin AM, Garbarg M Palacios JM, Quach TT, Rose C. Histamine receptors in brain: characterization by binding studies and biochemical effects. In *Receptors for Neurotransmitters and Peptide Hormones.* Pepeu G, Kuhar MJ, Enna SJ (Eds.). New York: Raven Press, 1980, pp. 169-182.
41. Schwartz JC. Minireview: Histamine receptors in brain. Life Sci 25:895-911, 1979.
42. Palacios JM, Schwartz JC, Garbarg M. High affinity binding of ^{3}H-histamine in rat brain. Eur J Pharmacol 50:443-44, 1978.
43. Hill SJ, Emson PC, Young JM. The binding of (^{3}H) mepyramine to histamine H_1 receptors in guinea-pig brain. J Neurochem 31:997-1004, 1978.
44. Quach TT, Duchemin AM, Rose C, Schwartz JC. *In vivo* occupation of cerebral histamine H_1 receptors evaluated with ^{3}H-mepyramine may predict sedative properties of psychotropic drugs. Eur J Pharmacol 60:391-92, 1979.
45. Burkard WP. Histamine H_2 receptor binding with ^{3}H-cimetidine in brain. Eur J Pharmacol 50:449-50, 1978.
46. Badger AM, Young J, Poste G. Inhibition of phytohemagglutinin-induced proliferation of human peripheral blood lymphocytes by histamine and histamine H_1 and H_2 agonists. Clin Exp Immunol 51:178-84, 1983.
47. Clark RAF, Gallin JI, Kaplan AP. The selective eosinophil chemotactic activity of histamine. J Exp Med 142:1462-76, 1975.

48. Tung R, Kagey-Sobotka A, Plaut M, Lichtenstein LM. H_2 antihistamines augment antigen-induced histamine release from human basophils *in vitro*. J Immunol 129:2113-5, 1982.
49. Rocklin RE. Modulation of cellular-immune responses *in vivo* and *in vitro* by histamine receptor-bearing lymphocytes. J Clin Invest 57:1051-58, 1976.
50. Plaut M, Lichtenstein LM, Gillespie E, Henney CS. Studies on the mechanism of lymphocyte-mediated cytolysis. IV. Specificity of the histamine receptor on effector T cells. J Immunol 111:389-94, 1973.
51. Schwartz A, Askenase PW, Gershon RK. Histamine inhibition of the *in vitro* induction of cytotoxic T-cell responses. Immunopharmacology 2:179-90, 1980.
52. Fallah HA, Maillard JL, Voison GA. Regulatory mast cells. I. Suppressive action of their products on an *in vitro* primary immune reaction. Ann Immunol (Paris) 126:669-82, 1975.
53. Melmon KL, Bourne HR, Weinstein Y, Shearer GM, Kram J, Bauminger S. Hemolytic plaque formation by leukocytes *in vitro*. J Clin Invest. 53:13-21, 1974.
54. Lima M, Rocklin RE. Histamine modulates *in vitro* IgG production by pokeweed mitogen-stimulated human mononuclear cells. Cell Immunol 64:324–36, 1981.
55. Casale TB, Wescott S, Rodbard D, Kaliner M. Characterization of histamine H-1 receptors on human mononuclear cells. Int J Immunopharmacol 7:639–645, 1985.
56. Wescott SL, Kaliner M. Histamine H_1 binding site on human polymorphonuclear leukocytes. Inflammation 7:291–300, 1983. □

Chapter III

Abnormalities in the Histamine-Induced Suppressor Cell Network in Atopic Subjects*

Dennis J. Beer, M.D.

ABSTRACT

Antibody responses of the IgE isotype, like other immunoglobulin classes, are regulated by a finely- tuned network of complex positive and negative regulatory factors. This paper reviews studies concerning abnormalities of histamine-induced suppressor T cell activity in atopic subjects. In atopic subjects, there is a reduction in the generation of histamine-induced suppressor cell activity which positively correlates with decreased phenotypic expression of histamine-type 2 receptors on T lymphocytes. Nonatopic control subjects with systemic mastocytosis have normal functional and phenotypic data, suggesting that chronic in vivo activation by histamine of T cells from atopics does not explain the abnormal histamine-induced suppressor response. Proper functioning of the histamine-induced suppressor cell system involves obligatory interactions between lymphocytes and monocytes. Monocytes from atopic subjects produced significantly less prostaglandin E_2 in response to exogenous histamine-induced suppressor factor. A new immunostimulatory drug, Fanetizole mesylate, partially corrects the abnormal histamine-induced suppressor response. Clinical application of this information may lead to new treatments of the atopic diathesis.

Assistant Professor of Medicine, Pulmonary Center, Evans Memorial Department of Clinical Research, Boston University School of Medicine, Boston, MA

Antibody responses of the the IgE isotype, like other immunoglobulin classes, are regulated by a finely-tuned network of complex cellular and molecular interactions. The relevent cells in this immunologic network consist of B lymphocyte precursors of IgE antibody secreting cells, macrophages, and T lymphocytes. In this scheme, the T lymphocyte plays the most sophisticated regulatory role. Thus, there are helper and suppressor T cells capable of mutually interacting with one another as well as with IgE antibody secreting cells. Suppressor T cells may interfere with IgE production at one or more sites along the immunologic network including: (a) the activation of helper T cells; (b) the function of helper T cells in facilitating B cell function; (c) the differentiation of the precursor B lymphocyte to an effector cell and; (d) the production of antibody by a fully mature antibody-secreting cell.

The atopic state is characterized by hyperactivity of IgE-synthesizing B cells.[1-3] Several observations in humans suggest that suppressor T cell dysfunction may contribute to the atopic diathesis. These observations include the following: (a) IgE levels are elevated in recipients of bone marrow transplants during acute graft-versus-host disease - a situation in which suppressor T cells are severely deficient;[4] (b) IgE levels are often elevated in patients with pan-T-cell deficiency;[5,6] numbers of T lymphocytes are decreased in patient with eczema and in infants of atopic parents;[7] and (c) the percentage of membrane-receptor-bearing T cells for the Fc portion of IgG (Tγ) - the T cell populations encompassing suppressor cells - is decreased in atopic subjects.[8]

*This work was supported by a USPHS grant HL-00898 and a grant from the American Lung Association.

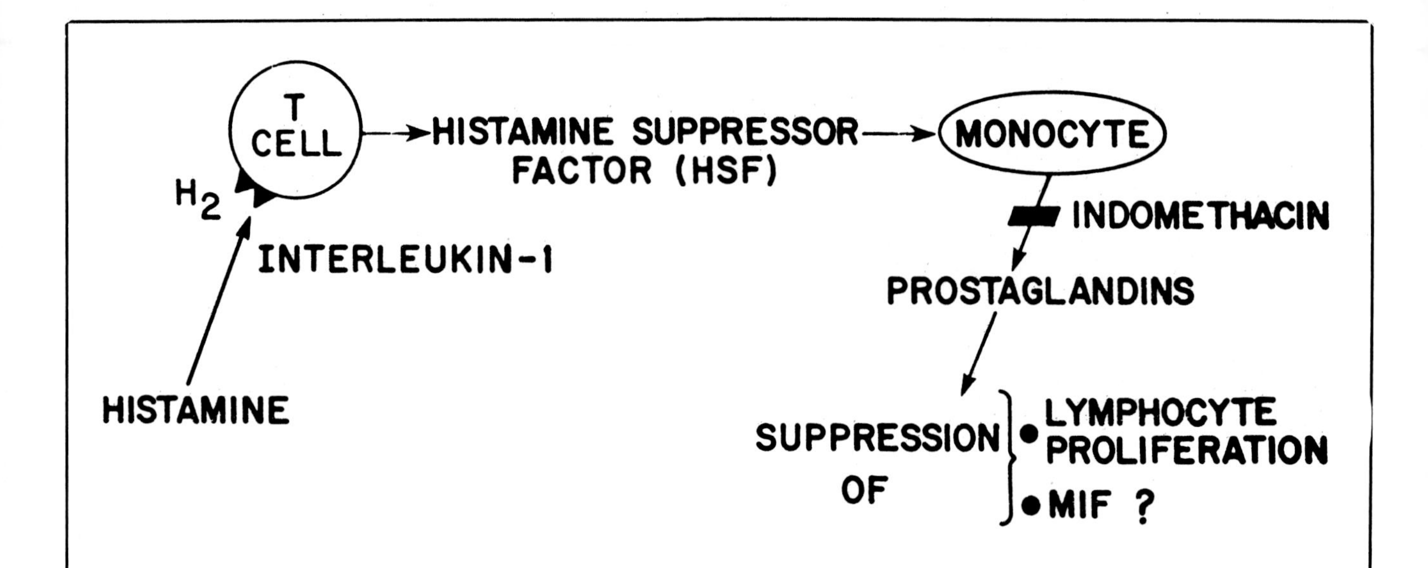

Figure 1. A Proposed Model of the In Vitro Monocyte-Lymphocyte Interactions Required for the Generation and Expression of Histamine-Induced Suppression.

Histamine, in the presence of monocytes or their secretory products, activates a subpopulation of T lymphocytes to elaborate histamine-induced suppressor factor which is capable of stimulating mononuclear phagocytes to synthesize prostaglandins that subsequently suppress lymphocyte proliferation and lymphokine production.

Functionally distinct subsets of T cells with suppressor capabilities have been defined both serologically with monoclonal antibodies directed at stable cell surface glycoproteins[9] and by the presence of functional histamine-type 2 (H_2) receptors.[10-12] Models of immune-induced inflammation have demonstrated that histamine induces an inhibitory signal to leukocytes which participate in inflammatory reactions.[13-15] In particular, histamine interaction with H_2 receptor-bearing lymphocytes induces the elaboration of a suppressor lymphokine (histamine-induced suppressor factor, HSF), which results in the dampening of both T and B cell effector functions.[16-18] Proper functioning of the histamine-induced suppressor cell system involves obligatory interactions between lymphocytes and monocytes.[19] A monokine, interleukin-1 (IL-1) has been shown to augment suppressor lymphocyte activation in response to histamine[20] (Fig. 1). In addition, H_2 receptor-bearing T lymphocytes when activated with histamine in the presence of IL-1, elaborate the lymphokine HSF which augments the production of prostaglandins by monocytes[19,21] (Fig. 1). These latter compounds are thought to be intimately involved in the effector stage of this reaction and may directly suppress T cell function, or further activate suppressor T cells. Recent investigations have provided insights into apparent defects of this immunoregulatory network in atopic subjects.

Figure 2A depicts the results of activating mononuclear cells by histamine (10^{-5}M to 10^{-3}M) and 20μg of concanavalin A (ConA) for 24 hours and coculturing of these cells with autologous mitogen-stimulated indicator cells. As a group, the atopic subjects had cells that were less able to generate histamine-induced suppressor activity than those of a normal control group; however, there was overlap between individual subjects in both groups. At each of the three concentrations of histamine, mononuclear cells from the atopic subjects generated significantly less suppressor activity than did mononuclear cells from normal controls. A histamine concentration of 10^{-3}M was required in the atopic group to induce the same degree of suppressor activity as that produced by 10^{-5}M histamine in the normal control group. The factors of age, sex, presence of asthma, and severity of symptoms did not differentiate the atopic subjects with regard to their ability to generate histamine-induced suppressor activity. This defect in suppressor cell response appeared to be specific for histmine since ConA-induced suppressor activity in these subjects was not statistically different from such activity in the normal controls. Another control group of patients (nonatopic subjects with systemic mastocytosis) had histamine-induced and ConA-induced suppressor activity that was indistinguishable from that of the normal control group.[22]

Although the atopic group had a lower percentage of T cells bearing H_2 receptors than did the normal control population, the percentages of H_2 receptors overlapped between individual subjects in both goups (Fig. 2B). The percentage of T cells possessing the H_1 receptor was the

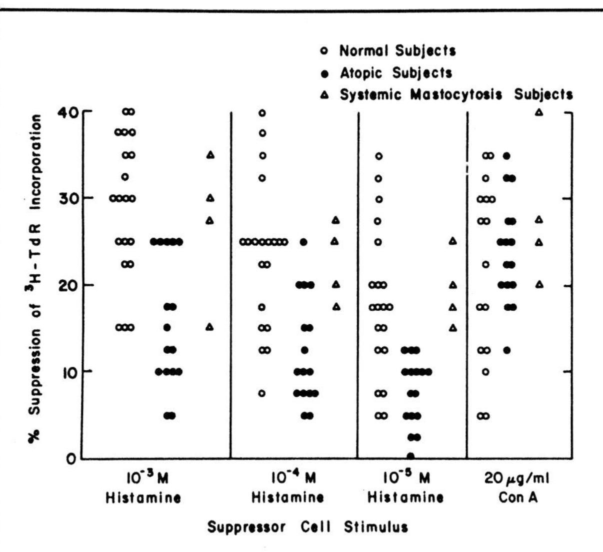

Figure 2A. Suppressor Activity Induced by Histamine and Concanavalin A (ConA) in Atopic Subjects and Controls.

Activity was expressed as the percentage of suppression of tritiated thymidine (^3H-TdR) incorporated into cellular DNA. ConA-induced suppressor activity was similar in all three groups. Despite the overlap of the percentages of histamine-induced suppression in individual subjects in the atopic population with percentages in the normal group, the atopic population as a whole had reduced histamine-induced activity ($p < 0.005$). Suppressor activity in the control group of patients (nonatopic patients with systemic mastocytosis) was similar to that in the normal-control group.

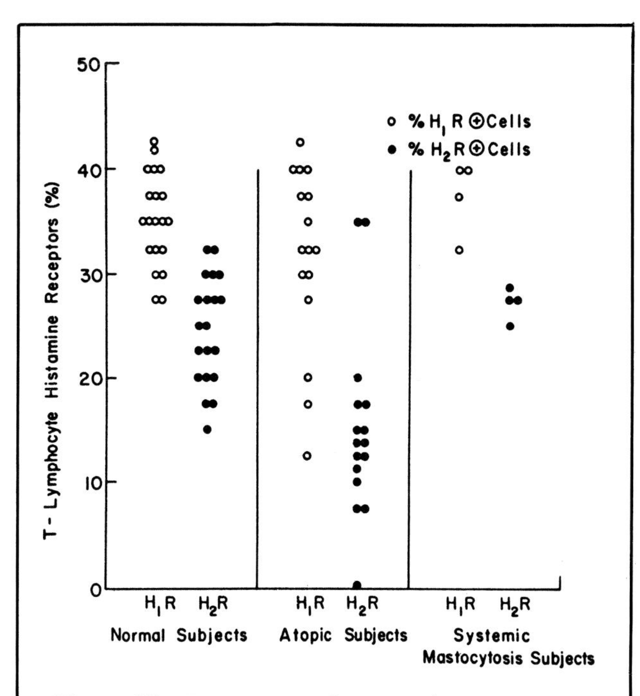

Figure 2B. Percentage of T Lymphocytes Bearing H_1 and H_2 Receptors.

The percentage of T cells bearing H_1 receptors was similar in all three populations. Despite the overlap of percentages of T lymphocytes bearing H_2 receptors in individual subjects in the atopic population with those in the normal group, the atopic population as a whole had a reduced percentage of these T cells ($p<0.001$). Expression of the H_2 receptor in the control mastocytosis patients was similar to that in the normal controls.

same in all three groups. In the atopic group, the results regarding T cell receptors, like those regarding suppressor activity, did not correlate with the clinical features of the subjects. The control group of mastocytosis patients had essentially the same percentage of T cells expressing histamine H_2 receptors as did the normal control subjects.[22] The abnormality in H_2 receptor expression in the atopic population may reflect either a reduction in the number of T lymphocytes bearing the receptor or an abnormality in the binding affinity for histamine of the receptors themselves.

It is of particular interest that regression analysis (Fig. 3) showed a significant correlation between the degree of histamine (10^{-4}M)-induced suppressor cell activity and the phenotypic expression of H_2 receptors in the atopic population.[22] The observations of normal histamine-induced suppressor activity and normal phenotypic expression of H_2 receptors on T lymphocytes of systemic mastocytosis patients (a disease characterized by elevated levels of circulating histmine) mitigates against the observed abnormalities in atopic subjects as being secondary to *in vivo* "desensitization". Rather, the suppressor cell abnormalities observed in allergic subjects may reflect a primary defect inherent in the atopic diathesis.

A subsequent study[23] investigating lymphocyte-monocyte dysfunction in atopic subjects provided further evidence for an underlying defect in the immunoregulatory system of mononuclear cells of atopic patients. As discussed in an earlier section of this review, proper functioning of the histamine-induced suppressor cell system involves obligatory interactions between lymphocytes and monocytes.[19] A monokine, IL-1, has been shown to augment suppressor lymphocyte activation in response to histamine[20] (Fig. 2). In addition, H_2 receptor-bearing T lymphocytes when activated with histamine in the presence of IL-1, elaborate the lymphokine histamine-induced suppressor factor which augments the production of prostaglandins by monocytes[21] (Fig. 1). These latter compound are thought to be intimately involved in the effector stage of this reaction and may

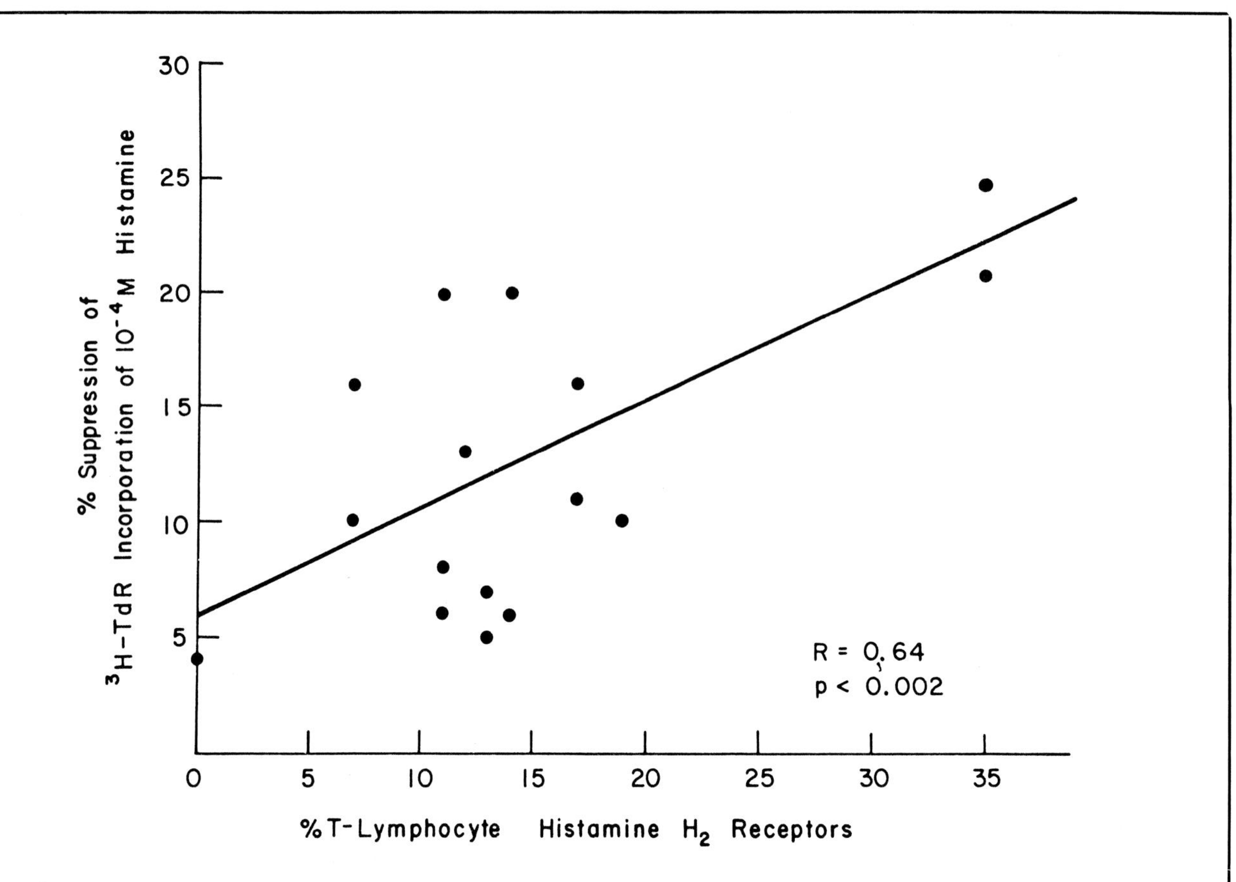

Figure 3. *Regression Analysis of Histamine-Induced Suppression and Percentage of T Lymphocytes Possessing H_2 Receptors in the Atopic Subjects. The line of best fit has a y intercept of 3.8 and a slope of 0.47. The correlation coefficient (r=0.64) is statistically significant (p<0.002).*

directly suppress lymphocyte proliferation or lymphokine production, or further activate suppressor T cells.[24] Mononuclear cells from asymptomatic atopic subjects generated significantly less histamine-induced suppressor activity than cells from nonatopic controls, and mean suppressor factor production was also significantly reduced. The latter two responses were not corrected by the addition of exogenous IL-1. Monocytes from atopic subjects produced significantly less prostaglandin E_2 (PGE_2) in response to exogenous suppressor factor, compared to monocytes from controls (Figs. 4A and B). The atopic group had normal numbers of T-helper and T-suppressor cells. These data indicate that despite having a proper T-helper/T-suppressor cell ratio, T-suppressor cells from atopics produced less suppressor signal than cells from nonatopics, and their monocytes produced less PGE_2 even if the suppressor signal was provided. The reason for the decrease production of PGE_2 by monocytes from atopic subjects is unknown, but may reflect differences in the way in which arachidonic acid is metabolized.

A new immunostimulating drug, Fanetizole mesylate, significantly increased *in vitro* histamine-induced suppressor cell activity of atopic individuals.[25] In the presence of the drug (2.5 x 10^{-4}M), HSF activity in supernatants derived from histamine stimulation of lymphocytes from atopic subjects increased to equal that of normal control values. *In vitro* IgE synthesis by mononuclear cells from atopics (asthma and/or rhinoconjunctivitis) was significantly reduced in the presence of Fanetizole mesylate. Of note, this immunostimulator did not significantly alter pokeweed-induced IgG synthesis by atopic or control cells. These results suggest that Fanetizole mesylate could partially correct an *in vitro* immunoregulatory defect in atopic individuals which may result in reduced *in vitro* IgE synthesis. Clinical application of this drug in symptomatic allergic subjects is currently under way.

In summary, lymphocytes from atopic individuals have a reduced capacity to produce a suppressor factor (HSF) when stimulated by histamine. This defect is not corrected by the exogenous addition of IL-1, but is reversed by the addition of the immunostimulating drug Fanetizole mesylate which also reduced the synthesis of

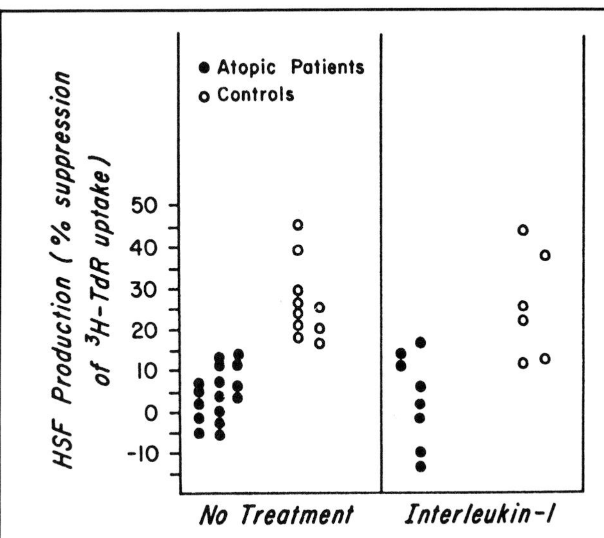

Figure 4A. *HSF Production by Mononuclear Cells from Atopic Patients* (•) and Controls (○). *The mean amount of HSF activity was lower ($p<0.01$) in atopic patients compared to controls. IL-1 added to the cultures did not augment the production of HSF by mononuclear cells from atopic subjects.*

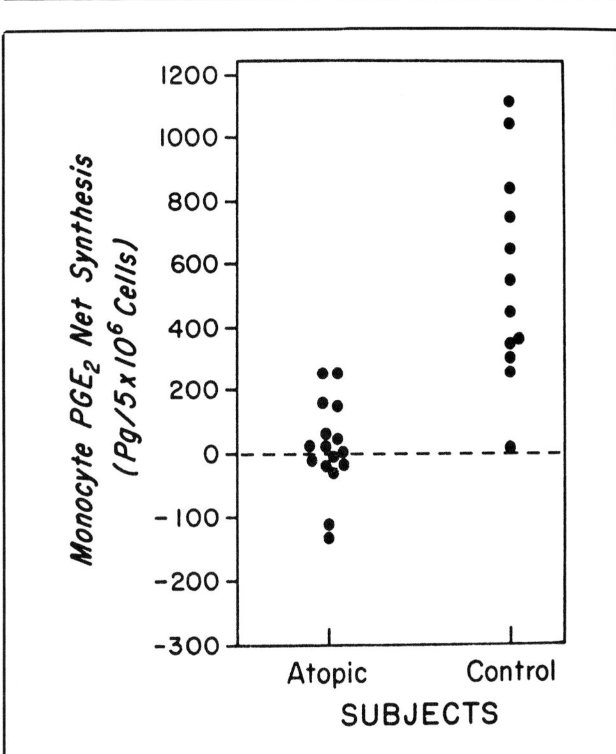

Figure 4B. *PGE_2 Production by HSF-Stimulated Monocytes Obtained from Atopic Patients and Normal Subjects. The mean net synthesis of PGE_2 by monocytes from atopic subjects was significantly reduced ($p<0.01$) compared to that of monocytes from normal controls.*

IgE. This reduction in the generation of HSF is correlated with a decreased phenotypic expression of H_2 receptors of T lymphocytes. Further, if the suppressor factor is exogenously provided to a culture of monocytes from atopic individuals, their production of PGE_2 is reduced compared to the response of monocytes from normal subjects. Collectively, these data provide insight into an apparent defect in immunoregulation in atopic subjects.

It must be stated that the relation between histamine-induced suppressor cell dysfunction and the *in vivo* regulation of IgE biosynthesis is not clear at present. However, in view of the T cell dependence of IgE antibody production, hyperproduction of specific IgE observed in reagenic allergic disease might be a consequence of altered regulatory function. In humans, it has been demonstrated that atopic individuals have reduced proportions of T cells with surface membrane receptors for the Fc portion of IgG and that after successful immunotherapy, the proportion of these T cells reached normal values.[8] Cells within the latter subpopulation are known to regulate immunoglobulin synthesis by suppressing T-dependent B cell differentiation. In the context of the above studies,[22,23,25] it has been shown that T lymphocytes bearing H_2 receptors and expressing suppressor activity following stimulation with histamine also possess receptors for IgG.[26] It is possible then that the observed abnormalities in atopic subjects reflect a global *in vivo* deficiency in antigen-nonspecific and/or antigen-specific suppressor cell activity, either or both of which may be necessary for the dampening of IgE antibody production.

Indirect evidence for this hypothesis is provided by a recent study[27] in which it was demonstrated that ragweed antigen-specific suppressor T lymphocytes could be detected in ragweed allergic individuals after six and twelve months of immunotherapy, but not prior to therapy. When lymphocytes were taken from treated patients and passed over columns containing insolubilized histamine, antigen-specific suppressor T cells that could be activated by ragweed antigen were deleted. These results indicate that antigen-specific suppressor T cells belonging to the subpopulation of lymphocytes bearing histamine receptors were generated during antigen desensitization, and failure to detect these cells in untreated patients may be a reflection of the basic defect leading to the atopic diathesis.

REFERENCES

1. Tada T. Regulation of reagenic antibody formation in animals. Prog Allergy 19:122-94, 1975. (206 Ref.)
2. Ishizaka K, Ishizaka T. Mechanisms of reagenic hypersensitivity and IgE antibody response. Immunol Rev 41:109-48, 1978. (88 Ref.)

3. Katz D.H. Control of the IgE antibody production by suppressor substances. J Allergy Clin Immunol 62:44-55, 1978.
4. Geha RS, Rappaport JM, Twarog FJ, Parkman R, Rosen FS. Increased serum immunoglobulin E levels following allogeneic bone marrow transplantation. J Allergy Clin Immunol 66:78-81, 1980.
5. Waldman TA, Polmar SH, Balestra ST, et al. Immunoglobulin E in immunologic deficiency diseases. II. Serum IgE concentration of patients with acquired hypogammaglobulinemia, thymoma, and hypogammaglobunemia, myotonic dystrophy, intestinal lymphangiectasia and Wiscott-Aldrich syndrome. J Immunol 109:304-10, 1972.
6. Kikkawa Y, Kamimura K, Hamajima T, et al. Thymic alymphoplasia with hyper-IgE-globulinemia. Pediatrics 51:690-96, 1973.
7. Strannegård O, Strannegård IL. T lymphocyte numbers and function in human IgE-mediated allergy. Immunol Rev 41:149-70, 1978. (128 Ref.)
8. Canonica GW, Mingari ML, Melioli G, Colombatti M, Moretta L. Imbalances of T cell subpopulations in patients with atopic diseases and effect of specific immunotherapy. J Immunol 123:2669-72, 1979.
9. Reinherz EL, Schlossman SF. The differentiation and function of human T lymphocytes. Cell 19:821-27, 1980. (38 Ref.)
10. Shearer GM, Melmon KL, Weinstein Y, Sela M. Regulation of antibody response by cells expressing histamine receptors. J Exp Med 136:1302-07, 1972.
11. Rocklin RE. Modulation of cellular-immune responses *in vivo* and *in vitro* by histamine receptor-bearing lymphocytes. J Clin Invest 57:1051-58, 1976.
12. Lima, M, Rocklin RE. Histamine modulates *in vitro* IgG production by pokeweed mitogen-stimulated human mononuclear cells. Cell Immunol 64:324-36, 1981
13. Plaut M, Lichtenstein LM, Gillespie E, Henney CS. Studies on the mechanism of lymphocyte-mediated cytolysis. IV. Specificity of the histamine receptor on effector T cells. J Immunol 111:389-94, 1973.
14. Rocklin RE, Greineder D, Littman BH, Melmon KL. Modulation of cellular immune function *in vitro* by histamine receptor-bearing lymphocytes: Mechanism of action. Cell Immunol 37:162-73, 1978.
15. Beer DJ, Rocklin RE. Histamine and immune modulation, in Advances in Internal Medicine, (Stollerman GH, ed), vol. 28. Chicago, 1983, Year Book Medical Publishers, Inc. p. 225.
16. Rocklin RE. Histamine-induced suppressor factors (HSF): Effect on migration inhibitory factor (MIF) production and proliferation. J Immunol 118:1734-38, 1977.
17. Garovoy MR, Reddish MA, Rocklin RE. Histamine-induced suppressor factor (HSF): Inhibiton of helper T cell generation and function. J Immunol 130:357-61, 1983.
18. Plaut M, Lichtenstein LM. Histamine and immune responses, in: Pharmacology of Histamine Receptors, (Ganelin CR, Patsons E, eds), London, 1982, John Wright and Sons, p. 392.
19. Beer DJ, Rosenwasser LJ, Dinarello CA, Rocklin RE. Cellular interactions in the generation and expression of histamine-induced suppressor activity. Cell Immunol 69:101-12, 1982.
20. Beer DJ, Dinarello CA, Rosenwasser LJ, Rocklin RE. Human monocyte-derived soluble product(s) has an accessory function in the generation of histamine-and concanavalin A-induced suppressor T cells. J Clin Invest 70:393-400, 1982.
21. Rocklin RE, Kiselis I, Beer DJ, Rossi P, Maggi F, Bellanti JA. Augmentaion of prostaglandin and thromboxane production *in vitro* by monocytes exposed to histamine-induced suppressor factor (HSF). Cell Immunol 77:92-98, 1983.
22. Beer DJ, Osband ME, McCaffrey RP, Soter NA, Rocklin RE. Abnormal histamine-induced suppressor-cell function in atopic subjects. N Engl J Med 306:454-58, 1982.
23. Matloff SM, Kiselis IK, Rocklin RE. Reduced production of histamine-induced suppressor factor (HSF) by atopic mononuclear cells and decreased prostaglandin E_2 output by HSF-stimulated atopic monocytes. J Allergy Clin Immunol 72:359-64, 1983.
24. Goodwin JS, Webb DR. Regulation of the immune response by prostaglandins. Clin Immunol Immunopath 15:106-22, 1980. (104 Ref.)
25. Rocklin RE, Hemady Z, Matloff S, et al. Correction of an *in vitro* immunoregulatory defect in atopic subjects by the immunostimulating drug Fanetizole mesylate (CP-48,810). Internatl J Immunopharm In press.
26. Rocklin RE, Breard J, Gupta S, et al. Characterization of the human blood lymphocytes that produce a histamine-induced suppressor factor (HSF). Cell Immunol 51:226-37, 1980.
27. Rocklin RE, Sheffer AL, Greineder DK, Melmon KL. Generation of antigenspecific suppressor cells during allergy desensitization. N Engl J Med 302:1213-19, 1980. □

Chapter IV

Anaphylaxis

Michael A. Kaliner, M.D.

ABSTRACT

Anaphylaxis is an acute medical emergency caused by systemic mast cell degranulation in response to diverse stimuli. The etiology of anaphylaxis ranges from IgE-mediated allergic reactions to anaphylactoid responses caused by infusions of radiocontrast media. The common thread in the spectrum of causes is mast cell degranulation with systemic release of mediators, particulary histamine. As histamine is one of the predominant causes of the clinical changes occurring in anaphylaxis, treatment of anaphylaxis requires both H_1 *and* H_2 *histamine receptor antagonists in addition to epinephrine.*

Porter and Richet employed the word *anaphylaxis* to describe the fatal reaction induced by the introduction of minute amounts of antigen into dogs which had been previously sensitized.[1] The dramatic and unexpected fatal response was the opposite (ana =Greek: back, backwards) of protection (phylax = Greek: guard). Our knowledge and comprehension of anaphylaxis has paralleled our understanding of the components of the immune system and, while there are still areas of uncertainty, is now rather complete.

Anaphylaxis is the syndrome elicited in a hypersensitive subject upon subsequent exposure to the sensitizing antigen. The spectrum of *anaphylactic responses* ranges from localized to systemic. Systemic anaphylaxis can cause *anaphylactic shock* and death. The necessary components of the anaphylactic response are 1) a sensitizing antigen, usually administered parenterally; 2) an IgE class antibody response resulting in systemic sensitization of mast cells (and basophils); 3) reintroduction of the sensitizing antigen, usually systemically; 4) mast cell degranulation with mediator release and/or generation; and 5) production of a number of pathologic responses by the mast cell-derived mediators and manifested as anaphylaxis.

Because anaphylaxis is caused by the mediators that are released or generated by mast cells, any event associated with mast cell activation may produce the same clinical disease. Anaphylaxis usually refers to IgE-mediated, antigen-stimulated mast cell activation, while *anaphylactoid* reactions denote other, non-IgE-mediated responses such as may be produced by chemical agents capable of causing mast cell degranulation (e.g., opiates).

The common causes of anaphylaxis are summarized on Table 1. The most frequent causes include penicillin reactions (causing 400-800 deaths), *Hymenoptera* stings (causing 100 or more deaths), and radiocontrast dye reactions (causing 250-1000 deaths).

Regardless of cause, the symptoms of anaphylaxis are quite similar. The primary organs that express anaphylactic shock in humans are in the cutaneous, gastrointestinal, respiratory, and cardiovascular systems (Table 2). Characteristically, patients describe an immediate sense of impending doom coincident with flushing, tachycardia, and oftentimes pruritus (either diffuse, localized to

---

Allergic Diseases Section, Laboratory of Clinical Investigation, National Institute of Allergy and Infectious Diseases, National Institutes of Health, Building 10, Room 11C205, Bethesda, Maryland 20205

Table I

Causes of Anaphylaxis/Anaphylactoid Reactions

I. **IgE-mediated reactions**
   Antibiotics and other drugs
   Foreign proteins (horse serum, chymopapain)
   Foods
   Immunotherapy
   Hymenoptera stings
   Seminal plasma
II. **Complement-mediated reactions**
   Blood, blood products
III. **Nonimmunologic mast cell activators**
   Opiates (narcotics)
   Muscle depolarizing agents
   Radiocontrast media
IV. **Modulators of arachidonic acid metabolism**
   Nonsteroidal anti-inflammatory agents
   Tartrazine (possible)
V. **Idiopathic recurrent anaphylaxis**
VI. **Others, as yet unclassified**
   Sulfiting agents
   Exercise
   Many drugs and chemicals

the palms and the soles of the feet, and/or noted particulary in the genital and inner thigh areas). These initial symptoms rapidly evolve to urticaria, angioedema, rhinorrhea, bronchorrhea, nasal congestion, asthma, laryngeal edema, abdominal bloating, nausea, vomiting, cramps, arrhythmias, faintness, syncope, prostration, and even death. The organ systems involved are the richest sources of mast cells.[2] Since anaphylaxis is caused by mast cell degranulation, it is predictable that the "shock organs" involved would be those richest in mast cells. Thus, knowledge of mast cell-derived mediators, the pathologic responses to mediator release, and the organs involved should permit anticipation of all of the changes seen in anaphylaxis.

When the larynx and cardiovascular systems are involved, mortality becomes a significantly greater concern. The most common causes of death are cardiovascular collapse and laryngeal edema with asphyxiation. In most cases, laryngeal edema is preceded by "a lump in the throat," hoarseness, and difficulty in breathing. Hypotension due to anaphylactic shock is usually preceded by diffuse flushing, urticaria, light-headedness, faintness, and syncope.

The usual progression of symptoms begins within minutes of exposure to the inciting agent, peaks within 15-30 min. and is complete within hours. Anaphylaxis may be complicated by myocardial infarction or stroke, resulting in death.

PATHOGENESIS

Mast cells and their mediators have been extensively reviewed elsewhere.[2,3] When mast cells degranulate, preformed and rapidly generated mediators are released into the connective tissue along with the molecules which constitute the granular matrix. While many of these mediators induce dramatic local effects, few, other than histamine, are capable of entering the circulation in an active state. Thus, the symptoms of anaphylaxis can be attributed primarily to the local actions of the many mast cell mediators and the circulating effect of histamine. As summarized in Table 3, the majority of the changes occurring in anaphylaxis can be attributed to histamine (acting through H1 and H2 receptors), prostaglandins, and leukotrienes.

DIFFERENTIAL DIAGNOSIS

Given the constellation of an acute exposure to a provocative condition followed within minutes by the evolution of multisystem manifestations including flushing, urtication, pruritus, and angioedema, there is usually not much difficulty in diagnosing anaphylaxis. The diagnosis which might be most easily confused with anaphylaxis is a vasovagal reaction. In deciding between these diagnoses, the clearest differential features are the presence in vasovagal reactions of pallor, extreme diaphoresis, and bradycardia or normal sinus rhythm, and the absence of flushing, urticaria, angioedema, pruritus and asthma.

The correct diagnosis is much more difficult in a syncopal patient. The usual differential diagnoses include cardiac arrhythmias, myocardial infarction, pulmonary embolism, seizures, asphyxiation, hypoglycemia, and stroke. In analyzing the syncopal subject, anaphylaxis should be considered if urticaria, angioedema, or asthma are present or if the history suggests an acute exposure to conditions associated with anaphylaxis (e.g., *Hymenoptera* stings).

If laryngeal edema is the presenting problem, hereditary angioedema (HAE) must be considered. This disorder is usually inherited (although a smaller portion of the affected population may acquire the defect) and is accompanied by painless (and pruritus-free) angioedema, GI cramps and distension, recurrent attacks, and usually a family history of similar attacks and/or sudden death. HAE, which is not associated with flushing, asthma, or urticaria, is of slower onset and, in the absence of severe airway obstruction, is not a cause of hypotension.

Serum sickness differs from anaphylaxis in that it is characterized by fever, lymphadenopathy, macular-papular and urticarial rashes, arthralgias and arthritis,

Table II

Clinical Findings in Anaphylaxis

System	Signs	Symptoms
Cutaneous	Flushing, urticaria, angioedema	Flushing, pruritus
Cardiovascular	Tachycardia, hypotension, shock, syncope, arrhythmias	Faintness, palpitations, weakness
Gastrointestinal	Abdominal distension, vomiting, diarrhea	Bloating, nausea, cramps, pain
Respiratory	Rhinorrhea, laryngeal edema, wheezing, bronchorrhea, asphyxiation	Nasal congestion, shortness of breath, difficulty breathing, choking, cough, hoarseness, lump in throat
Others	Diaphoresis, fecal or urinary incontinence	Feeling of impending doom, conjunctival pruritus and edema, sneezing, disorientation, hallucinations, genital burning, headaches, metallic taste

and less frequently with nephritis and neuritis. Serum sickness generally develops 5-10 days after antigen exposure and may persist for 2-3 weeks.

Systemic mastocytosis, another diagnostic possibility, is a widespread hyperplasia of mast cells, usually of a benign or very low grade malignancy. Urticaria pigmentosa is a more frequently encountered benign growth of mast cells restricted to the skin. In either disease, it is possible for the mast cells to degranulate, generally producing local effects or more rarely causing systemic effects exactly like anaphylaxis. Degranulation of these lesions can occur spontaneously, and after exposure to nonsteroidal anti-inflammatory drugs, alcohol, or narcotics (as well as other nonimmunologic mast cell-degranulating agents). The diagnosis should be suggested by the recognition of the classic fawn-colored macular-to-low-papular skin lesions which urticate on trauma (Darier's sign), the history of flushing attacks, evidence of bone involvement (pain or abnormalities revealed by bone scans and X-rays), GI pain and peptic ulcers, histaminurea, histaminemia and increased urinary PGD_2 metabolites.

Other conditions which might also be considered include overdoses of medications, cold urticaria, pheochromocytoma, carcinoid tumors, and sulfite or monosodium glutamate ingestion in sensitive subjects.

TREATMENT OF ACUTE ANAPHYLAXIS

Anaphylaxis is an acute medical emergency requiring prompt and appropriate attention (Table 4). If possible, remove the source of antigen or retard its systemic circulation. Carefully remove the stinger if a *Hymenoptera* bite is responsible, tourniquet the extremity and inject epinephrine (0.1-.2 ml, 1:1000) directly into the antigen source in order to reduce the local circulation. Epinephrine (1:1000, 0.3-0.5 ml SQ) is the mainstay of the treatment plan. This drug maintains the blood pressure, antagonizes many of the adverse actions of the mediators of anaphylaxis, and reduces the subsequent release of mediators through its action on mast cells and basophils.

In moderate-to-severe cases where epinephrine alone is not adequate therapy, administer both H1 and H2 antihistamines, diphenhydramine 25-50 mg IM and cimetidine 300 mg *slowly* IV (over 3-5 min). If upper airway obstruction is evident (lump in the throat, hoarseness, stridor), have the patient spray *epinephrine* from a

Table III

Processes Involved in the Symptoms of Anaphylaxis

Pathologic Process	Sign or Symptom	Putative Mediator Responsible
Vascular permeability	Urticaria, angioedema, laryngeal edema, abdominal swelling, cramps	Histamine (H1), leukotrienes, prostaglandins
Vasodilation	Flushing, headache	Histamine (H1 and H2), leukotrienes, prostaglandins
Smooth muscle contraction	Wheezing (asthma), GI cramps, diarrhea	Histamine (H1), leukotrienes, prostaglandins
Tachycardia	Palpitations	Histamine (H1), leukotrienes
Reduced peripheral vascular resistance	Faintness, syncope	Histamine (H1 and H2)
Mucus secretion	Rhinorrhea, bronchorrhea	Histamine (H2), prostaglandins, leukotrienes

metered-dose inhaler against a closed glottis in order to try to reduce the local swelling. If the obstruction is progressing, *immediately* place a nasopharyngeal airway or perform a tracheostomy. Once laryngeal edema has developed, it is impossible to place a nasopharyngeal tube! One of our subjects developed severe recurrent laryngeal edema during recurrent anaphylaxis from idiopathic causes and was effectively treated only after opening a tracheal fenestration.

Blood pressure should be maintained with fluid, plasma expanders and pressors, as needed. Asthma that has not responsed to diphenhydramine should be treated with aminophylline (loading dose = 5.6 mg/kg/20 min followed by 0.9-1 mg/kg/hr) and inhaled β_2-adrenergic agonists. Corticosteroids have no immediate effect but should be administered to prevent prolonged or recurrent sequelae. The usual dose is 100 mg of hydrocortisone every 6 hr.

A recent complexity in the treatment of anahylaxis has developed with the increased use of β-adrenergic blocking agents in many subjects (e.g., headaches, hypertension, heart failure, glaucoma). It appears that β-adrenergic receptor antagonists potentiate allergic reactions, possibly by reducing the normal homeostatic influences induced by circulating catecholamines. Treatment of anaphylaxis in the presence of β-adrenergic blockade should be essentially unchanged, recognizing the fact that agents such as epinephrine that ordinarily stimulate both α- and β-adrenergic receptors will act predominantly upon α-receptors under these circumstances. Asthma developing as part of the spectrum of anaphylaxis should not be treated solely with β-adrenergic agonists as they are likely to be ineffective. When searching for underlying causes of unexplained anaphylaxis, attention should be directed at topical β-adrenergic antagonists used in the treatment of glaucoma.

PREVENTION AND PROPHYLAXIS OF ANAPHYLAXIS

Subjects with known sensitivity should avoid reexposure if possible. For instance, insect sting-sensitive individuals should avoid areas with the increased likelihood of insect encounters, should always wear shoes when walking in grass, avoid smelling like a flower (hair sprays, perfumes, after-shaving lotion, etc.), avoid looking like a flower (flowered or brightly colored clothing), and carry an anaphylaxis emergency treatment kit at all times. The so-called "stinging-insect emergency kit" usually con-

Table IV

Treatment of Acute Anaphylaxis (adult)

1) When possible, tourniquet the draining blood flow from the source of the antigen or inciting medication. Remove the stinger if an insect bite. Remove the tourniquet every 15 min.

2) Place patient in recumbent position, elevate legs, keep warm, provide 0_2.

3) Epinephrine aqueous 1:1,000, 0.3-0.5 ml SQ; from this amount inject epinephrine 1:1,000, 0.1-0.2 ml directly into source of antigen to reduce blood flow.

4) Diphenhydramine 25-50 mg IM or IV over 3 min.

5) Cimetidine 300 mg IV over 3-5 min.

6) Establish and maintain airway; administer racemic epinephrine metered-dose inhaler to closed airway if laryngeal edema present.

7) Maintain blood pressure with fluids, volume expanders or pressors: dopamine hydrochloride 2-10 μg/kg/min or norepinephrine bitartrate, 2-4 μg/min.

8) If wheezing is a problem, administer aminophylline 5.6 mg/kg over 20 min, initiate maintenance dose of 0.9 mg/kg/hr thereafter.

9) For prolonged reactions, repeat epinephrine every 20 min x 3, provide hydrocortisone, 100 mg IV every 6 hr.

tains injectable epinephrine and a rapidly-absorbed antihistamine. Certain epinephrine preparations are available in a spring-loaded form that facilitates injection. Anyone who is given such a kit should be carefully instructed in its use, *including injecting themselves* with epinephrine while under the direct observation of a physician. Consideration of desensitizing such patients with venom is certainly warranted.

When there is doubt about the appropriate therapeutic material or when a medication is required despite likely reactivity, the subject may be treated with prophylactic H1 and H2 antihistamines - hydroxyzine 25 mg QID and cimetidine 300 mg QID - for several doses before exposure. Subjects at increased risk, e.g., previous reactors to iodinated contrast media, should in addition be pretreated with prednisone (50 mg every 6 hr x 3) before reexposure.

CONCLUSION

Anaphylaxis is a dramatic, major medical emergency. Comprehension of the pathogenesis, emergency treatment, and subsequent prophylaxis can reduce both morbidity and mortality. The most important component in the avoidance of anaphylaxis is a conscientious physician who carefully weighs each therapeutic decision and ferrets out possible warnings of prior exposures/reactions. Prompt medical attention to subjects experiencing anaphylaxis should reduce mortality.

Initiating a carefully considered therapeutic or diagnostic maneuver only to elicit anaphylaxis remains one of the major misfortunes of medicine. This result, which is truly the opposite of prophylaxis, reveals the terrible potency that allergic reactions can muster.

REFERENCES

1. Richet C. Des effets anaphylactiques de l'actinotoxine sur la pression arterielle. Comptes Rend Scan Soc Biol 54:832-837, 1902.
2. Metcalfe DD, Kaliner M, Donlon MA. The mast cell. CRC Crit Rev Immunol 3:23-74, 1981. (456 Ref.)
3. Wasserman SI. Mediators of immediate hypersensitivity. J Allergy Clin Immunol. 72:101-119, 1983. (185 Ref.) □

HISTAMINE RECEPTORS IN TISSUES

Chapter V

Nasal Neural-Chemical Receptors

Guy A. Settipane, M.D.

ABSTRACT

Nasal neural-chemical receptors of the nose play an important role in the physiology of both the upper and lower airways. The H_1 histamine receptor initiates significant reactions while the H_2 histamine receptor is essentially nonfunctional in the nose. Other major nasal receptors are the alpha and beta$_2$ adrenoceptor, cholinoceptor, and the irritant receptor. Understanding the characteristics of these receptors both in terms of agonistic and inhibiting drugs is important in the proper treatment of rhinitis, sinusitis, and asthma.

There are six neural-chemical receptors identified in the nose. Five of these are highly functional and play an important role in the physiology of the nose.[1] These nasal receptors are as follows: Alpha adrenoceptor, beta$_2$ adrenoceptor, cholinoceptor, H_1 histamine receptor, H_2 histamine receptor (essentially nonfunctional), and the irritant receptor, Table I.

The H_1 histamine receptor is stimulated by histamine, which causes a direct and indirect increase in nasal airway resistance. If histamine is placed in one nasal canal, both canals will have an increased nasal resistance to airflow, but the side without histamine will be congested only about 60%, as much as the side with histamine.[2] Therefore, it is postulated that about 60% of nasal congestion is indirectly produced by histamine through neural reflex action. Repeated application of histamine to the nasal mucosa will produce tachyphylaxis of this neural reflex but will not inhibit the direct action of histamine on the mucosa.[2] H_1 antihistamines block the H_1 receptors, greatly diminishing the effect of histamine. H_1 antihistamines do not improve nasal airway resistance but do suppress sneezing, itching, and hypersecretion.

The H_2 histamine receptor is essentially nonfunctional in the nose.[3] The anatomical location, description, function, and physiology of this receptor will be described in detail in other parts of this symposium. Essentially, it is stimulated by histamine and is blocked by cimetidine and other newer types of H_2 antihistamines. H_1 antihistamines have no effect on the H_2 histamine receptors.

The alpha adrenoceptor is stimulated by neosynephrine and norepinephrine-like drugs causing a decreased nasal airway resistance. Most topical nasal medications are directed toward the alpha adrenoceptor. Reserpine and reserpine-like drugs deplete natural occurring norepinephrine from neural junctions, causing an increased nasal airway resistance.

Unlike its effect on the lung, stimulation of the Beta$_2$ adrenoceptor increases airway resistance in the nose. Isoproterenol application to the nose causes an increased airway resistance, which is blocked by propranolol.[4] One hypothesis for this opposite action on the nose compared to the lung is that Beta$_2$ adrenoceptor agonists cause relaxation of smooth muscles. In the lung, this action results in bronchial dilation. The only smooth muscle present in the nose is associated with the blood capillary walls, and relaxation of these muscles result in dilation of

Clinical Associate Professor, Brown University and Director, Division of Allergy, Department of Medicine, R.I. Hospital

Table I

Nasal Receptors

	Type of Receptor	Drug	Action	Nasal Airway Resistance	Remarks
1	Histamine (H_1) Receptor	Histamine	Stimulation	Increased	60% of action is through neuro-reflexes, H_1 receptor blocked by H_1-antihistamines
2	Histamine (H_2) Receptor	Histamine	Stimulation	Slightly increased	H_2 receptor blocked by cimetidine which has slight to no effect
3	Alpha Adrenoceptor	Neosynepherine Norepinephrine	Stimulation	Decreased	Reserpine depletes nor-epinephrine causing increased nasal airway resistance
4	$Beta_2$ Adrenoceptor	Isoproterenol	Stimulation	Increased	Blocked by propranolol
5	Cholinoceptor	Methacholine	Stimulation	Increased	Causes profuse rhino-rrhea blocked by atropine
6	Irritant Receptor	Non specific (dust, histamine, NH_3, SO_2, etc)	Stimulation	Increased	Reflex abolished by atropine. Antihista-mines have no effect

Antihistamines do not improve nasal airway resistance, but do suppress sneezing, itching and hypersecretion.

Table II

Drugs That Have Different Affect On Nose and Lungs

DRUGS	NOSE	LUNGS
Isoproterenol	↑ NAR	Bronchodilation
Methacholine	↑ NAR in normals, ↑ rhinitis, asthma	↑ Sensitivity in asthma
Histamine	↑ NAR in normals, ↑ rhinitis, asthma	↑ Sensitivity in asthma

NAR = Nasal Airway Resistance

the capillaries, engorgement of blood vessels, and extravasation of fluid. The end result being nasal congestion.

Besides isoproterenol, other drugs have different effects on the nose compared to the lungs, Table II. Methacholine and histamine cause a worsening of normal function both in the nose and lungs;[4] topical application or inhalation of these drugs cause an increase in nasal airway resistance and bronchospasm, respectively. However, inhalation challenges of histamine and methacholine to the lungs differentiates between an asthmatic patient and a normal individual. Asthmatic patients respond with bronchospasm to these drugs at a significantly lower dose than normal individuals. On the other hand, both of these drugs produce increased nasal airway resistance to the same degree so that patients with allergic rhinitis and normal individuals are not differentiated with this procedure.

The cholinoceptor is part of the parasympathetic system and is stimulated by methacholine which causes profuse rhinorrhea. The cholinoceptor is blocked by atropine. Antihistamines have no effect on this receptor.

The irritant receptor is an extremely important receptor, whose significance has been appreciated only recently. This receptor is stimulated by nonspecific chemicals such as dust, histamine, NH_3, and SO_2. Most of the action of this receptor is through neural reflex action and is inhibited by atropine. Local anesthetics to the nose, such as lidocaine, will also inhibit this reflex. Antihistamines, both H_1 and H_2, do not inhibit actions initiated by the irritant receptor.

The irritant receptor plays an important role in the rhinobronchial reflex. Stimulation of neural receptors in the nose, pharyngeal and sinus areas can produce bronchospasm through neural reflexes. The receptors involved are the histamine (H_1) and irritant receptors which send afferent neural impulses through the Trigeminal, Facial and Glossopharyngeal nerve to the medulla oblongata where the vagal nucleus is stimulate. The efferent arm of this reflex is the vagal nerve with its ramifications sending neural impulses to the bronchial tree causing bronchospasm in much the same way as a methacholine inhalation challenge. Kaufman and Wright[5] demonstrated that increased airway resistance produced by exposing the nasal and nasopharyngeal area to silica particles, which stimulate the irritant receptors, was prevented by pre-treatment with atropine. Ogura et al[6] reported that functional compliance in the lung is increased by the use of nasal sprays (vasoconstrictors) or following nasal surgery where an airway obstruction is removed. They also noted that functional lung compliance, measured through the mouth, decreased with increasing grades of nasal obstruction.

In dogs, Whicker et al[7] found that nasal stimulation typically produced marked changes in breathing patterns such as a large transient increase (150%) in pulmonary air flow resistance. This response could also be produced by stimulation of the nasal branches of the trigeminal or the vagus nerves.

In normal human males, Wyllie et al[8] produced nasal obstruction by bilateral placement of petrolatum nasal packing and found a statistically significant increase in pulmonary airway resistance. These individuals also complained of sleeplessness and increasing fatigue. Both of these symptoms are frequently associated with patients who have allergic rhinitis. Mistakenly, fatigue may be attributed to antihistamines that patients may be taking, rather than this intrinsic characteristic of allergic rhinitis.

Recently, Yan and Salome[9] tested 12 subjects with perennial allergic rhinitis and stable asthma with increasing doses of histamine sprayed bilaterally on the nasal mucosa. All subjects experienced a greater than six-fold increase in inspiratory nasal flow resistance. Six subjects out of 12 had a dose-related fall of greater than 20% in FEV_1. These results suggest that only some asthmatic patients are affected by the rhinobronchial reflex.

It is not clear whether a cold stimulus to the nose produces a response through the irritant receptor or that a separate cold receptor exists. Nolte and Berger[10] reported that in 27 asthmatic patients, a single cold stimulus into the nose resulted in a sudden increase in pulmonary airway resistance. This effect could be blocked by previous intrabronchial application of an anticholinergic drug. They stated that in laryngectomised patients, who no longer have a connection between the upper and lower airways, a cold stimulus into the nose also caused bronchoconstriction, thus, confirming a reflex mechanism.

Clinically, the treatment of acute or chronic sinusitis with antibiotics, decongestants or surgical procedures (both removal of polyps or sinus operations) has been found to diminish asthmatic episodes in certain cases to such a degree that corticosteroids were able to be discontinued or greatly reduced.[11-14] As far back as 1947, Robert A. Cooke[15] suggested that sinusitis may aggravate an existing asthma and improvement of the sinus condition may improve the asthma. He was so convinced of this association that he had an extensive operation done on his own diseased sinuses in order to control his asthma. A subsequent painting of Dr. Cooke displays a prominent scar over his right frontal sinus as a result of this operation. Now, his clinical observations have been confirmed by objective scientific data using modern technology.

Since acute or chronic sinusitis or rhinitis aggravates asthma probably through the rhinopulmonary reflex, it becomes extremely important to treat the nose and sinus areas in patients with asthma, especially since chronic sinusitis and rhinitis frequently co-exist with asthma.

The irritant receptor in the nose and pharynx also plays an important role in metabisulfite reactions. The main symptoms of this reaction are flushing, acute bronchospasm, and hypotension occurring within minutes of ingesting foods sprayed with this preservative (foods and drugs containing this antioxidant are listed in the NER Allergy Proc. 5: 243, 1984). These patients are usually asthmatics and only about 10% of them experience this reaction.[16,17] The pathogenic mechanism is through the rhinobronchial reflex. Sulfites or an immediate breakdown product such as SO_2 stimulates the irritant receptor,

Table III

Nasal Reflexes

TYPE	ACTION
1. Rhinobronchial	Bronchospasm
2. Sneezing (5th nerve)	Clears nasal passages
3. Rhinosalivary	↑ Salivation
4. Rhinogastric	↑ Gastric Secretion
5. Exercise (hypothalamus)	↓ Nasal resistance (↑ sympathetic tone)
6. ↑ CO_2 (arterial chemoreceptors)	↓ Nasal resistance
7. ↓ CO_2 (arterial chemoreceptors)	↑ Nasal resistance
8. Vasomotor rhinitis (parasympathetic overactivity)	↑ Nasal resistance
9. Pain/Fear (adrenalin)	↓ Nasal resistance
10. Recumbent position	↑ Nasal resistance
11. Lateral recumbent position	↑ Nasal resistance (on down side)
12. Submersion reflex	Apnea, bradycardia, and ↑ BP

causing a cholinergic efferent response resulting in symptoms. Anticholinergic drugs prevent sulfite reactions.[18]

In challenge studies,[19] sulfites administered through a nasogastric tube will not cause adverse reactions in sensitive patients, but sulfites in solutions or inhalants will cause symptoms. Also, subcutaneous injections of sulfites in sensitive individuals will not cause adverse reactions, thus eliminating an IgE mechanism.[20] In addition, most studies[21] have reported a negative skin test to sulfites in these patients.

Despite the fact that a sulfite oxidase deficiency has been reported in these patients,[22] the irritant receptor, the rhinobronchial reflex, and the cholinergic efferent response appear to be the logical mechanism for metabisulfite adverse reactions.

Other important neural reflexes involving the nose are listed in Table III. The most common is the sneezing reflex. An extremely important reflex is the submersion reflex, which results in apnea, bradycardia, and increased blood pressure. This reflex is related to that of aquatic mammals and is responsible for saving the lives of many children who otherwise would have been accidental drowning cases.

In summary, nasal receptors and reflexes play an important role in the physiology of the nose, lower respiratory system, and in our general well being.

REFERENCES

1. Settipane GA. (Ed) Rhinitis, 1st ed., NER Allergy Proc, Prov., R.I., 1984.
2. Mygind N. Mediators of nasal allergy. J Allergy Clin Immunol 70:149-159, 1982.
3. Brooks CD, Butler D, Metzler C. Effect of H_2 blockade in the challenged allergic nose. J Allergy Clin Immunol 70:373-376, 1982.
4. Mclean JA. Nasal rhinomanometry and experimental nasal challenges. N Engl Reg Allergy Proc 3:397-404, 1982.
5. Kaufman J, Wright GW. The effect of nasal and nasopharyngeal irritation on airway resistance in man. Amer Rev Resp Dis 100:626-30, 1969.
6. Ogura JH, Nelson JR, Dammkoehler R, Kawasaki M, Togawa K. Experimental observations of the relationships between upper airway obstruction and pulmonary function. Trans Amer Laryng Ass. 85:40-64, 1964.
7. Whicker JH, Kern EG, Hyatt RE. Nasopulmonary relflex: Evaluation in the nonparalyzed and paralyzed anesthetized dog. Ann Otol 87:91-98, 1978.
8. Wyllie JW 3rd, Kern EB, O'Brien, PC, Hyatt, RE. Alteration of pulmonary function associated with artificial nasal obstruction. Surg Forum 27:535-537, 1976.
9. Yan K, Salome C. The response of the airways to nasal stimulation in asthmatics with rhinitis. Eur J Respir Dis 64:105-109, 1983.
10. Nolte D, Berger D. On vagal bronchoconstriction in asthmatic patients by nasal irritation. Eur J Respir Dis 64:110-115, 1983.
11. Slavin RG. Relationship of nasal disease and sinusitis to bronchial asthma. Ann Allergy 49:76-79, 1982.
12. Slavin RG, Linford PA, Friedman WH. Sphenoethmoidectomy (SE) in the treatment of nasal polyps, sinusitis and bronchial asthma. J Allergy Clin Immunol 71:(Part 2) 156, 1983. (abstract).

13. Friedman R, Ackerman M, Wald E, Friday G, Reilly J, Casselbrant M, Fireman P. Bacterial sinusitis exacerbating asthma. J Allergy Clin Immunol 71(Part 2) 155, 1983, (abstract).
14. Rachelefsky G, Siegel S, Katz R. Chronic sinus disease with associated induced reactive airways disease in children. J Allergy Clin Immunol 71: (Part 2) 156, 1983, (abstract).
15. Cooke RA (Ed). Allergy in theory and practice. W.B. Saunders Co., Philadelphia and London, 1947.
16. Freedman BJ. Asthma induced by sulfur dioxide, benzoate and tartrazine contained in orange drinks. Clin allergy 7:407-415, 1977.
17. Simon RA, Green L, Stevenson DD. The incidence of ingested metabisulfite sensitivity in an asthmatic population. J Allergy Clin Immunol 69:118, 1982 (abstract).
18. Simon RA, Goldfarb G, Jacobsen D. Blocking studies in sulfite sensitive asthmatics (SSA). J Allergy Clin Immunol 73:136, 1984 (abstract).
19. Delohery J, Castle W, Simmul R, Allen D. Metabisulfite and SO_2 reactivity in asthmatics. J Allergy Clin Immunol 73:136, 1984 (abstract).
20. Goldfarb G, Simon R. Provocation of sulfite sensitive asthma. J Allergy Clin Immunol 73:135, 1984 (abstract).
21. Settipane, GA. Metabisulfite in Drugs. NER Allergy Proc 4:304-306, 1983.
22. Jacobsen DW, Simon RA, Singh M. Sulfite oxidase deficiency and cobalamin protection in sulfite-sensitive asthmatics (SSA). J Allergy Clin Immunol 73:135, 1984 (abstract). □

Chapter VI
Airway Receptors and Asthma

Peter J. Barnes, D.M. (England)

ABSTRACT

Airway caliber is determined by a balance between many constrictor and dilator agents, which bring about their effects on the various target cells of the airway by activating specific cell surface receptors. Asthma and bronchial hyperresponsiveness may be viewed as an imbalance between excitatory and inhibitory receptor-mediated effects on the various target cells in the airway. Airway receptors can be grouped into those mediating the effects of the autonomic nervous system on the airways or those mediating the effects of the various mediators which may be generated in asthma. There is no convincing evidence that a fundamental defect in receptor function is involved in the pathogenesis of asthma, although minor abnormalities have been described. Recently there has been a considerable increase in our understanding of receptor function and control, which should throw light on the pathogenesis of airway obstruction and may lead to advances in asthma therapy. This may also lead to the development of novel drugs for treating asthma in the future.

INTRODUCTION

Airway caliber is influenced by many hormones, neurotransmitters, drugs and mediators, which produce their effects by binding to specific recognition sites or receptors on the external surface of the various target cells in the airway. It is therefore possible to view bronchoconstriction and bronchodilation in terms of receptor activation or blockade. There have recently been considerable advances in our understanding of receptor function and many new selective drugs which interact with receptors have been developed. A great impetus to research into basic mechanisms of receptor function has been provided by the technique of radioligand binding, in which a radiolabelled agonist or antagonist permits direct study and isolation of receptors. Most bronchodilators in current use produce their effects by interacting with airway receptors, so that a knowledge of receptor function is fundamental to understanding their mechanism of action.

Much emphasis has been placed on contraction of airway smooth muscle as the cause of airflow obstruction in asthma, but airway narrowing may also be due to edema of the bronchial wall (resulting from microvascular leakiness) and to plugging of the airway lumen by viscous mucus secretions. These pathological events may be produced by mediators released from inflammatory cells, including mast cells, macrophages, neutrophils and eosinophils. In discussing airway receptors in asthma it is therefore important to consider not only the receptors on airway smooth muscle, but also receptors on other target cells, such as submucosal glands, airway epithelium, microvascular endothelium, mast cells and other inflammatory cells.

Cell receptors relevant to airway function may be broadly grouped into autonomic receptors, which mediate the effects of the autonomic nervous system on the airways, and mediator receptors, which are activated

Department of Clinical Pharmacology, The Cardiothoracic Institute, Brompton Hospital, London SW3, UK

by the various inflammatory mediators implicated in asthma.

RECEPTORS AND CELL FUNCTION

Recent advances in molecular pharmacology have shed light on the mechanisms by which receptor activation may lead to cellular responses. Cells are exposed to many neurotransmitters, hormones and mediators, which bind to specific receptors which then generate second messengers, such as cyclic AMP or calcium. This leads to the characteristic response of the cell, such as contraction or relaxation in the case of airway smooth muscle. There appear to be two major signalling systems:

1. Some receptors are linked to adenylate cyclase (AC) which activates the response by changes in intracellular concentrations of cyclic AMP. The linking of a receptor to AC involves a coupling protein which is regulated by guanine nucleotides (nucleotide regulatory protein or N), which may be stimulatory (N_s) or inhibitory (N_i).[1] Some receptors stimulate AC, including β-receptors, VIP-receptors and PGE_2-receptors which leads to relaxation of airway smooth muscle, whereas others such as muscarinic receptors inhibit AC and cause bronchoconstriction (Fig 1).

2. Other receptors are associated with a rise in intracellular calcium and recent evidence suggests that the transducing mechanism may involve breakdown of phosphatidylinositol (PI) in the cell membrane which leads to release of calcium from intracellular stores.[2] Although this has not been extensively investigated in airways, there is now evidence that cholinergic receptor activation in airway smooth muscle causes PI breakdown which leads to contraction.[3] The changes in cyclic GMP which are associated with cell activation are now thought to be secondary to changes in PI or intracellular calcium. Since PI breakdown may be involved in contraction of airway smooth muscle and also mucus secretion and inflammatory cell activation, this biochemical pathway may be very important in understanding the pathogenesis of asthma and bronchial hyperresponsiveness. Furthermore interactions with PI turnover may lead to advances in therapy.

AUTONOMIC RECEPTORS

Autonomic Control of Airways

Autonomic innervation of the airways is complex.[4] In addition to classical cholinergic pathways which cause bronchoconstriction and adrenergic mechanisms which are usually bronchodilator, there is a more recently recognized component of autonomic control which is neither cholinergic nor adrenergic.[5] These nervous pathways influence airway caliber by activating specific receptors on target cells in the airways (Fig 2). For cholinergic pathways, acetylcholine released from postganglionic nerve endings stimulates muscarinic cholinergic receptors on target cells. Adrenergic mechanisms comprise sympathetic nerves, which release norepinephrine and circulating epinephrine secreted from the adrenal medulla; these catecholamines then activate α- or β-adrenoceptors on target cells. The neurotransmitter of the non-adrenergic non-cholinergic (NANC) nerves in airways is not certain, but the most likely candidate for the non-adrenergic inhibitory nerves is vasoactive intestinal polypeptide (VIP), whereas that of non-cholinergic excitatory nerves is probably substance P (SP) or a related peptide. These neuropeptides also interact with specific receptors on target cells.

Autonomic Abnormalities in Asthma

Asthma is characterized by exaggerated bronchoconstrictor responses to a wide variety of apparently unrelated stimuli, which has suggested that there may be an abnormality in autonomic control mechanisms. This might be an exaggeration of excitatory mechanisms (cholinergic, α-adrenergic or non-cholinergic excitatory) or a deficiency in inhibitory mechanisms (β-adrenergic or non-adrenergic inhibitory).[4] The idea that there may be an imbalance between cholinergic and adrenergic mechanisms was first proposed more that 60 years ago[6] and there have been many studies which have examined the possibility that autonomic receptor function may be abnormal in asthma.[7]

Beta-adrenoceptors

Localization and function. Radioligand binding studies have demonstrated a high density of β-receptors in lung of many species, including man.[8] More recent autoradiographic techniques have revealed that β-receptors are localized to many different cell types within lung.[9] β-Receptors are found in airway smooth muscle from all airways, as expected, since β-agonists are potent relaxants of bronchial smooth muscle, bronchioles and peripheral lung strips.[10] β-Agonists also stimulate secretion of mucus and active ion transport across airway epithelium in several species, including humans. Autoradiographic studies confirm a high density of β-receptors in human airway glands and epithelium.[9] β-Agonists potently inhibit antigen-induced release of mast cell mediators from human lung fragments and isolated lung mast cells *in vitro*,[11] suggesting the presence of inhibitory β-receptors on human mast cells. Whether this contributes to the bronchodilator effect of β-agonists in asthma is not certain, however. Histamine-induced microvascular leakiness in airways of guinea pigs is reduced by prior treatment with β-agonists, suggesting

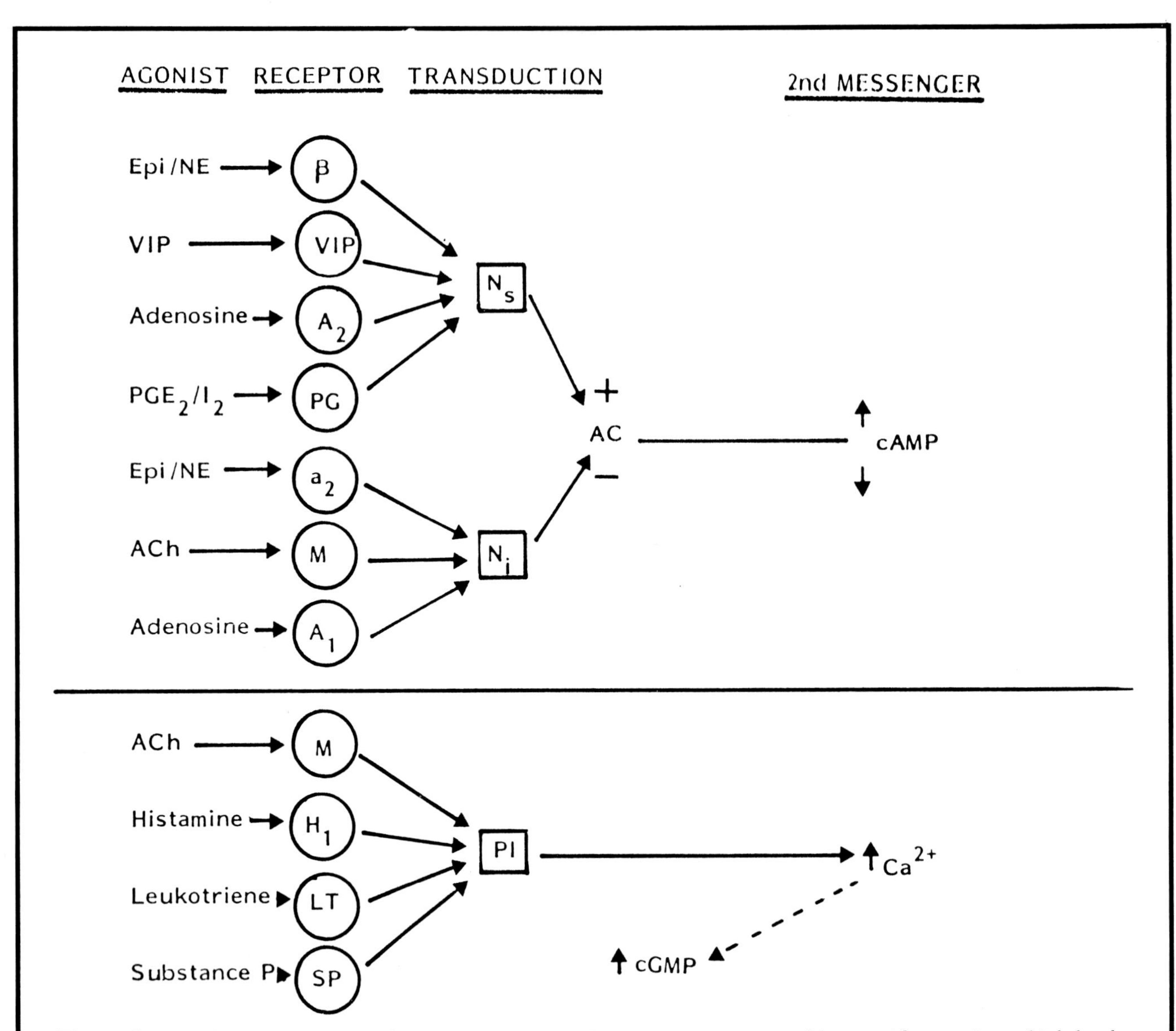

Figure 1. *Signal transduction mechanisms in airways. Receptors are activated by specific agonists which lead to the response either by changing intracellular cAMP or by increasing intracellular calcium. Receptors which involve cAMP activate or inhibit adenylate cyclase (AC), involve a linking protein, nucleotide regulatory protein which either stimulates (N_s) or inhibits (N_i) the enzyme. Other receptors which result in increases in intracellular Ca^{2+} cause hydrolysis of phosphatidyl inositol (PI) in the membrane.*

that β-receptors also regulate bronchial microvascular permeability. β-Agonists also modulate cholinergic neurotransmission in animals, either at the level of cholinergic ganglia or at postsynaptic nerve terminals.

β-Agonists therefore have several beneficial actions on airway obstruction. In addition to relaxing airway smooth muscle they also reduce release of mediators from mast cells, reduce cholinergic tone and possibly reduce mucosal edema and increase clearance of airway mucus.[8]

Beta-receptor Subtypes

Although originally β-receptors of airway smooth muscle were classified as β_2-receptors, later studies showed that in several species relaxation of tracheal smooth muscle was intermediate between a β_1- and β_2-mediated response, suggesting the presence of β_1 in addition to β_2-receptors. Using direct receptor binding techniques and selective β-antagonists the coexistence of β_1 and β_2 receptors was confirmed in animal and

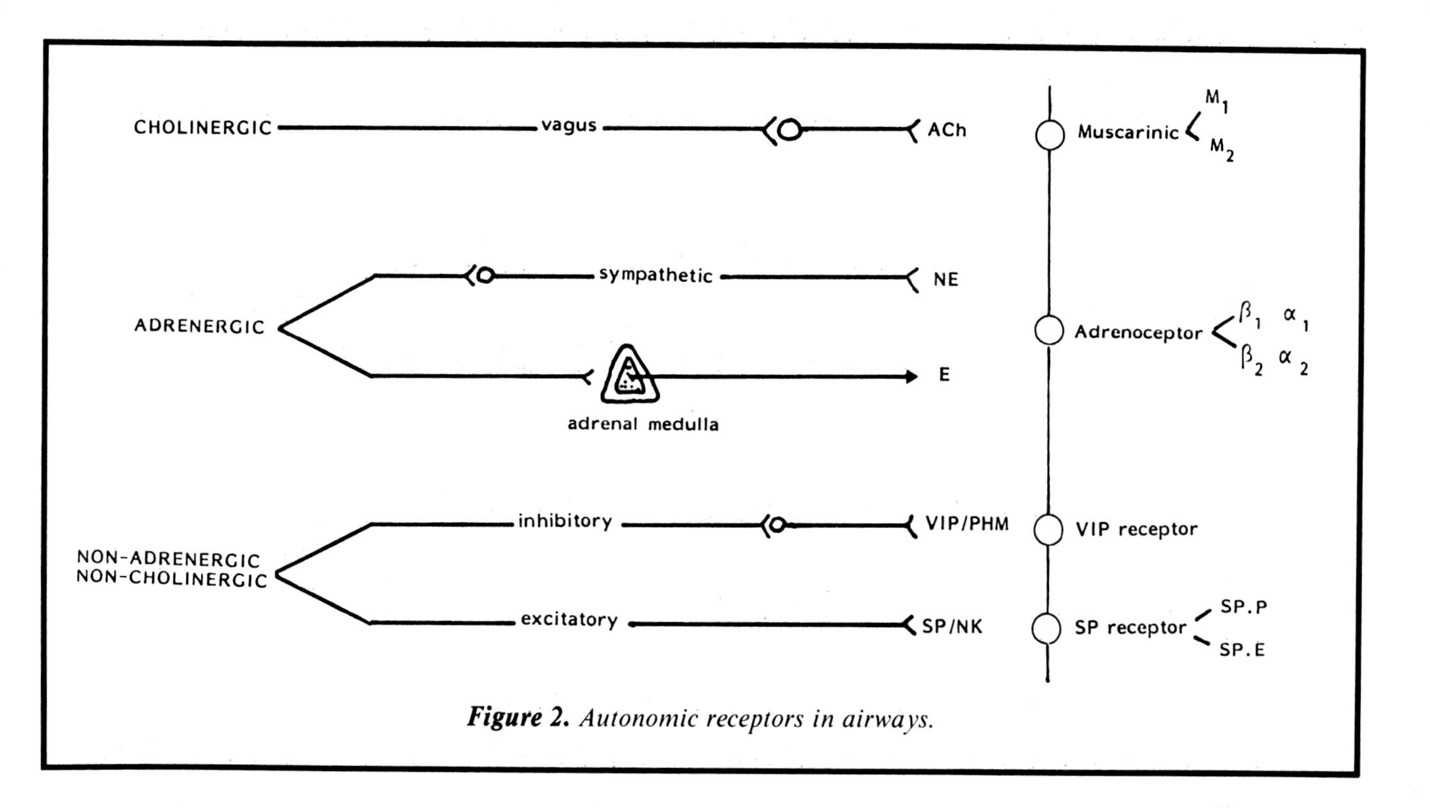

Figure 2. *Autonomic receptors in airways.*

human lung.[12] In dog tracheal smooth muscle, while β_2 receptors predominate, 20% of receptors are of the β_1-subtype.[13] Functional studies of the same airways show that relaxation to exogenous β-agonists is mediated by β_2-receptors, but relaxation to sympathetic nerve stimulation is mediated by β_1-receptors. These findings are consistent with the view that β_1-receptors are regulated by sympathetic nerves ('neuronal β-receptors'), whereas β_2-receptors are regulated by circulating epinephrine ('hormonal β-receptors'). In human airway smooth muscle, which has no sympathetic innervation, no β_1-receptor mediated effects would be expected. This has been confirmed in functional studies *in vitro*, in which relaxation of central and peripheral airways is mediated only by β_2-receptors.[10] Our recent autoradiographic studies of β-receptor subtypes in human lung have confirmed that the β-receptors of human airway smooth muscle from bronchi to terminal bronchioles are entirely of the β_2-subtype.[9]

Submucosal glands, which receive a sparse sympathetic nerve supply have a small population of β_1-receptors (approximately 10% of total determined by autoradiography), and functional studies show that mucus secretion is mediated by β_1 and β_2-receptors, whereas epithelial β-receptors, which are not adrenergically innervated, are entirely of the β_2-subtype.[9].

Beta-receptor function in asthma. Because β-agonists reverse the bronchospasm in asthmatic airways it was logical to suggest that there might be a defect in β-receptor function underlying asthma. There is unlikely to be a fundamental defect in β-receptor function in asthma however, since blockade of β-receptors does not produce asthma or bronchial hyperresponsiveness in normal individuals. However there is still debate about whether there may be impaired β-receptor function in asthma which is secondary to the disease.[14] A defect in β-receptors would not only apply to airway smooth muscle (tipping the balance in favour of cholinergic and possibly α-adrenergic constriction), but may also increase mediator release and bronchial wall edema.

Early studies showed that cardiovascular, metabolic and leukocyte responses to β-agonists were impaired in asthmatic patients when compared with normal controls and that there was a decreased number of β-receptors on circulating leukocytes. These changes could be explained by tolerance as a result of prior adrenergic therapy. Studies of β-receptor function in untreated asthmatics are conflicting, some studies showing no significant differences compared with normal subjects, whereas others have shown impaired cardiovascular or metabolic responses to β-agonists, although the magnitude of the changes is very small. It has been suggested that the cause of this impairment in β-receptor function might be autoantibodies to β_2-receptors, which have been detected in the serum of asthmatic patients,[15] but these antibodies have been detected in only a small proportion of asthmatic patients and also occur in normal subjects. A reduction in leukocyte β-receptor density and responses has also been detected in asthmatics after antigen challenge, suggesting that any defect in β-receptors might be secondary to the disease.[16] It is possible that mediators released in asthma may impair β-adrenergic function, possibly by an effect on the cell membrane.

Studies of cardiovascular, metabolic and leukocyte β-receptors may not reflect on abnormality of airway β-receptors. It has been difficult to determine whether airway β-receptor function is impaired in asthma however. No significant difference in bronchodilator dose-response curves to inhaled β-agonist was found in mild asthmatics,[17] but more severe asthmatics appeared less sensitive to β-agonists than normal subjects, the reduction in sensitivity being related to the initial bronchoconstriction.[18] This could be explained by functional antagonism, due to greater initial bronchoconstriction, rather than a defect in β-receptor function per se. It is difficult to make comparisons between dose response curves *in vivo* when there are differences in baseline lung function and when differences in delivered dose of inhaled β-agonist may occur, and some of these difficulties may be overcome by studying β-receptor function in isolated airways. Asthmatic airways are only rarely available, but in three asthmatics who died during an attack, an apparent reduction in isoproterenol responsiveness was found, although in another study no impairment in β-receptor responses could be detected.[14]

Because airway β-receptor function has been difficult to study in asthma, various animal models have been used, although none closely mimics human disease. In a guinea pig model of asthma, while a 20% reduction in pulmonary β-receptor density has been found, there is no change in β-agonist induced adenylate cyclase activation, suggesting no significant functional defect.[19]

The question of whether β-receptor function is impaired in asthma has not yet been resolved, although such a defect would have little clinical significance, since asthmatics bronchodilate so readily to β-agonists. Any apparent failure to respond to β-agonists during acute exacerbations is more likely to be explained by other factors, such as bronchial edema or luminal mucus plugging. In one such patient who died, the airways were subsequently found to respond normally to β-agonists *in vitro*.

Alpha-adrenoceptors

Localization and function. α-Receptors which mediate contraction of airway smooth muscle have been demonstrated in many species, including man,[20] although it may only be possible to demonstrate their presence under certain conditions. Autoradiographic studies in ferret have shown a very low density of α-receptors in smooth muscle of large airways, although there is an unexpectedly high density of small bronchioles.[21] α-Agonists stimulate mucus secretion and α_1-receptors have been demonstrated autoradiographically on serous cells of submucosal glands α-Agonists also facilitate mediator release from human lung fragments,[7] suggesting the presence of α-receptors on human lung mast cells.

Alpha-receptor subtypes. With the development of selective α-antagonists two subtypes of α-receptor have been recognized. α_1-Receptors are the classical α-receptors mediating contractile effect and are selectively blocked by prazosin, whereas presynaptic α-receptors mediating negative feedback of norepinephrine and selectively blocked by yohimbine are termed α_2-receptors. More recently α_2-receptors have also been found postsynaptically. It was suggested that α_1-receptors were regulated physiologically by norepinephrine and α_2-receptors by epinephrine, but there is now little evidence to support this. There have been few studies on α-receptor subtypes in airways; in dog tracheal smooth muscle the contractile response to both sympathetic nerve stimulation and to exogenous α-agonists is mediated almost entirely by α_2-receptors, and radioligand binding studies confirm that the majority of α-receptors in this tissue are α_2-receptors.[22]

Alpha-receptor function in asthma. There is some evidence that α-adrenergic responses may be increased in asthma and may therefore contribute to bronchial hyperreactivity.[4] The α-agonist methoxamine causes bronchoconstriction in asthmatic but not in normal subjects, even in the absence of β-blockade.[23] This suggests that α-adrenergic responses are increased in the airways of asthmatics, and there is also evidence for α-adrenergic hyperresponsiveness of pupillary and vascular responses in asthmatics.[7]

No α-adrenergic response can be demonstrated in normal canine or human airway smooth muscle *in vitro*, even after β-blockade, but with diseased human airways or pretreatment of normal canine airways with histamine or serotonin a marked α-adrenergic contractile response is found,[20,24] suggesting activation of α-adrenergic responses by mediators or disease. This is not an artefact of the *in vitro* situation, as similar activation of α-adrenergic responses can also be demonstrated in dogs *in vivo*.[25] This suggests that inflammatory mediators may 'turn on' α-adrenergic mechanisms in asthma. This enhanced responsiveness does not involve any change in airway α-receptor density or affinity,[24] and is therefore likely to be a post-receptor mechanism (possibly involving voltage-operated calcium channels). In a guinea pig model of asthma the density of pulmonary α_1-receptors is doubled,[19] although functional studies have shown no increase in α-adrenergic responsiveness.

If exaggerated α-responses were an important factor

in bronchial hypereactivity, then α-blockers should be beneficial in asthma. α-Antagonists, such as phentolamine and thymoxamine, inhibit bronchoconstriction induced by histamine, allergen and exercise, but such drugs lack specificity and their protective effects may be explained by other pharmacological actions such as antihistamine activity. The specific α_1-blocker prazosin given by inhalation has no bronchodilator effect in asthmatics, who readily bronchodilate with a β-agonist, suggesting that α-adrenergic hyperresponsiveness does not contribute to resting bronchomotor tone in asthma.[26] Similarly prazosin has no effect on histamine-induced bronchoconstriction, although it does have a weak protective effect against exercise-induced bronchospasm,[27] suggesting that under some circumstances α-receptor activation may contribute to bronchoconstriction, but it is unlikely to be of major significance. The effects of specific α_2-blockers on airway function have not yet been reported.

Cholinergic Receptors

Localization and function. In normal human airways there is a small amount of resting tone due to vagal motor activity with release of acetylcholine in the vicinity of airway smooth muscle, and it has been suggested that cholinergic mechanisms may be increased in asthma. Acetylcholine causes contraction of airway smooth muscle by activating muscarinic receptors, which are blocked by atropine.

Direct receptor binding studies have demonstrated a high density of muscarinic receptors in smooth muscle of large airways, and this has been confirmed autoradiographically.[21] The density of muscarinic receptors decreases as airways become smaller, so that terminal bronchioles are almost devoid of muscarinic receptors. This is consistent with physiological studies in dogs using tantalum bronchography, showing that vagal stimulation has a marked effect on large airways but little effect on bronchioles.[4] Similarly in humans anticholinergic drugs have more effect on large than on small airways, as measured by helium-oxygen flow-volume curves, whereas β-agonists relax all airways.[28]

Vagus nerve stimulation and cholinergic agonists potently stimulate mucus secretion in animals and man, and submucosal glands have a high density of muscarinic receptors. Cholinergic agonists are also reported to stimulate histamine secretion from human lung fragments,[7] suggesting that there may be muscarinic receptors on human lung mast cells.

Muscarinic receptor function in airway obstruction. Atropine and related drugs, such as ipratropium bromide, cause bronchodilation in normal subjects, by blocking vagal tonic contraction. If increased vagal activity or cholinergic hyperresponsiveness were contributing to bronchoconstriction in asthma, these drugs should be effective bronchodilators. Although they have some bronchodilator effect in asthma, they are less effective than β-agonists, presumably because in asthma bronchospasm is due to additional mechanisms, such as the direct effect of mediators such as histamine and leukotrienes on airway smooth muscle. The increased bronchoconstrictor responses to cholinergic agonists seen in asthmatic subjects is not evidence of abnormal cholinergic airway receptors, but a manifestation of nonspecific hyperresponsiveness to any contractile agent. Anticholinergic drugs appear to be more effective in chronic bronchitis, probably because they block vagal tone, which has a greater effect in already narrowed airways for geometric reasons.[29]

Muscarinic receptor subtypes. There is some evidence from binding and functional studies that muscarinic receptors may be subclassified into at least two subtypes, based on the development of selective blocking drugs such as pirenzipine.[30] In gut M_1-receptors, which are selectively blocked by pirenzipine, are localized to nerve terminals, ganglia and secretory cells, whereas M_2-receptors are localized to smooth muscle. The functional significance of muscarinic receptor subtypes in airways has not yet been determined.

Non-adrenergic Non-cholinergic (NANC) Receptors

The demonstration that there is a third component of the autonomic nervous system in airways is of considerable interest, particularly as it may function abnormally in airway disease.[5] A non-adrenergic inhibitory nervous pathway has been found in airways of several species, and in human airways it is the only inhibitory nervous mechanism. In guinea pigs a non-cholinergic excitatory pathway has also been described.[31] Until specific blockers are developed it is difficult to know whether there may be abnormalities in NANC mechanisms in asthma.

Non-adrenergic inhibitory receptors. The neurotransmitter of non-adrenergic inhibitory nerves is not yet certain, but VIP is the most likely candidate. VIP-immunoreactive nerves are found in human airways, and VIP and a closely related peptide (peptide histidine methionine), are potent relaxants of human bronchi *in vitro*, mimicking the effect of non-adrenergic nerve stimulation.[32] VIP activates a specific receptor, which has been identified in homogenized lung by direct binding techniques,[33] and activation of this receptor stimulates adenylate cyclase.

VIP also stimulates mucus secretion and fluid transport across airway epithelium[34,35] and immunocytochemical studies have demonstrated that VIP increases the cyclic AMP content in submucosal glands, airway epithelium and airway smooth muscle, indicating the presence of VIP receptors on these cells.[36]

Non-cholinergic excitatory receptors. Electrical stimulation of the vagus causes bronchoconstriction in guinea pigs which is not entirely blocked by atropine,[31] but the residual contraction is blocked by an antagonist of substance P (SP). SP is localized to afferent nerves in the airway and may be released by antidromic conduction. Substance P causes contraction of airway smooth muscle, increased mucus secretion, mucosal edema and may increase mediator release from mast cells.[5] Its actions are mediated by specific SP receptors and using a series of related peptides (tachykinins), which have been isolated from non-mammalian species, it has been possible to differentiate at least two types of receptor. For SP.P receptors SP is more potent than eledoisin, whereas for SP.E receptors eledoisin is more potent than SP. In airway smooth muscle the receptors appear to be SP.E subtype,[37] and we have recently confirmed this in human airways. Recently an endogenous tachykinin which is active at SP.E receptors (neurokinin A/substance K) has been isolated from mammalian tissues, and is present in airway nerves. A recently described peptide, calcitonin gene-related peptide, has also been found in human airway nerves which is a potent constrictor of human airways and appears to act through specific receptors.[38]

MEDIATOR RECEPTORS

Several inflammatory mediators have now been implicated in asthma, although certain evidence of their contribution to asthmatic bronchoconstriction is often lacking. These mediators have several actions on the airways which contribute to bronchial obstruction, including contraction of airway smooth muscle, mucus hypersecretion, chemotaxis of inflammatory cells, which themselves then release further mediators. The cellular origin of the various mediators is uncertain. Mast cells, macrophages, eosinophils and neutrophils are all probably involved. Mediators produce their effects by activating specific receptors on target cells in the airway and there is increasing information about the characteristics of these receptors and their antagonism. Because many mediators are involved in asthma, it seems unlikely that antagonism of a single mediator receptor will produce significant clinical benefit, however. Furthermore there is likely to be complex interaction between the different mediators. Bronchial hyperreactivity in asthma is characterized by exaggerated bronchoconstrictor responses to many mediators, including histamine, leukotrienes and bradykinin. This argues against an abnormality in any specific mediator receptor in asthma.

Histamine Receptors

Histamine may produce its effects by activation of H_1- and H_2-receptors. Inhaled histamine causes bronchoconstriction *in vivo* and contraction of large and small human airways *in vitro* by activating H_1-receptors, which are antagonized by the classical antihistamines, such as chlorpheniramine.[39] Studies with radiolabelled H_1-antagonists have demonstrated a high density of H_1-receptors in guinea pig lung, but these receptors have not yet been localized.[40] In human airways there is little evidence for H_2-receptor mediated bronchodilatation, as has been reported in other species.[39,41] Histamine also causes bronchial edema by an H_1-mediated contraction of bronchial venule endothelial cells, thus increasing microvascular permeability. Histamine increases bronchial mucus production in human airways by an H_2-mediated effect,[42] and increases lung epithelial permeability (and therefore perhaps airway mucosal permeability) via H_2-receptors.[41] Antihistamines have been disappointing in asthma, and even in high doses given by inhalation have little protective effect against various bronchial challenges, presumably because other mediators are also involved.

Leukotriene Receptors

There is evidence that leukotriene B_4 and the sulfidopeptide leukotrienes C_4, D_4 and E_4 (which comprise slow-reacting substance of anaphylaxis) are involved in asthmatic bronchoconstriction and there is increasing evidence that they produce their effects by activating specific and probably distinct receptors. LTB_4 has potent chemotactic activity, particularly for neutrophils, and using $(^3H)LTB_4$ specific binding sites have been identified on human neutrophils.[43] Functional studies with LTC_4 and LTD_4 indicate that there are probably discrete receptors for each leukotriene and the leukotriene antagonist FPL 55712 appears to selectively inhibit the LTD_4 receptor. This is confirmed by binding studies which show specific, stereoselective and distinct binding sites for $(^3H)LTC_4$ and $(^3H)LTD_4$ in guinea pig lung membranes[44] and autoradiographic studies have indicated that the receptors are differentially distributed.[45] The sulfidopeptide leukotrienes are potent bronchoconstrictors in human airways *in vivo* and *in vitro* and potent stimulants of mucus secretion in human airways *in vitro* and in guinea pigs they produce microvascular leakiness and bronchial edema.

Prostaglandin Receptors

Several prostaglandins have effects on airways, although their role in asthma is uncertain since inhibition of cyclooxygenase (by drugs such as aspirin and indomethacin), which blocks their synthesis, usually has no beneficial effect and there are a few individuals (approximately 4% of asthmatics) who develop bronchoconstriction. Prostaglandin receptors have not been well characterized since no specific blockers are available. Specific prostacyclin receptors have been identified in guinea pig lung by radioligand binding, although they are probably localized to vessels rather than to airways.[46] PGD_2 (which is the major prostaglandin produced by human lung mast cells) and $PGF_{2\alpha}$ are both potent bronchoconstrictors of human airways, whereas PGE_2 may be a bronchodilator. These prostaglandins presumably produce their effects by activating specific receptors on airway smooth muscle. Thromboxane A_2, which is also a cyclooxygenase product, is also a potent bronchoconstrictor which activates specific receptors, for which selective antagonists have recently been developed. Prostaglandins have a variety of other actions on the respiratory tract including mucus secretion, production of bronchial edema (by increasing bronchial blood flow) and chemotaxis.

Adenosine Receptors

Adenosine is produced under conditions of hypoxia and its concentration increases in plasma after antigen challenge. At least two specific adenosine receptors have been recognized, with the development of a series of adenosine analogues: A_1-receptors are usually excitatory and associated with a fall in intracellular cyclic AMP, whereas A_2-receptors are inhibitory and associated with a rise in cyclic AMP. Adenosine given by inhalation causes bronchoconstriction in asthmatic subjects,[47] but has little effect on isolated human airways *in vitro*,[48] suggesting that its bronchoconstrictor action is indirect, possibly involving a reflex mechanism. Adenosine may potentiate mast cell mediator release, probably via an A_2-receptor. Theophylline is a specific antagonist of both A_1 and A_2-receptors at concentrations which are within its therapeutic range, but there is good evidence against this as its mechanism of bronchodilatation, since an analogue of theophylline, enprofylline, is a more potent bronchodilator, without significant adenosine antagonism.

PAF Receptors

Platelet activating factor (PAF) is a potent bronchoconstrictor in animals, causes bronchial edema and produces long-lasting bronchial hyperresponsiveness. These effects are produced by release of factors from platelets and probably also from other cells such as neutrophils. Specific receptors for PAF have been identified in human neutrophils and lung.[49] Specific receptor antagonists such as gingkolide B have now been developed.

Bradykinin Receptors

Bradykinin is generated in inflammatory processes by the action of enzymes derived from inflammatory cells on a high molecular weight plasma kininogen. Bradykinin has potent bronchoconstrictor effects and may activate specific bradykinin receptors, which have been identified in other tissues by radioligand binding.[50] Bradykinin has little effect on human bronchi *in vitro*, suggesting that its bronchoconstrictor effect may be indirect (Cuss F, Barnes P J: unpublished). Bradykinin is also potent at causing bronchial edema and airway secretions.

CONCLUSIONS

There have been many recent advances in our understanding of receptor structure and function. This information has been applied to the study of airway function and has given fresh insights into possible defects in receptor function in airway diseases, particularly asthma. Autonomic receptors regulate airway tone and several such receptors have now been well characterized; in the case of β-receptors and muscarinic receptors this has elucidated how bronchodilators work. Inflammatory mediators produce their effects on the airway by interacting with specific receptors, but inhibition of a single receptor is unlikely to be of great clinical benefit, since many interacting mediators are presumably involved in asthma.

REFERENCES

1. Stiles GL, Caron MG, Lefkowitz RJ. β-Adrenergic receptors: biochemical mechanisms of physiological regulations. Physiol Rev. 64:661–743, 1984.
2. Berridge MJ, Irvine RF. Inositol trisphosphate, a novel second messenger in cellular signal transduction. Nature 312:315–21, 1984.
3. Baron CB, Cunningham M, Strauss JF, Coburn RF. Pharmacomechanical coupling in smooth muscle may involve phosphatidylinositol metabolism. Proc Natl Acad Sci USA 81:6899–6903, 1984.
4. Nadel JA, Barnes PJ. Autonomic regulation of the airways. Annu Rev Med 35:451–67, 1984.
5. Barnes PJ. The third nervous system in the lung: physiology and clinical perspectives. Thorax 39:561–67, 1984.
6. Alexander HL, Paddock R. Bronchial asthma: response to pilocarpine and epinephrine. Arch Int Med 27:184–91, 1921.
7. Kaliner M, Shelhamer J, Davis PB, Smith LJ, Venter JC. Autonomic nervous system abnormalties and allergy. Ann Intern Med 96:349–57, 1982.
8. Barnes PJ. Beta-adrenoceptors in lung tissue. In: Morley J, ed. Beta-adrenoceptors in asthma. London: Academic Press 67–90, 1984.
9. Carstairs JR, Nimmo AJ, Barnes PJ. Autoradiographic visualization of beta-adrenoceptor subtypes in human lung. Am Rev Respir Dis 132:541–47, 1985.
10. Zaagsma J, van der Heijden PJCM, van der Schaar MW, Bank CM. Comparison of function β-adrenoceptor heterogeneity in central and peripheral airway smooth muscle of guinea pig and man. J Recept Res 3:89–106, 1983.

11. Peters SP, Schulman ES, Schleimer RP, Macglashan DW, Newball HH, Lichtenstein LM. Dispersed human lung mast cells. Pharmacologic aspects and comparison with human lung tissue fragments. Am Rev Respir Dis 126:1034–1039, 1982.
12. Engel G. Subclasses of beta-adrenoceptors—a quantitative estimation of β_1- and β_2-adrenoceptors in guinea pig and human lung. Postgrad Med J 57(suppl 1):77–83, 1981.
13. Barnes PJ, Nadel JA, Skoogh BE, Roberts JM. Characterization of beta-adrenoceptor subtypes in canine airway smooth muscle by radioligand binding and physiological responses. J Pharmacol Exp Ther 225:456–61, 1983.
14. Barnes PJ, Ind PW, Dollery CT. Beta-adrenoceptors in asthma and their response to agonists. In: Kay AB, Austen KF, Lichtenstein LM, eds. Asthma: London, New York: Academic Press, 339–58, 1984.
15. Venter JC, Fraser CM, Harrison LC. Autoantibodies to β_2-adrenergic receptors: a possible cause of adrenergic hyporesponsiveness in allergic rhinitis and asthma. Science 207:1361–1363, 1980.
16. Meurs H, Koëter GH, De Vries K, Kauffman HF. The beta-adrenergic system and allergic bronchial asthma: changes in lymphocyte beta-adrenergic receptor number and adenylate cyclase activity after an allergen-induced attack. J Allergy Clin Immunol 70:272–280, 1982.
17. Harvey JE, Tattersfield AE: Airway response to salbutamol: effect of regular salbutamo inhalations in normal, atopic and asthmatic subjects. Thorax 37:280–87, 1982.
18. Barnes PJ, Pride NB. Dose-response curves to inhaled beta-adrenoceptor agonists in normal and asthmatic subjects. Br J Clin Pharmacol 15:677–82, 1983.
19. Barnes PJ, Dollery CT, MacDermot J. Increased pulmonary α-adrenergic and reduced β-adrenergic receptors in experimental asthma. Nature 285:569–571, 1980.
20. Kneussl MP, Richardson JB. Alpha-adrenergic receptors in human and canine tracheal and bronchial smooth muscle. J Appl Physiol 45:307–11, 1978.
21. Barnes PJ, Basbaum CB, Nadel JA. Autoradiographic localization of autonomic receptors in airway smooth muscle: marked differences between large and small airways. Am Rev Respir Dis 127:758–62, 1983.
22. Barnes PJ, Skoogh BE, Nadel JA, Roberts JM. Postsynaptic alpha$_2$-adrenoceptors predominante over alpha$_1$-adrenoceptors in canine tracheal smooth muscle and mediate neuronal and hormonal alpha-adrenergic contraction. Mol Pharmacol 23: 570–575, 1983.
23. Black JL, Salome CM, Yan K, Shaw J. Comparison between airways response to an α-adrenoceptor agonist and histamine in asthmatic and no-asthmatic subjects. Br J Clin Pharmacol 14:464–6, 1982.
24. Barnes PJ, Skoogh BE, Brown JK, Nadel JA. Activation of alpha-adrenergic response in tracheal smooth muscle: a post-receptor mechanism. J Appl Physiol 54:1469–76, 1983.
25. Brown JK, Shields R, Jones C, Gold WM. Augmentation of alpha-adrenergic contractions in trachealis muscle of living dogs. J Appl Physiol 54:1558–66, 1983.
26. Barnes PJ, Ind PW, Dollery CT. Inhaled prazosin in asthma. Thorax 36:378–81, 1981.
27. Barnes PJ, Wilson NM, Vickers H. Prazosin an alpha$_1$-adrenoceptor antagonist partially inhibits exercise-induced asthma. J Allergy Clin Immunol 68:411–15, 1981.
28. McFadden ER, Ingram RH, Haynes RL, Wellman JJ. Predominant site of flow limitation and mechanisms of postexertional asthma. J Appl Physiol 42:746–52, 1977.
29. Gross NJ, Skorodin MS. Anticholinergic, antimuscarinic bronchodilators. Am Rev Respir Dis 129:856–70, 1984.
30. Hammer R, Berrie CP, Bridsall NJM, Burgen AS, Hulme EC. Pirenzipine distinguishes between different subclasses of muscarinic receptors. Nature 283:90–92, 1980.
31. Andersson RG, Grundström N. The excitatory non-cholinergic, non-adrenergic nervous system of the guinea-pig airways. Eur J Respir Dis 131:141–157, 1983.
32. Palmer JB, Cuss FM, Barnes PJ. The effect of vasoactive intestinal peptide and related peptides on isolated human airway smooth muscle. Am Rev Respir Dis 131:A97, 1985.
33. Robberecht P, Tatemoto K, Chatelain P, Waelbroeck M, Delhaye M, Taton G, De Neef P, Camus JC, Heuse D, Christophe J. Effects of PHI on vasoactive intestinal peptide receptors and adenylate cyclase activity in lung membranes. A comparison in man, rat, mouse and guinea pig. Regul Pept 4:241–50, 1982.
34. Peatfield AC, Barnes PJ, Bratcher C, Nadel JA, Davis B. Vasoactive intestinal peptide stimulates tracheal submucosal gland secretion in ferret. Am Rev Respir Dis 128:89–93, 1983.
35. Nathanson I, Widdicombe JH, Barnes PJ. Effect of vasoactive intestinal peptide on ion transport across dog tracheal epithelium. J Appl Physiol 55:1844–48, 1983.
36. Lazarus SC, Basbaum CB, Barnes PJ, Gold WM. Mapping of VIP receptors by use of an immunocytochemical probe for the intracellular mediator cyclic AMP. Am J Physiol 1985 (in press).
37. Karlsson JA, Finney MJB, Persson CGA, Post C. Substance P antagonists and the role of tachykinins in non-cholinergic bronchoconstriction. Life Sci 35:2681–91, 1984.
38. Palmer JBD, Cuss FMC, Mulderry PK, Ghatei MA, Bloom SR, Barnes PJ. Calcitonin gene-related peptide is a potent constrictor of human airway smooth muscle. Thorax (in press).
39. White J, Eiser NM. The role of histamine and its receptors in the pathogenesis of asthma. Br J Dis Chest 77:215–26, 1983.
40. Carswell H, Nahorski SR. Distribution and characteristics of histamine H_1-receptors in guinea-pig airways identified by (^3H) mepyramine. Eur J Pharmacol 81:301–7, 1982.
41. Braude S, Royston D, Coe C, Barnes PJ. Histamine increases lung permeability by an H_2-receptor mechanisms. Lancet 2: 372–4, 1984.
42. Shelhamer JH, Marom Z, Kaliner M. Immunologic and neuropharmacologic stimulation of mucous glycoprotein release from human airways in vitro. J Clin Invest 66:1400–8, 1980.
43. Goldman DW, Goetzl E-J. Specific binding of leukotriene B to receptors on human polymorphonuclear leukocytes. J Immunol 129:1600–4, 1982.
44. Bruns RT, Thomsen WJ, Pugsley TA. Binding of leukotrienes C_4 and D_4 to membranes from guinea pig lung: regulation by ions and guanine nucleotides. Life Sci 33:645–53, 1983.
45. Barnes PJ, Carstairs JR, Norman P, Abram TS. Autoradiographic localization of leukotriene receptors in guinea pig lung and trachea. Am Rev Respir Dis 131:A29, 1985.
46. MacDermot J, Barnes PJ, Waddell K, Dollery CT, Blair IA. Prostacyclin binding to guinea pig pulmonary receptors. Eur J Pharmacol 75:127–30, 1981.
47. Cushley MJ, Tattersfield AE, Holgate ST. Adenosine-induced bronchoconstriction in asthma: antagonism by inhaled theophylline. Am Rev Respir Dis 129:380–84, 1984.
48. Finney MJB, Karlsson J-A, Persson CG. Effects of bronchoconstrictors and bronchodilators on a novel human small airway preparation. Br J Pharmac 85:29–36, 1985.
49. Hwang SB, Lam MH, Shen TY. Specific binding sites for platelet activating factor in human lung tissues. Biochem Biophys Res Commun 128:972–9, 1985.
50. Odya CE, Goodfriend TL, Peña C. Bradykinin receptor-like binding studied with iodinated analogues. Biochem Pharmacol 29:175–85, 1980. □

Chapter VII

Histamine Receptors in the Lung

Sidney S. Braman, M.D.

ABSTRACT

The availability of specific histamine receptor antagonists has provided evidence that human airways have both H_1 and H_2 receptors. H_1 receptors, which mediate bronchoconstriction, predominate. H_1 receptor antagonism can produce significant bronchodilatation in some asthmatics, block bronchoconstriction induced by antigen and histamine inhalation challenge, and have some protective effect against exercise and aspirin-induced bronchoconstriction. H_2 receptors mediate bronchodilatation, but this effect is relatively weak in man.

The role of classic antihistamines (H_1 receptor antagonists) in the treatment of asthma has not been established. Since factors that precipitate asthma are quite varied, these agents may provide benefit in select patients. The availability of new, nonsedating H_1 receptor antagonists show some promise in this regard. Future studies may more precisely define their use in asthma therapy.

INTRODUCTION

There are a number of animal and human experiments that demonstrate histamine receptors in the lung. Early in this century Dale and Laidlaw[1] injected guinea pigs with intravenous histamine and produced bronchospasm and other consequences of anaphylaxis. In 1928, Weiss[2] gave intravenous histamine to asthmatic subjects and reproduced the clinical features of asthma, but not the anaphylactic shock previously observed in the animal studies. In 1946 Curry[3] showed that inhaled as well as intravenously administered histamine could produce bronchospasm in asthmatics. He demonstrated a fall in the vital capacity of asthmatics after histamine challenge, but no change in the lung function of normal subjects. These early studies provided some of the first evidence to support the idea that there are histamine receptors in human airways, that they mediate bronchoconstriction, and in some way may be implicated in the pathogenesis of asthma. This report will describe the evidence for the existence of histamine receptors in the airways, the role these receptors might play in the pathogenesis of asthma and whether histamine receptor antagonists might be useful in the treatment of asthma.

Associate Professor of Medicine, Brown University Director, Division of Pulmonary and Critical Care Medicine Rhode Island Hospital, Providence, Rhode Island

H_1 AND H_2 AIRWAY RECEPTORS

After an intense search for specific histamine antagonists, the classic "antihistamines" were introduced in the 1940's. In 1966 Ash and Schild[4] observed that the effects of histamine in the guinea pig ileum and bronchus could be inhibited by the classic "antihistamine", mepyramine, but that several other actions of histamine such as stimulation of gastric acid secretion and inhibition of uterine contraction could not be blocked by this histamine antagonist. As a result of these observations, it was postulated that histamine acts on two different types of receptors: H_1 or classic antihistamine sensitive and H_2 or classic antihistamine resistant. These speculations were subsequently confirmed after the discovery of H_2 receptor antagonists.

Dunlop and Smith[5] were the first to show the presence of both H_1 and H_2 receptors in human airways. In their experiments, passively sensitized preparations of human bronchus were exposed to histamine and antigen challenge following the exposure of these airways to mepyramine, an H_1 receptor antagonist, and to metiamide, an H_2 receptor antagonist. Histamine alone induced bronchial muscle contraction. In the presence of the H_1 blocking agent, dose related relaxation occurred, but after adding the H_2 blocker, the mepyramine-induced relaxation was abolished. The antigen challange, also caused smooth muscle constriction. Mepyramine reduced this response while metiamide caused a significant increase in the response to a submaximal antigen challenge. This experiment, therefore suggested that both H_1 and H_2 receptors are present in human airways and that H_1 receptors stimulate and H_2 receptors inhibit bronchial smooth muscle contraction. Subsequent *in vivo* experiments have supported these conclusions regarding the H_1 receptor. H_1 antagonists such as chlorpheniramine[6,7] diphenylhydramine[8] and clemastine[9–11] have all been shown to block the bronchoconstriction caused by inhaled histamine.

Subsequent studies regarding the role of the H_2 receptor in the human airway, however, have yielded more conflicting results. Some human studies showed that the H_2 blocker, cimetidine, potentiated the bronchoconstriction induced by histamine.[12–14] These studies have supported the *in vivo* work of Dunlop and Smith[5] suggesting that the H_2 receptor mediates bronchodilatation. Other researchers[7] using inhaled histamine and antigen have not shown the same effect from H_2 receptor blockade. While the role of the H_2 receptor in modulating airway tone must be further clarified, it is believed that its activity is trivial compared to the H_1 receptor site[15].

Since Dunlop & Smith's[5] results with the histamine and antigen challenge showed that the effects of H_1 and H_2 receptors cancelled one another out, the authors postulated that the mechanism of histamine-induced bronchospasm is more likely to be due to an indirect rather than to a direct action. Support for an indirect action for histamine on bronchial smooth muscle through vagally-mediated reflexes has come from studies in animals and man. Considerable controversy, however, has existed regarding the importance of parasympathetic reflex-mediated bronchoconstriction compared to a direct smooth muscle action by histamine. Some studies have shown that cholinergic agents can prevent histamine and antigen-induced bronchoconstriction[16,17]; others show no protection by these agents.[18–20] Since anticholinergic agents, like atropine, can by themselves bronchodilate, often it has been difficult to tell whether in some studies the apparent inhibitory effect was due to changes in baseline airway caliber or to inhibition of the vagal reflex. A recent study by Sheppard et al[21] reexamined this controversy. These authors showed that atropine caused a dose dependent inhibition of histamine-induced bronchoconstriction that was not a function of increased baseline airway caliber. In two subjects in the study, however, a neurally-mediated component of histamine-induced bronchoconstriction seemed minimal. The authors concluded that there may be a heterogeneity among asthmatic subjects regarding the direct versus the reflex mechanisms of histamine on airway smooth muscle with parasympathetic mechanisms predominating in some and non-parasympathetic or direct bronchoconstrictor mechanisms prevailing in others. Even more recently Popa[22] proposed an additional theory regarding the mechanism of histamine induced bronchoconstriction. In a study of both normal and asthmatic subjects, he concluded that the effects of histamine were mediated predominantly, but not exclusively, through cholinergic pathways and postulated that histaminergic and cholinergic responses were interrelated by anastomotic connections in the bronchi beyond the level of the muscarinic receptor.

While there is now considerable evidence showing a preponderance of H_1 receptors in human airways and that their stimulation results in bronchoconstriction, it is probable that several mechanisms of histamine-induced bronchial smooth muscle contraction are important. These include: (1) direct smooth muscle stimulation by the H_1 receptor, (2) neural receptor mediated reflex cholinergic bronchoconstriction, and (3) the release of secondary mediators (prostaglandins, thromboxanes, etc.) through activation of both H_1 and H_2 receptors[23].

HISTAMINE RECEPTORS AND ASTHMA

It has been accepted that histamine is important in the pathogenesis of allergy and nonallergy mediated bronchospasm. The immunologically mediated release of histamine following antigen challenge has been shown in preparations of sensitized lung tissue[24] and some *in-vivo* studies have demonstrated the release of histamine in antigen-induced[25] and exercise-induced[26] asthma. Histamine is a potent bronchoconstrictor and the airways of asthmatics are considerably more responsive to inhaled or parenterally administered histamine than normal subjects.[27] In fact, the degree of sensitivity to inhaled histamine correlates well with the clinical severity of asthma. Bronchial hyperresponsiveness to inhaled histamine and other constrictors is therefore a cardinal feature of asthma and is often incorporated into the definition of asthma.

The demonstration of a protective effect of H_1 receptor antagonists on experimentally induced bronchoconstriction with inhaled histamine and antigen has given further evidence for an important role for histamine receptors in bronchial asthma. After atopic asthmatics were pretreated with 10–15 mg. of intravenously administered chlorpheniramine, an H_1 blocker, the threshold dose of allergen that caused a greater than 10% drop in FEV_1 was doubled.[6] Eiser et al[7] showed a similar effect in antigen-induced bronchospasm with IV chlorpheniramine as did Phillips and co-workers[11] with an aerosolized H_1 blocking agent clemastine. Studies with histamine inhalation challenges have also been conducted following the administration of H_2 antagonists. Nathan and co-workers[12] have shown that orally administered cimetidine in asthmatic subjects produces a significant decrease in the threshold of histamine-induced bronchoconstriction. Schachter et al[14] also showed that asthmatic patients displayed significantly more bronchospasm to inhaled histamine when pretreated with cimetidine than with placebo. By contrast, healthy subjects showed no difference in response after the H_2 blocker. These authors concluded that H_2 receptors are important in mediating bronchial relaxation but that this effect is only significant in the asthmatic subject.

Based on a number of observations with H_1 and H_2 antagonists, a "theory" of histamine H_2 receptor deficiency in allergic asthma has been proposed by Chand.[23] An imbalance of H_1 and H_2 receptors has been suggested that is comparable to the beta-adrenoreceptor deficiency theory of asthma proposed by Szentivanyi.[28] While some observations, including those of Eiser et al[7] who found that intravenously administered cimetidine in asthmatics caused a slight increase rather than the expected decrease in responsiveness to inhaled histamine, do not support this theory, the idea is intriguing and provocative and deserves further consideration.

ANTIHISTAMINES IN THE TREATMENT OF ASTHMA

Early trials with the classic antihistamines for the treatment of asthma met with mixed results. Those showing improvement in asthma symptoms were poorly controlled and often lacked objective measurements of improved airway function. Nonetheless, a number of studies have established the H_1 antagonists as potential agents in the treatment of asthma. Booij-Nord et al[29] used intramuscular thiazinamium to show that a classic antihistamine could bronchodilate as well as two inhalations of the beta agonist, isoproterenol. Popa[30] showed that high doses of intravenously administered chlorpheniramine produced reproducible increases in the FEV_1 and other flow rates that lasted over several hours. Drowsiness, however, was a commonly associated side effect with this dose of the drug used. Karlin[31] studied 25 asthmatic children with low doses of four antihistamines usually used to control hayfever symptoms and high doses of two of these agents, diphenylhydramine (10 mg/kg/day) and chlorpheniramine (.70 mg/kg/day). In this study, which lasted over several weeks, the low dose antihistamines had no effect on symptoms, medication use, or peak expiratory flow rates (PEFR) when compared to a placebo. Some individual patients, however, had significantly higher PEFR during the drug period. The high dose H_1 antagonists often gave a significant improvement in the PEFR and asthma symptoms. This effect could not be predicted by the presence of concomitant allergic rhinitis symptoms or by skin test reactivity. The authors concluded that the classic antihistamines have no use in the treatment of asthma because any clinical improvement would be offset by severe CNS (sedation or jitteriness) or GI (dry mouth, nausea, vomiting) side effects. Similar pessimism has been expressed by Chai[32] who believes that the availability of a number of alternative anti-asthma agents has even more significantly limited the use of the H_1 antagonists.

Since H_1 antagonists held some promise as bronchodilators but were limited by their systemic side effects, delivery by inhalation route was attempted. Clemastine appears to offer the least bronchial irritant effects and is an effective bronchodilator in both adults[33] and children.[34] It has also been shown to afford a substantial degree of protection from exercise-induced asthma.[35] In a comparison with albuterol, 1 cc of .05% clemastine produced a mean change in FEV_1 of 21% compared to 29% with 0.5% albuterol when these agents were inhaled by asthmatics from a Wright's nebulizer.[33] However in a long-term study of inhaled clemastine as a maintenance treatment for asthma, the drug offered no more effect than placebo in controlling airflow obstruction and did not reduce the need for standard bronchodilator treatment.[36]

Popa[37], summarizing the bronchodilator effects of the H_1 antagonists, concluded that these agents 1) require high bronchial concentrations and therefore are most effected by intravenous or inhaled route, 2) are dose dependent, 3) can unpredictably bronchodilate some asthmatic patients and rarely normals, and 4) are effective when the degree of airflow obstruction is moderate rather than mild or severe.

Several new antihistamines, pharmalogically different from previous H_1 antagonists in that they poorly penetrate the blood brain barrier (and are therefore nonsedating) and offer no anticholinergic, antiadrenergic, or antiserotonin effects, hold some promise for the treatment of asthma. Astemizole[38,39] has been shown to be at least four times more potent in antagonizing histamine-induced bronchoconstriction than the pre-

Table I

Lung Histamine Receptors

Action	Receptor
Bronchoconstriction	H_1 (ref. 5, 23)
Bronchodilatation (weak)	H_2 (ref. 5, 23)
Pulmonary Vasoconstriction	H_1 (ref. 45)
Pulmonary Vasodilatation	H_2 (ref. 45)
Increases Vascular Permeability	H_1 (ref. 23, 37)
Increases Bronchial Mucous Production	H_2 (ref. 46)
Increases Bronchial Epithelial Permeability	H_2 (ref. 47–48)
? Mediates Hypoxic Pulmonary Vasoconstriction	H_1 (ref. 49)

viously available H_1 antagonists and afford some protection from the seasonal symptoms of asthma. Cetirizine, the principal human metabolite of hydroxyzine, is capable of affording acute dose-dependent bronchodilatation in mild asthmatics and also shows significant protection in exercise-induced asthma.[40] Finally, terfenadine has been shown in two independent studies to block the effects of exercise-induced bronchospasm. The effect of the drug appears to be dose dependent and long lasting since protection was still evident in all patients one week after discontinuing therapy.[41]

Another group of antihistamines include those agents which not only have the ability to antagonize the H_1 airway receptor but also the capability of antiallergic action by stabilizing mast cell membranes and thereby preventing degranulation and mediator release. These powerful antihistamines, such as ketotifen and oxatomide, are able to block histamine-induced bronchoconstriction.[42–44] The importance of the H_1 receptor blocking action of these agents and the newer non-sedentary pure H_1 antagonists for the long-term management of asthma must be established.

OTHER HISTAMINE RECEPTORS IN THE LUNG

It is clear that there are a number of other activities in the lung that are mediated by histamine receptors. A summary of the action of antihistamines through H_1 and H_2 receptors are listed in Table I.

SUMMARY

The availability of specific histamine receptor antagonists has provided evidence that human airways have both H_1 and H_2 receptors. H_1 receptors, which mediate bronchoconstriction, predominate. H_1 receptor antagonism can produce significant bronchodilatation in some asthmatics, block bronconstriction induced by antigen and histamine inhalation challenge, and have some protective effect against exercise and aspirin-induced bronchoconstriction. H_2 receptors mediate bronchodilatation, but this effect is relatively weak in man.

The role of classic antihistamines (H_1 receptor antagonists) in the treatment of asthma has not been established. Since factors that precipitate asthma are quite varied, these agents may provide benefit in select patients. The availability of new, nonsedating H_1 receptor antagonists show some promise in this regard. Future studies may more precisely define their use in asthma therapy.

REFERENCES

1. Dale HH and Laidlaw PO. Histamine Shock. J Physiol 41: 318–344, 1919.
2. Weiss S, Robb GP, Blumgart HL. The velocity of blood flow in health and disease as measured by the effect of histamine on the minute vessels. Am Heart J 4:664, 1928.
3. Curry JJ. The action of histamine on the respiratory tract in normal and asthmatic subjects. J Clin Invest 25:785–791, 1946.
4. Ash ASF and Schild HO. Receptors mediating some actions of histamine. Br J Pharmacol 27:427–439, 1966.
5. Dunlop LS and Smith AP. The effect of histamine antagonists in antigen-induced contractions of sensitized human bronchus in vitro. Br J Pharmaco (Proceedings) 59:475 1977.
6. Popa VT. Effect of an H_1 blocker, chlorpheniramine, on inhalation tests with histamine and allergen in allergic asthma. Chest 78:3, 442–451, 1980.
7. Eiser NM, Mills J, Snashall PD, Guz A. The role of histamine receptors in asthma. Clin Sci 60:363–370, 1981.
8. Casterline CL and Evans R. Further studies on the mechanism of human histamine-induced asthma: the effect of an aerosolized H_1 receptor antagonist (diphenhydramine). J Allergy Clin Immunol 59:6, 420–424, 1977.
9. Nogrady SG, Bevan C. Inhaled antihistamines-bronchodilatation and effects on histamine- and methacholine-induced bronchoconstriction. Thorax 33:700–704, 1978.
10. Thomson NC, Kerr JW. Effect of inhaled H_1 and H_2 receptor antagonists in normal and asthmatic subjects. Thorax 35:428–434, 1980.
11. Phillips MJ, Ollier S, Gould C, Davies RJ. Effect of antihistamines and antiallergic drugs on responses to allergen and histamine provocation tests in asthma. Thorax 39:345–351, 1984.
12. Nathan RA, Segall N, Glover GC, Schocket AL. The effects of H_1 and H_2 antihistamines on histamine inhalation challenges in asthmatic patients. Am Rev Respir Dis 120:1251–1258, 1979.
13. Nathan RA, Segall N, Schocket AL. A comparison of the actions of H_1 and H_2 antihistamines on histamine-induced bronchoconstriction and cutaneous wheal response in asthmatic patients. J Allergy Clin Immunol 67:3, 171–177, 1981.
14. Schachter EN, Brown S, Lach E, Gerstenhaber B. Histamine blocking agents in healthy and asthmatic subjects. Chest 82: 2, 143–147, 1982.
15. White J and Eiser NM. The role of histamine and its receptors in the pathogenesis of asthma. Br J Dis Chest 77:215–226, 1983.
16. Yu DYC, Galant SP, Gold WM. Inhibition of antigen-induced bronchoconstriction by atropine in asthmatic patients. J Appl Physiol 32:6, 823–828, 1972.
17. Eiser MN and Guz A. The effects of atropine on histamine and antigen-induced bronchospasm. Prog Resp Res 14:75–77, 1980.

18. Casterline CL, Evans R, Ward GW. The effect of atropine and albuterol aerosols on the human bronchial response to histamine. J Allergy Clin Immunol 58:5, 607–613, 1976.
19. Rosenthal RR, Norman PS, Summer WR, Permutt S. Role of the parasympathetic system in antigen-induced bronchospasm. J Appl Physiol 42:4, 600–606, 1977.
20. Woenne R, Kattan M, Orange RP, Levison H. Bronchial hyperreactivity to histamine and methacholine in asthmatic children after inhalation of SCH 1000 and chlorpheniramine maleate. J Allergy Clin Immunol 62:2, 119–124, 1978.
21. Sheppard D, Epstein J, Skoogh BE, Bethel RA, Nadel JA, Boushey HA. Variable inhibition of histamine-induced bronchoconstriction by atropine in subjects with asthma. J Allergy Clin Immunol 73:82–87, 1984.
22. Popa V. The relationship between acetylcholine- and histamine induced constriction of large airways in normal subjects and subjects with asthma: A possible role for postreceptor mechanisms. J Allergy Clin Immunol 78:4, 601–614, 1986.
23. Chand N. Distribution and classification of airway histamine receptors: the physiological significance of histamine H_2-receptors. Adv Pharmacol Chemother 17:103–131, 1980.
24. Schild HO, Hawkins DF, Mongar JL, Herxheimer H. Reactions of isolated human asthmatic lung and bronchial tissue to a specific antigen; histamine release and muscular contractions. Lancet 2:376–382, 1951.
25. Atkins PC, Rosenblum F, Dunskey EH, et al. Comparison of plasma histamine and cyclic nucleotides after antigen and methacholine inhalation in man. J Allergy Clin Immunol 66: 478–486, 1980.
26. Anderson SD, Bye PTP, Schoeffel RE, Seale JP, Taylor KM, Ferris L. Arterial plasma histamine levels at rest, and during and after exercise in patients with asthma: effects of terbutaline aerosol. Thorax 36:259–267, 1981.
27. Cockcroft DW, Killian DN, Mellon JJA, Hargreave FE. Bronchial reactivity to inhaled histamine: a method and clinical survey. Clin Allergy 7:235–243, 1977.
28. Szentivanyi A. The beta adrenergic theory of the atopic abnormality in bronchial asthma. J Allergy 42:203–232, 1968.
29. Booij-Nord H, Orie NGM, Berg W, deVries K. Protection tests on bronchial allergen challenge with disodium cromoglycate and thiazinamium. J Allergy 46:1–11, 1970.
30. Popa VT. Bronchodilating activity of an H_1 blocker, chlorpheniramine. J Allergy Clin Immunol 59:1, 54–63, 1977.
31. Karlin JM. The use of antihistamines in asthma. Ann Allergy 30:342–347, 1972.
32. Chai H. Antihistamines and asthma. Do they have a role in therapy? Chest 78:3, 420–422, 1980.
33. Nogrady SG, Hartley JPR, Handslip PDJ, Hurst NP. Bronchodilatation after inhalation of the antihistamine clemastine. Thorax 33:479–482, 1978.
34. Hodges IGC, Milner AD, Stokes GM. Bronchodilator effect of two inhaled H_1-receptor antagonists, clemastine and chlorpheniramine, in wheezy school-children. Br J Dis Chest 77: 270–275, 1983.
35. Hartley JPR, Nogrady SG. Effect of an inhaled antihistamine on exercise-induced asthma. Thorax 35:675–679, 1980.
36. Partridge MR & Saunders KB. Effect of an inhaled antihistamine (clemastine) as a bronchodilator and as a maintenance treatment in asthma. Thorax 34:771–776, 1979.
37. Popa VT. The classic antihistamines (H_1 blockers) in respiratory medicine. Resp Pharmacol, Clinics in Chest Med 7:3, 367–382, 1986.
38. Holgate ST, Emanuel MB, Howarth PH. Astemizole and other H_1-antihistaminic drug treatment of asthma. J Allergy Clin Immunol 76:2, 375–380, 1985.
39. Clee MD, Ingram CG, Reid PC, Robertson AS. The effect of astemizole on exercise-induced asthma. Br J Dis Chest 78: 180–183, 1984.
40. Brik A, Tashkin DP, Gong H, Dauphinee B, Lee YE. Effectiveness of cetirizine, a new histamine H_1-antagonist, in causing bronchodilation and providing protection against histamine-induced bronchospasm in mild asthmatics. Chest 89:532S, 1986.
41. Patel KR. Terfenadine in exercise induced asthma. Br Med J 288:1496–1497, 1984.
42. Mattson K, Poppius H, Nikander-Hurme R. Preventative effect of ketotifen, a new antiallergic agent, on histamine-induced bronchoconstriction in asthmatics. Clin Allergy 9:411–416, 1979.
43. Gozalo Reques FG, Sanz CC, Sanchez CS, Sotes MR, Lopez TH, De Barrio Fernandez M. Long-term modification on histamine-induced bronchoconstriction by disodium cromoglycate and ketotifen versus placebo. Allergy 40:242–249, 1985.
44. Richards DM, Brogden RN, Heel RC, Speight TM, Avery GS. Oxatomide. A review of its pharmacodynamic properties and therapeutic efficacy. Drugs 27:210–231, 1984.
45. Marshall R. Pharmacologized and pathologized responses of the human pulmonary circulation to drugs. *In:* Widdencombe J (Ed): Resp Pharmacol, Oxford, Pergamon, 1981.
46. Shelhamer JH, Marom Z, Kaliner M. Immunologic and neuropharmacologic stimulation of mucous glycoprotein release from human airways in vitro. J Clin Invest 66:1400–1408, 1980.
47. Braude S, Royston D, Coe C, Barnes PJ. Histamine increases lung permeability by an H_2-receptor mechanism. Lancet 2, 372–374, 1984.
48. Rees PJ, Shelton D, Chan TB, Eiser N, Clark TJH & Maisey MN. Effects of histamine on lung permeability in normal and asthmatic subjects. Thorax 40:603–606, 1985.
49. Fishman AP. Hypoxia on the pulmonary circulation. How and where it acts. Circ Res 38:4, 221–231, 1976. □

Chapter VIII

Histamine and the Gut

Basil I. Hirschowitz, M.D.

ABSTRACT

The role of histamine in the gut is reviewed in relation to gastric secretion of acid, pepsin and intrinsic factor. Species-dependence of some of these actions are also discussed. Interactions with other agonists and antagonists in intact and isolated systems provide the basis for models of the role of histamine in control of gastric secretion. This review deals further with histamine H_1 and H_2 effects on gastrointestinal circulation and musculature including sphincters.

The most dramatic application of the development of histamine H_2 antagonists has been in the treatment of duodenal ulcer. The use of H_2 antagonists in the treatment of duodenal and gastric ulcer, gastrinoma, gastritis, and esophagitis is critically evaluated.

Much of the impetus for the new resarch in histamine in the last 10 years has come from the discovery in 1974 by James Black and his team at SKF of a specific H_2 histamine agonist and antagonist[1], and the phenomenal success of cimetidine in treating duodenal ulcer. A series of new agonists and antagonists specific for H_1 and H_2-receptors has provided the tools for study of histamine involvement, it seems, in every system of the body.[2] This brief review deals with histamine and the GI tract under the following headings:

Division of Gastroenterology, University of Alabama in Birmingham, Birmingham, Alabama 35294.

Submitted to Proceedings of the National Symposium on Histamine Receptors, Brown University, Providence, RI, December 1983

A. **Physiology**
   1. Gastric secretion of acid, pepsin, electrolytes and intrinsic factor — actions and interactions with non-histamine stimuli
   2. Gastric and intestinal circulation and capillary permeability
   3. Gastrointestinal musculature
      — Esophageal
      — Gastric & pyloric
      — Sphincter of Oddi
      — Gall Bladder
      — Intestinal

B. **Pathophysiology and treatment**
      — Duodenal ulcer, treatment
      — Gastric ulcer, treatment
      — Zollinger-Ellison syndrome
      — Systemic mastocytosis
      — Esophagitis
      — Gastritis

GASTRIC ACID SECRETION

Histamine is ubiquitously distributed in the animal kingdom, being present in all chordates. Though there is great variability in histamine content from tissue to tissue, only the gastric mucosa of all vertebrates is relatively rich in histamine; that is, there is a selective accumulation of histamine related to acid secretory cells. Gastric acid secretion is strongly stimulated by histamine and by a number of methyl histamine analogs - n(Me)histamine, n'n'dimethyl histamine,[3] 4-(Me)histamine[4] — with equal molar potency, and by analogs with a modified imidazole ring (triazole and betazole) with lesser molar potency.[3]

Histamine thus seems to serve a specific function relative to acid secretion. The definition[1] of gastric secretory effects of histamine as acting via the H_2 subset of receptors has been amply supported in the last decade by a wide range of studies of the stomach in man and animals with a broad selection of specific H_1 and H_2 agonists and antagonists. With few exceptions, the H_2 antagonists have been potent inhibitors of acid secretion in all species tested, and with all stimuli. This implies a critical role for histamine acting via an H_2 receptor pathway in the stimulation or secretion of HCl, but one that has so far been imperfectly defined.

The structure of the gastric H_2 receptor agonists, at first thought to depend on the 4-(Me) imidazole configuration, was later extended by the development of an even more specific H_2 agonist, dimaprit[5], which lacks the imidazole configuration and is as potent as histamine in stimulating acid secretion[6] and in its actions on H_2 receptors in other organs. Impromidine, an even more specific H_2 agonist, (H_2:H_1 = 10^3) is almost 100 times more potent than histamine in stimulating gastric acid secretion and in increasing heart rate than histamine,[7] but none of this potency is dependent upon lack of an H_1 effect. While impromidine is a full H_2 agonist in man[8] and dog,[7] it is a partial agonist in the rat[9] and, surprisingly, an inhibitor of histamine-stimulated acid secretion in the frog,[10] where H_1 agonists were more efficacious than dimaprit. The species differences offer important challenges to the understanding of the actions of histamine.

The stimulation by histamine of gastric acid secretion is mediated in all species by H_2 receptors. In the cat[11,12] and rabbit,[13] but not in man, dog, mouse, rat or guinea pig,[14] there is some evidence that H_1 receptors mediate an inhibitory effect, since acid secretion is greater with histamine in the presence of an H_1 antagonist or with 4(Me)-histamine a more specific H_2 agonist. In the rabbit, at least, H_1 inhibition of acid secretion is due to reduction in blood flow.[13]

Histamine stimulation of acid secretion is mediated via cAMP[14, 15] and this effect is blocked by very small amounts of prostaglandin E_2.[14] In intact animals, inhibition by PGE_2 is most effective against histamine.[16] Both stimulation of acid secretion and cAMP production are enhanced by the phosphodiesterase inhibitor isobutylmethylxanthine (IBMX)[14] and mimicked by cAMP analogs. Species differences are exemplified by more pronounced acid and cAMP responses to histamine in rabbit than dog parietal cells.[14]

Histamine induces an extensive morphologic change in canine parietal cells prior to the onset of secretion.[17] Similar changes in frog oxyntic cells have been induced by cAMP in both secreting and secretion-inhibited cells.[18] It is likely, though not definitely proved, that the many effects of histamine on the parietal cell — morphologic change, cAMP increase, increased respiration, acid secretion and electrolyte transport — all follow from a single interaction between histamine and H_2 receptors of the parietal cell.

Histamine interacts with other stimuli of gastric acid secretion. In isolated canine parietal cells, there is a 3-way potentiation (i.e. greater-than-additive effects) between histamine, acetylcholine and gastrin,[14] while in the intact dog there is potentiation of histamine and of gastrin by acetylcholine, while histamine and gastrin effects are only additive.[19] The basis for potentiation, whether at the receptor or post-receptor level is poorly understood. Acetylcholine is thought to act via a Ca^{++} dependent mechanism,[14] while the mechanism of the action of gastrin has not yet been elucidated.

In a wide variety of species and preparations of acid-secreting tissue, competitive antagonism by specific H_2 antagonists[2] has clearly defined the effect of histamine and various other analogs on acid secretion as well as on electrolytes, Na^+, K^+, Cl^-,[20] as being H_2 receptor mediated. Since the effects of agonists and antagonists are the same in isolated cells[14] as they are in the intact animal, one may conclude that histamine acts directly on receptors in the parietal cell. However, H_2 antagonists inhibit acid secretion in the intact animal stimulated by non-histamine stimuli, including food, gastrin, vagal,[2] caffeine and cholinomimetics.[21] In the isolated mouse stomach and in isolated glands or cells, H_2 antagonists do not inhibit cholinergic muscarinic stimuli.[14] The broad effects of H_2 antagonists in the intact animal suggest that non-histamine stimuli act via release of histamine from a histamine source in the stomach while the data in isolated stomach cells clearly point to separate histamine and muscarinic receptors on the parietal cell. However, the synergistic interaction between stimuli on the isolated parietal cell suggest that there must be interaction at or beyond the receptor level. Figure 1 attempts to reconcile the interaction data in the intact and isolated systems. While mast cells are present in the stomach of all species, it is not clear exactly what paracrine role they play — thus in the rat there is prominent histamine formation in the stomach, while in the dog stomach this is hard to demonstrate.

PEPSINOGEN SECRETION

Major species differences exist in histamine stimulation of pepsinogen secretion. In man, histamine stimulates pepsin coequally with acid and the effect on both is unaffected by H_1 antagonists and equally inhibited by H_2 antagonists. In the rat, histamine also stimulates pepsin secretion, while in the cat and dog, histamine stimulates pepsinogen secretion at low doses and inhibits dose responsively at doses above about 50 nMol/kg. hr. We have shown that both actions, the stimulant (low dose,

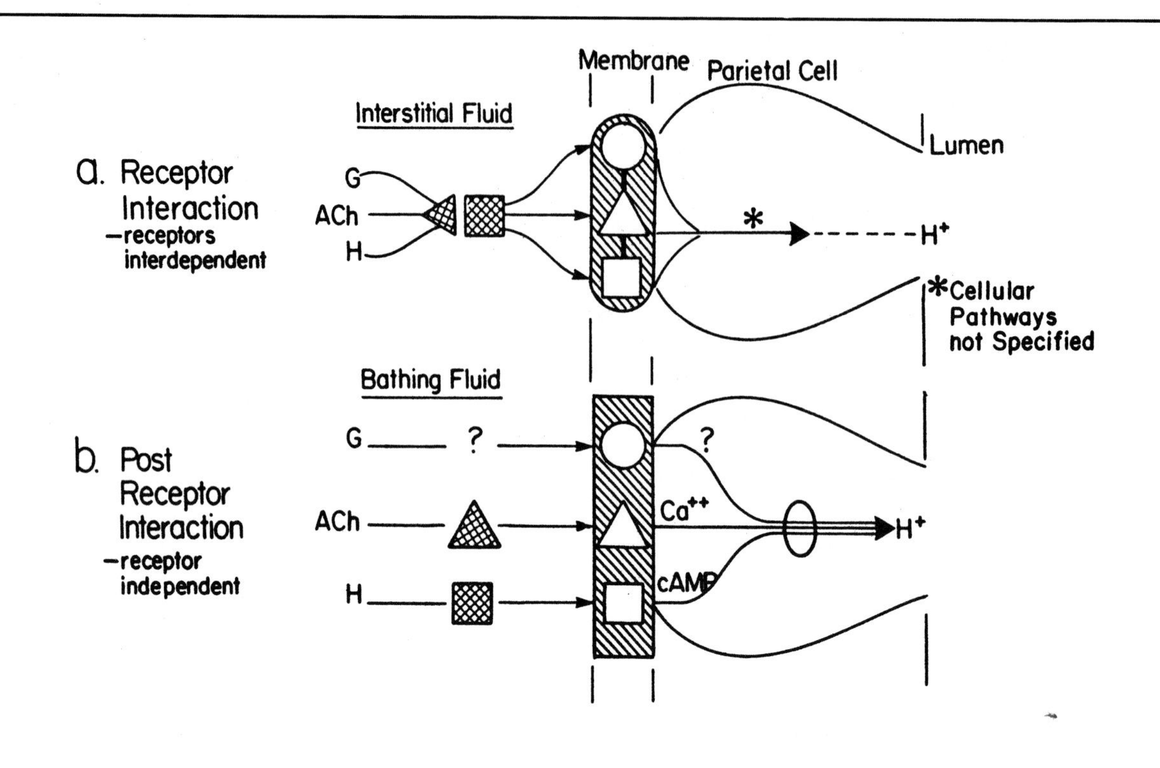

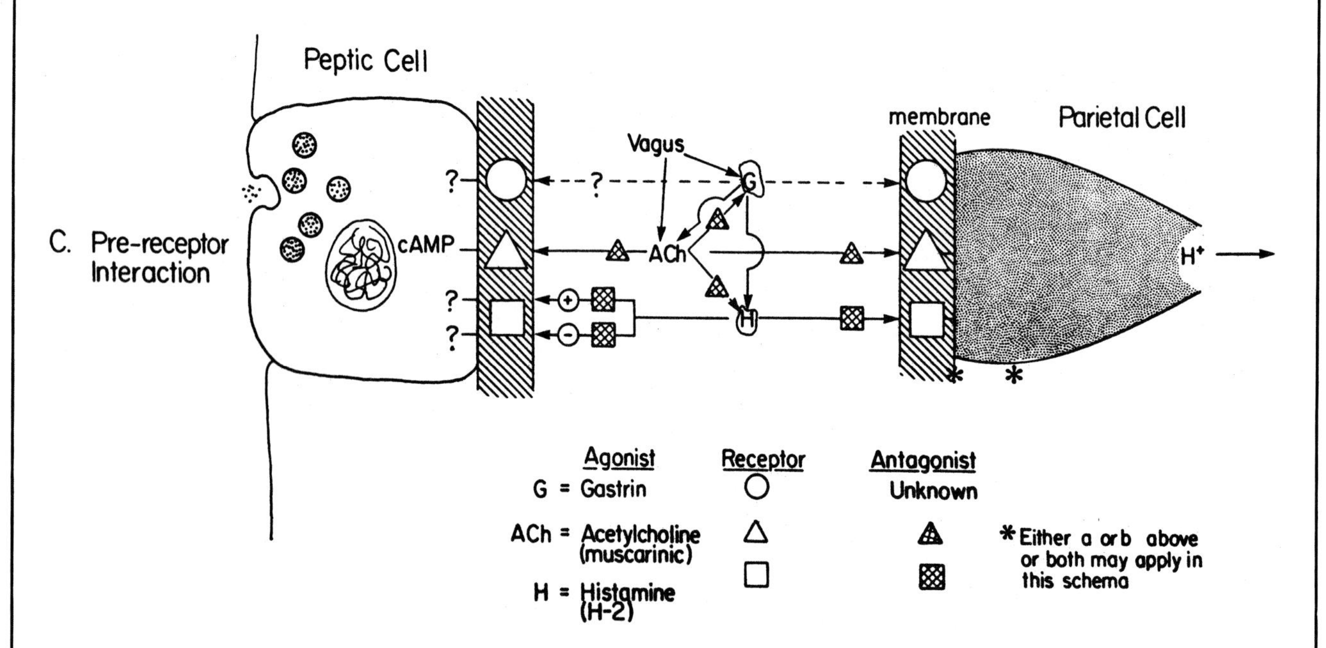

Figure 1. *Three models which could account for observed actions and interactions between the vagus, gastrin (G), acetylcholine (AcH), and histamine (H) on acid. The models also attempt to reconcile the effects of specific antagonists of gastric secretagogues. In the intact animal, model c could be coupled to either or both models a or b. In the isolated gastric membrane or parietal cells, which exhibit synergism between agonists without crossover effect of antagonist, model b would best apply. The model for pepsin secretion is shown for only the intact animal (model c) as there are no adequate data for pepsin secretion in isolated mammalian systems. Histamine is capable of both stimulating (+) and inhibiting (−) pepsin secretion. (Ref. 21).*

Reprinted with permission of the Journal of Pharmacology & Exp. Therapeutics

high affinity) as well as the predominant inhibitory (high dose, low affinity) action are H_2 mediated.[22] We have also shown that other H_2 agonists (impromidine, 4(Me)histamine) also have the dual action on pepsin, whether that secretion is stimulated by histamine or by cholinergic stimuli.[23] The inhibitory effect can be partly antagonized by H_2 antagonists.

In birds[24] and in amphibia in which both acid and pepsin are secreted by one cell, histamine stimulates both products, while the frog esophageal peptic glands are insensitive to histamine.[25]

Intrinsic factor (IF): IF is apparently secreted from parietal cells and characteristically upon acid stimulation, say with betazole,[26] exhibits a sharp early peak lasting about 15 min and then is secreted at a low steady rate. The nature of the secretion suggests that IF is synthesized and accumulates very slowly in the parietal cell. The early peak is not eliminated by pretreatment with cimetidine,[26] but the low, sustained secretion of IF in pentagastrin-stimulated secretion is reduced by cimetidine given I.V. at the same time.[27]

Gastrin: The H_2 antagonists have no direct effect on serum gastrin in animals[28] or man,[29,30,31] nor does treatment with cimetidine for six weeks change serum gastrin.[32] By preventing gastric acidification, cimetidine delays the normal acid-induced fall in serum gastrin 2-3 hours after food,[33,34] but does not increase the initial response to food.

Other secretions: Parotid — Histamine and analogs in the presence of IBMX increase parotid cAMP dose responsively, suggesting a histamine effect on canine parotid.[35]

Pancreas — In an isolated blood-perfused whole pancreas preparation arterial infusion of histamine or 4(Me)-histamine stimulated bicarbonate and enzyme secretion via H_2 receptors.[72]

BLOOD FLOW

Gastric circulation: Gastric blood flow increases with all stimuli of acid secretion, more so with histamine (presumably via H_1 receptors) than with pentagastrin or feeding at the same rate of acid secretion.[36,37] When histamine-induced acid stimulation in the rat is inhibited by cimetidine or prostaglandin, blood flow is unimpaired;[37] 2-pyridylethylamine (PEA), an H_1 agonist, stimulates blood flow. In the rabbit, dog and cat, H_2 but not H_1 receptors mediate the gastric vasodilation.[38,39] In the rabbit gastric blood flow is reduced by histamine via H_1 receptors[40] while the rat exhibits both H_1 and H_2-mediated vasodilation of gastric vessels. A number of agents including PEA and prostaglandin E_2 dilate gastric vessels independently of acid secretion in the dog.[41] It is not clear whether the vasodilation that accompanies stimulation of acid secretion by secretagogues other than histamine is due to local histamine release or to other mechanisms, e.g. a prostaglandin effect.[42]

Intestinal blood flow: Mesenteric blood flow in the anesthetized cat is increased by histamine and at the same time the vascular permeability is increased. Vasodilation is via H_1 receptors[43] with a maximum dose ratio shift of 16 by H_1 antagonists.[36,38] Permeability increases are mediated via H_2 receptors and are reversed by metiamide.[43] Initial dilation by H_1 receptors is accompanied by an increased O_2 uptake and redistribution of blood flow to the muscularis.[44]

Hepatic blood flow: In anesthetized dogs, hepatic portal blood flow is decreased by an H_1 mediated vasoconstriction and hepatic arterial flow is increased at the same time, also by an H_1 mediated effect;[45] neither is affected by metiamide.

MUSCULATURE

Esophagus: While a variety of histamine effects have been demonstrated on lower esophageal sphincter (LES) muscle in various preparations and in different species, there is little or no evidence to support a physiologic role for histamine in the control of the LES.

Stomach: Gastric muscle *in vivo*[1] or *in vitro*[46] contracts with H_1 receptor stimulation and relaxes with H_2;[47] the acetylcholine contracted stomach of guinea pig is also relaxed via H_2 effects.

Gastric emptying of solids and liquids is unaffected by cimetidine.[34, 48] The effect of histamine on gastric emptying has not to my knowledge been appropriately studied.

Pylorus: Acting via neural and myogenic H_1 receptors, histamine produces high amplitude phasic contractions in the cat pyloric sphincter.[49] Histamine, also via H_1 receptors, *reduces* the frequency and amplitude of the phasic (7.3 contractions/min, 83 $\pm$ 4 mm Hg) contractions of the opossum *sphincter of Oddi.*

Intestine: Ileal contraction with histamine is a classic H_1 effect.[1,50,51] The adult guinea pig ileum is more sensitive than the rabbit ileum, which is only sensitive to histamine before 11 days of age.[52]

Using implanted monopolar electrodes along the small intestine of conscious dogs, Konturek et al[53] showed that the interdigestive myoelectric complex (IMC) was stimulated by histamine via H_1 receptors. No H_2-mediated effect with either dimaprit or metiamide was seen in either fasted or fed dogs. Baker and Ebersole[54] suggest a histamine H_2-mediated release of a contractile substance from the myenteric plexus of guinea pig ileum *in vitro.*

Gallbladder: Waldman *et al*[55] have demonstrated that H_1 receptors mediate gallbladder contraction by histamine and that H_2 receptors mediate gallbladder relaxation. These observations were confirmed in baboon gallbladder.[56] Blockade of H_2 receptors augments the response to cholecystokinin, suggesting that histamine may modify the response to hormonal agents.

CLINICAL APPLICATIONS

The clinical applications of the H_2 antagonists have been the subject of numerous symposia and reviews, some of which are cited.[57,58] Despite the extensive list of actions of histamine on H_2 receptors of almost every tissue so far described there is only one practical clinical application of the H_2 antagonists: the suppression of gastric acid secretion. The H_2 antagonists are very effective in this action in the basal state and with all stimuli of gastric secretion including food, gastrin, histamine, caffeine, distension, vagal, and other cholinergic agonists. The obvious application of the antisecretory effect is to the treatment of those diseases of the gastrointestinal tract in which acid and pepsin are thought to be, if not causative, at least responsible for delayed healing or the failure to heal at all. These include duodenal, gastric and esophageal ulcer, recurrent ulcer after gastric surgery, and perhaps on less solid evidence, reflux esophagitis, erosive gastritis and duodenitis.

The first of the H_2 antagonists, metiamide, to be used in widescale testing resulted in a number of cases of agranulocytosis,[59-62] which in at least one of these cases, (a patient with systemic mastocytosis),[61] was fatal and led to its withdrawal from use. Its successor cimetidine has been free of hematological side effects, even when given to two patients who had had metiamide-induced agranulocytosis.[60,62] Cimetidine underwent extensive clinical trials in a number of countries prior to its release on the market in late 1976 abroad and in mid-1977 in the United States under the trade name Tagamet.

Since its release eight years ago, cimetidine has been used in perhaps 30 million patients and is the largest selling drug in the world. In the last two years ranitidine, another more potent H_2 antagonist, with a nitrofuran configuration, has also come into general use for the treatment of duodenal ulcer and hypersecretory states.

Duodenal Ulcer:

Worldwide endoscopically-controlled double-bind trials of cimetidine and ranitidine tested against each other or against placebo have demonstrated a healing rate of 76% at 4 weeks and 87% at 6 weeks with both drugs, compared to 40% and 45% respectively for placebo. The beneficial effect of the H_2 antagonists in duodenal ulcer, however, is not unique since equal efficacy has been demonstrated in similar trials by at least eight different non-H_2 antagonist types of drugs including several which have no effect on acid secretion.[63]

Upon withdrawal of H_2 antagonist treatment after healing, there is a recurrence rate of 50-90% in one year. This rate is the same whether the ulcer healed spontaneously without treatment or with any of the several effective treatments. Maintenance therapy with H_2 antagonists (generally a bedtime dose) has been reported as preventing symptomatic relapse in 87% of a collection of 15 controlled studies, compared to 53% for placebo.[4] Overall, if one adds asymptomatic recurrent ulcers discovered at routine endoscopy, relapse rates on treatment are 20-50% and without treatment 50-90% in 1 year after healing.

These findings clearly indicate that the natural history of duodenal ulcer is not materially altered by medicinal therapy, including H_2 antagonists. Cimetidine may heal ulcers but does not cure ulcer disease. This implies certain limitations on the rational use of ulcer treatments, including the use of surgery.[64]

Gastric Ulcer (GU):

The results of treatment of gastric ulcer are less well defined, and though cimetidine was recently approved by the F.D.A. for treatment of GU, the advantage of cimetidine over placebo is less uniformly reported than for duodenal ulcer. There are several factors which render GU less susceptible to healing including aspirin, alcohol, smoking, concomitant chronic renal, pulmonary, cardiovascular or neoplastic disease, old age and malnutrition. Since these factors are present in as many as 70% of all GU, the problem of GU treatment, especially in patients who carry these risk factors remains unsolved. Antacids and sucralfate are probably equally effective therapy for GU as H_2 antagonists.[65] The natural history of gastric ulcer is not well enough delineated yet to allow easy selection of the most effective form of treatment. Moreover, even malignant ulcers can become asymptomatic and heal on cimetidine.[66] Follow-up of all healed GU by endoscopy is essential. In a preliminary report on cimetidine, maintenance appears effective in preventing GU relapse.[67]

Zollinger-Ellison Syndrome:

Apart from the considerations of the malignancy itself, this condition presents the clearest rationale for the use of drugs that suppress the secretion of acid. Since H_2 antagonists effectively suppress the acid stimulation by gastrin, medical treatment has become a reasonable alternative to surgery, though this group of patients frequently require large doses of H_2 antagonists and, as a consequence also have a significant incidence of side-effects such as gynecomastia and impotence.[51] Ranitidine, which is 4-8 times more potent than cimetidine may be the choice between the two.[68] Occasionally treatment with H_2 antagonists has to be supplemented by antimuscarinic drugs; vagotomy may render these patients more susceptible to treatment by H_2 antagonists.[69] The most recent acid suppressing drugs, the benzimidazoles, which are H-K^+ATPase inhibitors may in fact be the treatment of choice in these patients. Non-ZE hypersecretors with normal gastrin values may be more susceptible to ranitidine than cimetidine.[70]

Systemic Mastocytosis and Basophil Leukemia:

These patients present another rational application for the use of H_2 antagonists to control acid secretion in those with hypersecretion. Not all such patients have a hypersecretory state and many symptoms persist despite combined H_1 and H_2 antagonist treatment including itching, rash, and diarrhea. This may indicate histamine actions which are not H_1 or H_2; or more likely the continued release of other biologically active amines.

Reflux Esophagitis:

Reflux esophagitis is another condition belonging to the group of acid/peptic diseases in which the results with cimetidine have been disappointing. Cimetidine does not affect LES pressure and its only effect could be through reduction in acid. Within the 8-week study period, those treated with cimetidine had fewer symptoms and consumed less antacid,[71] but there was no difference in endoscopically-judged esophagitis with 45% improved on cimetidine and 37% on placebo. It is obviously not enough only to reduce acid output in treating esophagitis or gastric ulcer. What we have learned is that our understanding of pathogenesis and pathophysiology of acid/peptic diseases is still fragmentary.

Erosive Gastritis:

There is contradictory evidence regarding the efficacy of cimetidine in the prevention or treatment of acute erosive (stress) gastritis.[2,57] The mechanism of erosive gastritis is not well understood. Several factors contribute to the development of gastritis — e.g. anoxia, disorders of microcirculation and sludging of red cells, reduction of the resistance or integrity of the mucosa in shock, sepsis, and severe anoxic states. The mucosa is subject to further trauma from lumenal acid, bile acids, and drugs such as aspirin. At what point the train of events becomes irreversible and leads to uncontrolled bleeding is unknown. In general, the improvements in managing the very sick patient in intensive care units has contributed more to the prevention of stress lesions of the stomach than can be attributed to gastric neutralization by antacids or H_2 antagonists. The routine use of intravenous cimetidine in all stressed and potentially stressed patients is not justified by experience.

REFERENCES

1. Black JW, Duncan WA, Durant CJ, Ganellin CR, Parsons EM. Definition and antagonism of histamine H_2-receptors. Nature 236:385-90, 1972.
2. Hirschowitz BI. H_2 histamine receptors. Ann Rev Pharmacol Toxicol 19:203-44, 1979. (250 Ref.)
3. Hirschowitz BI, Gibson R, Hutchison G. Stimulation of acid and pepsin secretion in the fistula dog by 4(5)-methyl histamine, a specific H_2 agonist. Am J Dig Dis 19:307-314, 1974.
4. Burland WL, Simkins MA, eds 1977. Cimetidine: 2nd int. symp. histamine H_2 receptor antagonists, 1976. Amsterdam. 1977 (published date) Oxford: R Coll Physicians Excerpta Med 392 pp.
5. Durant GJ, Ganellin CR, Parsons ME. Dimaprit, (S-[3-(N,N-dimethylamino) propyl]isothiourea). A highly specific histamine H_2-receptor agonist. Part 2. Structure-activity considerations. Agents Actions 7:39-43, 1977.
6. Hirschowitz BI, Rentz J, Molina E. Gastric and cardiac H_2-receptor effects of dimaprit and N'(Me),5(Me) histamine in conscious dogs. Eur. J. Pharmacol. 61(4):355-61, 1980.
7. Molina E, Rentz J, Hirschowitz B. Use of impromidine to define specific histamine H_2 effects on gastric secretion, heart rate and blood pressure in conscious dogs. J Pharmacol Exp Ther 214(3):483-7, 1980.
8. Hunt RH, Mills JG, Beresford J, Billings JA, Burland WL, Multon-Thompson GJ. Gastric secretory studies in humans with impromidine (SK and F 92676) — a specific histamine H_2 receptor agonist. Gastroenterology 78(3):505-11, 1980.
9. Parsons M, Sykes C. Impromidine SK and F 92676) acts as a partial agonist on the isolated whole stomach of the rat. Br J Pharmacol 69(1):6-7, 1980.
10. Hersey SJ. Histamine receptor in bullfrog gastric mucosa. Am J Physiol 241(2):G93-7, 1981.
11. Parsons ME, Owen DA, Ganellin CR, Durant GJ. Dimaprit-(S[3-(N,N-dimethylamino)propyl]i-sothiourea) — a highly specific histamine H_2-receptor agonist Part I. Pharmacology Agents Actions 7:31-37, 1977.
12. Impicciatore M, Bertaccini G, Mossini F, Hansen D, Grossman MI. N-methyl, 5-methyl histamine evokes a higher maximal rate of gastric acid secretion than histamine. Proc Soc Exp Biol Med 156:296-98, 1977.
13. Curwain BP, Turner NC. The involvement of histamine receptor subtypes in gasric acid secretion and mucosal blood flow in the anaesthetized rabbit. J Physiol (Lond) 311:431-42, 1981.
14. Soll, AH. Physiology of isolated canine parietal cells: Receptors and effectors regulating function. In *PHYSIOLOGY OF THE DIGESTIVE TRACT.* Johnson LR ed. Raven Press, New York, NY. Chapt 24, pp 673-91, 1981.
15. Bearer CF, Chang LK, Rosenfeld GC, Thompson WJ. Histamine stimulation of rat gastric parietal cell adenyl-cyclase: modulation by guanine nucleotides. Arch Biochem Biophys 207(2):325-36, 1981.
16. Mihas AA, Gibson RG, Hirschowitz BI. Inhibition of gastric secretion in the dog by 16,16-dimethyl prostaglandin E_2. Am J Physiol 230:351-356, 1976.
17. Helander HF, Hirschowitz BI. Quantitative ultrastructural studies on inhibited and on partly stimulated gastric parietal cells. Gastroenterology 67:447-52, 1974.
18. Carlisle KS, Chew CS, Hersey SJ. Ultrastructural changes and cyclic AMP in frog oxyntic cells. J Cell Biol 76:31-42, 1978.
19. Hirschowitz BI, Sachs G, Hutchison G. Lack of potentiation or synergism between histamine and pentagastrin in the fistula dog. Am J Physiol 224:509-513, 1973.
20. Hirschowitz BI, Molina E. Effect of cimetidine on histamine-stimulated gastric acid and electrolytes in dogs. Am J Physiol 244:G416-G420, 1983.
21. Hirschowitz BI, Molina E. Effects of four H_2 histamine antagonists on bethanechol-stimulated acid and pepsin secretion in the dog. J Pharmacol Exp Ther 224:341-345, 1983.
22. Hirschowitz BI, Hutchison GA. Evidence for a histamine H_2 receptor that inhibits pepsin secretion in the dog. Am J Physiol 233:E225-28, 1977.
23. Hirschowitz BI, Rentz J, Molina E. Histamine H_2 receptor stimulation and inhibition of pepsin secretion in the dog. J Pharmacol Exp Ther 218(3):676-680, 1981.
24. Burhol PG. A review: regulation of gastric secretion in the chicken. Scand J Gastro 17:321-323, 1982.
25. Simpson L, Goldenberg D, Hirschowitz BI. Pepsinogen secretion by the frog esophagus *in vitro*. Am J Physiol 238:G79-84, 1980.
26. Burland WL, Mills JG, Sharpe PC, Horton MA, Mollin DL. The effect of cimetidine on intrinsic factor secretion. In cimetidine: 2nd int symp histamine H_2 receptor antagonists, 1976. Burland WL, Simkins MA eds. Amsterdam and Oxford: R Coll Physicians Excerpta Med 392 pp, 1977.
27. Fielding LP, Chalmers DM, Chanarin I, Levi AJ. Inhibition of intrinsic factor secretion by cimetidine. Br Med J 1:818-19, 1978.

28. Barbezat, GO, Daniel M, Bank S, Grant B, Vinik A. The effect of histamine H-receptor blockade on fasting serum gastrin and fasting gastric acid secretion in the dog. Nature 249:666-68, 1974.
29. Hirschowitz BI, Danilewitz M, Molina E. Inhibition of basal acid, chloride and pepsin secretion in duodenal ulcer by graded doses of ranitidine and atropine with studies of pharmacokinetics of ranitidine. Gastroenterology 82:1314-1326, 1982.
30. Carter DC, Forrest JA, Logan RA, Ansell I, Lidgard G, Heading RC, Shearman DJC. Effect of histamine H_2-receptor antagonist, cimetidine, on gastric secretion and serum gastrin during insulin infusion in man. Scand J Gastroent 11:565-570, 1976.
31. Pounder RE, Hunt RH, vincent SH, Milton-Thompson GJ, Misiewicz JJ. 24-hour intragastric acidity and nocturnal acid secretion in patients with duodenal ulcer during oral administration of cimetidine and atropine. Gut 18:85-90, 1977.
32. Bank S, Barbezat GO, Vinik AI, Helman C. Serum gastrin levels before and after 6 weeks of cimetidine therapy in patients with duodenal ulcer. Digestion 15:157-61, 1977.
33. Richardson CT, Bailey BA, Walsh JH, Fordtran JS. The effect of an H_2-receptor antagonist on food-stimulated acid secretion, serum gastrin, and gastric emptying in patients with duodenal ulcers. Comparison with an anticholinergic drug. J Clin Invest 55:536-42, 1975.
34. Longstreth GF, Go VL, Malagelada JR. Postprandial gastric, pancreatic, and biliary response to histamine H_2 receptor antagonists in active duodenal ulcer. Gastroenterology 72:9-13, 1977.
35. Nishibori M. Cyclic AMP increase in canine parotid gland mediated by histamine H_2-receptors. Eur J Pharmacol 76(4):309-316, 1981.
36. Guth PH, Smith E. The effect of gastrointestinal hormones on the gastric microcirculation. Gastroenterology 71:435-38, 1976.
37. Main IH, Whittle BJ. A study of the vascular and acid-secretory responses of the rat gastric mucosa to histamine. J Physiol (Lond) 257:407-18, 1976.
38. Flynn SB, Johnston BM, Owen DA. The cardiovascular response to dimaprit, a selective histamine H_2-receptor agonist. Br J Pharmacol 61:101-7, 1977.
39. Johnston BM, Owen DA. Tissue blood flow and distribution of cardiac output in cats: changes caused by intravenous infusions of histamine and histamine receptor agonists. Br J Pharmacol 60:173-80, 1977.
40. Curwain BP, Turner NC. Histamine H_1- and H_2-receptors in the gastric vasculature of the rabbit. Eur J Pharmacol 71(4):515-9, 1981.
41. Gerber JG, Nies AS. Canine gastric mucosal vasodilation with prostaglandins and histamine analogs. Dig Dis Sci 27(10):870-4, 1982.
42. Gerkens JG, Flexner C, Oates JA, Shand DG. Prostaglandin and histamine involvement in the gastric vasodilator action of pentagastrin. J Pharmacol Exp Ther 201:421-26, 1977.
43. Mortillaro NA, Granger DN, Kvietys PR, Rutili G, Taylor AE. Effects of histamine and histamine antagonists on intestinal capillary permeability. Am J Physiol 240(5):G381-6, 1981.
44. Walus KM, Fondacaro JD, Jacobson ED. Mesenteric vascular reactivity to histamine receptor agonists and antagonists. Dig Dis Sci 26(5):438-43, 1981.
45. Richardson PD, Withrington PG. A comparison of the effects of bradykinin, 5-hydroxytryptamine, and histamine on the hapatic arterial and portal venous vascular beds of the dog: Histamine H_1- and H_2-receptor populations. Br J Pharmacol 60:123-33, 1977.
46. Nakazawa S, Ichikawa T, Naito Y, Tsukamoto Y. Effect of histamine on the gastric smooth muscles of guinea pig. Digestion 22(4):203-9, 1981.
47. Ercan ZS, Türker RK. Histamine receptors in the isolated rat stomach fundus and rabbit aortic strips. Pharmacology 15:118-26, 1977.
48. Heading RC, Logan RFA, McLoughlin GP, Lidgard G, Forrest JAH. Effect of cimetidine on gastric emptying. In cimetidine: 2nd int symp histamine H_2 receptor antagonists, 1976 Burland WL, Simkins MA, eds. Amsterdam and Oxford: R Coll Physicians Excerpta Med 392 pp, pp 145-54, 1977.
49. Biancani P, Cicalzi LK, McCallum RW. Mechanism of histamine-induced excitation of the cat pylorus. J Clin Invest 68(3):528-8, 1981.
50. Ash AS, Schild HO. Receptors mediating some actions of histamine. Br J Pharmacol 27:427-39, 1966.
51. Brimblecombe, RW, Duncan WAM. The relevance to man of pre-clinical data for cimetidine. In cimetidine: 2nd int symp histamine H_2 receptor antagonists, 1976. Burland WL, Simkins MA, eds. Amsterdam and Oxford: R Coll Physicians Excerpta Med pp 54-65, 1977.
52. Botting JH. Sensitivity of neonatal rabbit ileum to histamine. Br J Pharmacol 53:428-29, 1975.
53. Konturek SJ, Siebers R. Role of histamine H_1- and H_2-receptors on myoelectric activity of small bowel in the dog. Am J Physiol 238(1):G50-56, 1980.
54. Barker LA, Ebersole BJ. Histamine H_2-receptors on guinea pig ileum myenteric plexus neurons mediate the release of contractile agents. J Pharmacol Exp Ther 221(1):69-75, 1982.
55. Waldman DB, Zfass AM, Makhlouf GM. Stimulatory (H_1) and inhibitory (H_2) histamine receptors in gallbladder muscle. Gastroenterology 72:932-36, 1977.
56. Schoetz JR, Wise WE Jr, La Morte WW, et al. Histamine receptors in primate gallbladder. Dig Dis Sci 28(4):353-8, 1983.
57. Freston JW. Cimetidine. I. Developments, pharmacology, and efficacy. II. Adverse reactions and pattern of use. Ann Intern Med 97(4):573-80, 728-734, 1982.
58. Brogden RN, Carmine AA, Heel RC, Speight TM, Avery GS, et al. Ranitidine: a review of its pharmacology and therapeutic use in peptic ulcer disease and other allied diseases. Drugs 24:267-303, 1982. (198 Ref.)
59. Forrest JA, Shearman DJ, Spence R, Celestin LR. Neutropenia associated with metiamide. Lancet 1:392-93, 1975.
60. Burland WL, Sharpe PC, Colin-Jones DG, Turnbull PR, Bowskill P. [Letter]: Reversal of metiamide-induced agranulocytosis during treatment with cimetidine. Lancet 2:1085, 1975.
61. Feldman EJ, Isenberg JI. Effects of metiamide on gastric acid hypersecretion, steatorrhea and bone-marrow function in a patient with systemic mastocytosis. N Engl J Med 295:1178-79, 1976.
62. Fleischer D, Samloff IM. Cimetidine therapy in a patient with metiamide-induced agranulocytosis. (Letter) N Engl J Med 296:342, 1977.
63. Hirschowitz BI. Controls of gastric secretion. A roadmap to the choice of treatment for duodenal ulcer. Am J Gastroent 77:281-293, 1982.
64. Hirschowitz BI. Natural history of duodenal ulcer. (Editorial) Gastroenterology 85(4):967-970, 1983.
65. Hirschowitz BI. Gastric Ulcer. In current therapy in gastroenterology and liver disease. Bayless TM, ed. BC Decker, New York, NY. Chapt. 14, 1983.
66. Taylor RH, Menzies-Gow N, Lovell D, LaBrooy SJ, Misiewicz JJ. Misleading response of malignant gastric ulcers to cimetidine. Lancet 1:686-88, 1978.
67. Machell RJ, Ciclitira PJ, Farthing MJG, Rose JDR, Dick AD, Hunter JO. Maintenance cimetidine in the prevention of gastric ulcer relapse. Ann Br Soc Gastroent Abstr FA43, 1978.
68. Jensen RT, Pandol SJ, Collen MJ, Raufman JP, Gardner JD, et al. Diagnosis and management of the Zollinger-Ellison syndrome. J Clin Gastroenterol 5 (Suppl 1):123-131, 1983.
69. Richardson CT, Feldman M, McClelland RN, et al. Effect of vagotomy in Zollinger-Ellison syndrome. Gastroenterology 77:682-686, 1979.
70. Danilewitz M, Tim LO, Hirschowitz BI. Ranitidine suppression of gastric hypersecretion resistant to cimetidine. N Engl J Med 316:20-22, 1982.
71. Behar J, Brand DL, Brown FC, Castell DO, Cohen S, Crossley RJ, Pope CE II, Winans CS. Cimetidine in the treatment of sympotomatic gastroesophageal reflux: A double-blind controlled trial. Gatroenterology 74:441-48, 1978.
72. Nishibori M. Cyclic AMP increase in canine parotid gland mediated by histamineH_2-receptors. Eur J Pharmacol 76:309-316, 1981. □

Chapter IX

Histamine Receptors: Involvement in Cardiac Function and Dysfunction

Andrew A. Wolff, M.D., Steven S. Gross, Ph.D., Roberto Levi, M.D.

ABSTRACT

Cardiac manifestations of systemic anaphylaxis range from transient electrocardiographic changes to ventricular fibrillation with complete circulatory collapse. Many of these cardiovascular events are attributable to the stimulation of cardiac H_1- and H_2-receptors by histamine released during anaphylaxis. Indeed, the heart itself has been shown to contain high concentrations of histamine, which can be released not only by IgE-mediated hypersensitivity reactions, but by various drugs and chemicals, as well as ischemia. In man and guinea pig, release of cardiac histamine is accompanied by changes in rate, rhythm, contractility, and electrical conduction which can be reproduced by the administration of exogenous histamine H_2-receptors have been shown to mediate histamine-induced increases in sinus rate, myocardial contractility, and electrical automaticity, while decreases in contractility and atrioventricular conduction velocity are H_1-mediated. In the dog, cardiac histamine release may participate in the pathophysiology of early ischemic ventricular arrhythmias.

Early descriptions of anaphylaxis in various mammalian species all indicated profound cardiovascular involvement.[1-6] Although it was originally proposed that these cardiac effects were secondary phenomena resulting from bronchospasm and subsequent asphyxia,[3] observations of anaphylaxis in the rabbit and the dog, neither of which succumb to bronchoconstriction,[4,6] made this view untenable. Cesaris-Demel[7] proved that the heart is clearly capable of behaving as a primary target organ in anaphylaxis by showing that isolated hearts from immunized rabbits and guinea pigs would react specifically to very dilute solutions of antigens such as beef serum, horse serum, cow's milk and egg white. More recently, Zavecz and Levi[8] were able to separate the primary cardiac effects of anaphylaxis from secondary cardiac effects due to concomitant respiratory distress in the intact, sensitized guinea pig. Injection of antigen directly into the left ventricle, thus bypassing the lungs, resulted in increases in sinus rate and left ventricular and arterial pressures which preceded the rise in bronchial resistance by 60 seconds. Thus, evidence has been provided that the heart may serve as a target organ during systemic anaphylaxis.

After the isolation of histamine in 1910 by Barger and Dale,[9] the profound similarity between its effects on the heart and the cardiac responses to anaphylaxis began to be appreciated. When Bartosch and colleagues[10] showed the release of histamine from tissues undergoing anaphylaxis, the concept of histamine as a major mediator of anaphylaxis was well in place. Wilcox and Andrus[11] made a careful comparison of the cardiac responses to

---

Department of Pharmacology, Cornell University Medical College, New York, New York 10021

Corresponding Author: *Dr. Roberto Levi, Dept. of Pharmacology, Cornell University Medical College, 1300 York Avenue, New York, N.Y. 10021*

Supported by NHLBI grants HL 18828 and HL 34215, and by DANA TRUST.

anaphylaxis and to histamine. They found each to be characterized by an increase in the rate and force of contraction, a delay in atrio-ventricular conduction, the development of ectopic beats, and the appearance of intraventricular conduction defects. In 1939, Schild[12] demonstrated immunologic release of histamine from resting slices of guinea pig heart and later, Feigen *et al.*[13] showed histamine release from the isolated, whole guinea pig heart during anaphylaxis. In our laboratory, we have shown that the cardiac effects of anaphylaxis are indeed proportional to the amount of histamine released from the heart and are identical to the effects of pharmacologically-induced mast cell degranulation and exogenously administered histamine.[14] We have also defined the cardiac histamine receptors which mediate these effects.[14]

Exquisitely sensitive to histamine, the guinea pig has provided an excellent model for investigating cardiac dysfunction secondary to histamine. The guinea pig heart contains roughly 4 micrograms of histamine per gram of tissue;[15,16] assay of surgical specimens from human right atrial appendage yields values in the same range (2.81 ± 1.04 ug/g, nine specimens).[16,17] Furthermore, the human heart is as sensitive to histamine as is the guinea pig heart,[17] suggesting that results obtained from the animal model will prove applicable to humans. Histamine is found in greatest concentrations in the right atrium with decreasing amounts present in the left atrium, right ventricle and left ventricle, in that order.[18] Cardiac mast cells are similarly distributed throughout the chambers of the heart, implying that most cardiac histamine may be "mast cell histamine".[19] In fact, cardiac histamine can be released not only by the binding of antigen to specific, mast-cell bound IgE, but also by various chemicals known to cause mast cell degranulation.[14]

A variety of drugs and compounds have been shown to cause release of extra-cardiac histamine, some of them in common clinical use. These include morphine, D-tubocurarine, certain synthetic corticotropins, calcium ionophore and compound 48/80. We have shown them all to release histamine from the isolated guinea pig heart and the human atrium in a dose-dependent fashion.[14,20] Concurrent with the release of histamine, sinus tachycardia, idioventricular tachyarrhythmias, and atrio-ventricular conduction block of varying severity are seen. The more histamine released, the greater the increase in sinus rate and the longer the duration of the idioventricular tachyarrhythmias.[14,20] Isolated hearts from guinea pigs passively sensitized to dinitrophenol (DNP) also release histamine when challenged with that antigen. The quantity of histamine released is in direct proportion to the amount of sensitizing antibody previously administered. Again, the released histamine causes tachycardia and arrhythmias; the magnitude of these changes correlates with the amount of histamine released.[15,21]

That these changes in rate, rhythm and impulse conduction are due predominantly, if not exclusively, to released cardiac histamine, rather than to some other mast-cell product liberated during either immunologic or pharmacologic degranulation, can be shown in two ways. First, the increase in sinus rate is directly proportional to the total amount of histamine released; second, the effects are inhibited by antihistamines, i.e., the increase in sinus rate can be antagonized in a concentration-dependent fashion by treatment with burimamide, a specific H_2-receptor antagonist.[22] Similarly, the increase in ventricular automaticity seen during anaphylaxis is completely prevented by burimamide or by cimetidine, another H_2-receptor blocker.[22,23] "Classical" antihistamines, i.e., H_1-receptor blockers, prevent neither the increase in sinus rate nor the enhancement of ventricular automaticity during anaphylaxis.[23,24] However, the prolongation of atrio-ventricular conduction time, characteristic of anaphylaxis, is susceptible to pharmacologic blockade by H_1-receptor blockers, whereas, it is only weakly affected by drugs blocking the H_2-receptor.[25,26] That pharmacologic blockade of cardiac histamine receptors can greatly attenuate anaphylactic responses of the heart strongly suggests that they are mediated primarily, if not exclusively, by histamine.

All of the previously described changes in sinus rate, ventricular automaticity and atrio-ventricular conduction are reproduced by the administration of exogenous histamine, the effects of which can be prevented by blockade of the appropriate histamine receptors.[16,23,26] Thus, in the guinea pig and human, histamine H_2-receptors mediate increases in sinus rate and ventricular automaticity, but the slowing of atrioventricular conduction is H_1-mediated. Because acute myocardial ischemia is frequently accompanied by sinus tachycardia, ventricular ectopy and atrioventricular conduction block, it has been suspected to trigger cardiac histamine release. In turn, histamine has been proposed as a mediator of early ischemic ventricular arrhythmias,[27] which are responsible for the overwhelming majority of sudden cardiac deaths.[28] We have reported a mean ten-fold rise in the coronary sinus histamine concentration during the first 30 minutes after acute occlusion of the canine left anterior descending coronary artery.[29] This increase occurred simultaneously with the development of early ischemic ventricular arrhythmias and in proportion to their severity; however, attempts to prevent these arrhythmias by pre-treating dogs with the H_2-receptor antagonist ranitidine were associated with larger elevations of the coronary sinus histamine concentration and more severe ventricular arrhythmias.[30] These results are consistent with the physiologic role we have proposed for cardiac histamine, based on our observations that histamine is released from the guinea pig heart during sympathetic stimulation and acts to attenuate the car-

Table I

Summary Of The Effects Of Histamine On The Heart

Parameter	Guinea Pig	Human	Receptor
Automaticity	Increase	Increase	H_2
Sinoatrial Rate (direct)	Increase	Increase	H_2
Sinoatrial Rate (baroreceptor reflex)	Increase	Increase	H_1 and H_2
Contractile Force	Increase	Increase	H_2
Contractile Force	Decrease	Decrease	H_1
A-V Conduction Velocity	Decrease	?	H_1

diac responses to this adrenergic input.[31,32] Histamine release evoked by sympathetic stimulation appears to be subject to an autoinhibition mediated by H_2-receptors;[32] blockade by ranitidine may enhance release by this mechanism. Cardiac sympathetic tone increases dramatically after acute canine coronary occlusion and has been implicated in the pathogenesis of early ischemic ventricular arrhythmias.[33] Thus, while ischemia does indeed appear to release cardiac histamine, whether this reflects a physiologic response which has evolved to oppose sympathetic arrhythmogenesis during ischemia, or a pathologic role for histamine in the development of early ischemic ventricular arrhythmias is, as yet, undetermined.[34]

The ventricular myocardium of the guinea pig contains both H_1- and H_2- histamine receptors. Our studies with selective agonists and antagonists indicate that H_2-receptors mediate the positive inotropic effects of histamine which are superimposed upon and mask H_1-mediated negative inotropic effects.[35] Indeed, in the presence of H_1-blockers, histamine causes a pure positive inotropic response, whereas, in the presence of H_2-blockers, histamine causes a pure negative inotropic effect. Thus, H_1-agonists cause a decrease in contractility, while H_2-agonists cause an increase in contractility.[35]

This two-component inotropic effect of histamine also occurs in the human myocardium. Pectinate muscles obained from surgical specimens of human right atrial appendage exhibit a dose-dependent increase in contractile force in the presence of histamine. Much like the intact guinea pig hearts, when treated with cimetidine, the contractility of the pectinate preparations is depressed by concentrations of histamine which are insufficient to overcome the H_2-receptor blockade by cimetidine; under these conditions histamine causes only an H_1-mediated depression of inotropy. As its concentration is increased, histamine is able to compete successfully with cimetidine for occupancy of the H_2-receptors, and its positive inotropic effect becomes manifest.[16,36,37] The effects of histamine on the heart, and the specific receptors which mediate these effects, are summarized in Table I.

CONCLUDING REMARKS

We have demonstrated that: 1) guinea pig and human myocardium are about equally rich in histamine, 2) cardiac histamine can be released by the same mechanisms in the guinea pig and human, and 3) cardiac tissues from both species respond similarly to equivalent concentrations of histamine. Thus, it is likely that histamine-induced cardiac dysfunction in the guinea pig is paralleled by clinical situations in which histamine release occurs in humans, e.g., anaphylaxis or after intravenous bolus injection of certain anesthetics. In addition, we have raised important questions regarding the participation of histamine in the pathogenesis of ventricular arrhythmias during acute myocardial ischemia. It is our belief that therapy of human cardiac dysfunction in such states must eventually address the role of histamine. As investigations into the actions of histamine in the heart continue, it appears increasingly likely that drugs acting upon cardiac histamine receptors will find their rightful place in the cardiologic pharmacopoeia.

REFERENCES

1. Poitier D, Richet C. De l'action anaphylactique de certains venins. Compt Rend Soc Biol (Paris) 54:170, 1902.
2. Smith T. Degrees of susceptibility to diphtheria toxin among guinea pigs; transmission from parents to offspring. J. Med. Research 13:341-348, 1904-1905.
3. Auer J, Lewis PA. The physiology of the immediate reaction of anaphylaxis in the guinea-pig. J Exper Med 12:151-175, 1910

4. Auer J. Lethal cardiac anaphylaxis in the rabbit. J Exper Med 14:476-496, 1911.
5. Auer J, Robinson GC. An electrocardiographic study of the anaphylactic rabbit. J Expr Med 18:450-460, 1913.
6. Manwaring WH. The physiological mechanism of anaphylactic shock: A preliminary communication. Bull John Hopkins Hosp. 21:275-277, Sep 1910.
7. Cesaris-Demel A. Recherches sur l'anaphylaxie; sur le mode de se comporter du coeur isolé d'animaux sensibilisés. Arch. Ital. Biol. 54:141-152, 1910-1911.
8. Zavecz JH, Levi R. Separation of primary and secondary cardiovascular events in systemic anaphylaxis. Circ Res 40:15-19, 1977.
9. Barger G, Dale HH. The presence in ergot and physiological activity of β-imidazolethylamine. Proc Physiol Soc Lond 38-50, 1910.
10. Bartosch R, Feldberg W, Nagel E. Das Freiwerden eines histamin-ähnlichen Stoffes bei der Anaphylaxie des Meerschweinchens. Arch f. d. ges. Physiol.230: 129-153, 1932.
11. Wilcox HB, Andrus EC. Anaphylaxis in the isolated heart. J Exper Med 67:169-180, 1938.
12. Schild HO. Histamine release in anaphylactic shock from various tissues of the guinea-pig. J Physiol 95:393-403, April 14, 1939.
13. Feigen GA, Vaughan Williams EM, Peterson JK, Nielsen CB. Histamine release and intracellular potentials during anaphylaxis in the isolated heart. Circulat Res 8:713-23, 1960.
14. Levi R, Allan G. Histamine-mediated cardiac effects. *In*: Drug-Induced Heart Disease. Ed. by Bristow, M.R., Elsevier-North Holland Biomedical Press, 1980, pp. 377-395.
15. Capurro N, Levi R. The heart as a target organ in systemic allergic reactions: Comparison of cardiac anaphylaxis *in vivo* and *in vitro*. Circ Res 36:520-28, 1975.
16. Levi R, Guo ZG. Roles of histamine in cardiac dysfunction. *In*: Advances in the Biosciences, Vol.33: Advances in Histamine Research. Ed. by Uvnäs, B. and Tasaka, K. Pergamon Press, 1982, pp. 213.
17. Levi R, Zavecz JH, Lee CH, Allan G. Histamine-drug-disease interactions and cardiac function. *In*: Histamine Receptors:Proceedings of the A.N. Richards Symposium. Ed. by Yellin, T.O. Spectrum Publications, Inc., 1979, pp. 99.
18. Giotti A, Guidotti A, Mannaioni PF, Zilletti L. The influences of adrenotropic drugs and noradrenaline on the histamine release in cardiac anaphylaxis *in vitro*. J. Physiol. 184:924-41, 1966.
19. Beaven MA. Histamine: its role in physiological and pathological processes. Monogr Allergy, 13:1-113, 1978.
20. Levi R, Chenouda AA, Trzeciakowski JP, Guo ZG, Aaronson LM, Luskind RD, Lee CH, Gay WA, Alexander JC, McCabe JC, Subramanian VA. Dysrhythmias caused by histamine release in guinea pig and human hearts. Klin Wschr 60:965-71, 1982.
21. Levi R, Zavecz JH, Ovary Z. IgE-mediated cardiac hypersensitivity reactions. An experimental model. Int Arch Allergy Appl Immunol 57:529-34, 1978.
22. Capurro N, Levi R. Anaphylaxis in the guinea-pig isolated heart: selective inhibition by burimamide of the positive inotropic and chronotropic effects of released histamine. Br J Pharmacol 48:620-28, 1973.
23. Levi R, Zavecz JH. Acceleration of idioventricular rhythms by histamine in guinea-pig heart: mediation by H_2-receptors. Circ Res 44(6):847-855, Jun 1979.
24. Trendelenburg U. The action of histamine and 5-hydroxytryptamine on isolated mammalian atria. J Pharmacol Exper Ther 130:450-60, 1960.
25. Levi R, Kuye JO. Pharmacological characterization of cardiac histamine receptors: sensitivity to H_1-receptor antagonists. Eur J Pharmacol 27:330-38, 1974.
26. Levi R, Capurro N, Lee CH. Pharmacological characterization of cardiac histamine receptors: sensitivity to H_1- and H_2-receptor agonists and antagonists. Eur J Pharmacol 30:328-35, 1975.
27. Harris AS. Delayed development of ventricular ectopic rhythms following experimental coronary occlusion. Circulation 1: 1318-28, 1950.
28. Lown, B. Cardiovascular collapse and sudden cardiac death. In: Heart Disease. A Textbook of Cardiovascular Medicine. Ed. by Braunwald, E. W.B. Saunders Co., 1984, pp. 774–806.
29. Levi, R., Wolff A, Robertson DA, Graver LM. IgE-mediated hypersensitivity and ischemia as causes of endogenous cardiac histamine release. In: Advances in the Biosciences, Vol. 51: Frontiers in Histamine Research. Ed. by Ganellin, C.R. and Schwartz, J.-C. Pergamon Press, 1985, pp. 305–308.
30. Wolff AA, Levi R, Chenouda AA, Fisher VJ. Ventricular arrhythmias parallel cardiac histamine release after coronary artery occlusion in the dog: effects of ranitidine (abstr). Circulation 70(suppl II):225, 1984.
31. Gross SS, Guo Z-G, Levi R, Bailey WH, Chenouda AA. Release of histamine by sympathetic nerve stimulation in the guinea pig heart and modulation of adrenergic responses: a physiologic role for cardiac histamine? Circ Res 54:516–26, 1984.
32. Gross SS, Levi R. Histamine modulation of cardiac sympathetic responses. In: Advances in the Biosciences, Vol. 51: Frontiers in Histamine Research. Ed. by Ganellin, C.R. and Schwartz, J.-C. Pergamon Press, 1985, pp. 317–24.
33. Malliani A, Schwartz PJ, Zanchetti A. Neural mechanisms in life-threatening arrhythmias. Am Heart J 100:705–715, 1980.
34. Wolff A, Levi R. Histamine and cardiac arrhythmias. Circ Res 58:1–16, 1986.
35. Zavecz JH, Levi R. Histamine-induced negative inotropism: mediation by H_1-receptors. J Pharmacol Exp Ther 206:274–80, 1978.
36. Levi R, Guo ZG. Inotropic effects of histamine in human myocardium. Fed Proc 41:1719, 1982.
37. Guo ZG, Levi R, Graver LN, Robertson DA, Gay WA, Jr. Inotropic effects of histamine in human myocardium: Differentiation between positive and negative components. J Cardiovascular Pharmacol 6:1210–1215, 1984. □

Chapter X

Histamine Receptors in the Brain

Monique Garbarg, Dr. Sci., Jean-Charles Schwartz, Dr. Sci. (France)

ABSTRACT

In mammalian brain, neuronal histamine is likely to act as a neurotransmitter and is recognized by the two classes of histamine receptors (H_1 and H_2) previously characterized in peripheral organs. Cerebral H_1 receptors can be selectively labeled by a tritiated antagonist mepyramine, in particulate fractions or in the living animal. Cerebral H_1 receptors mediate the glycogen hydrolysis and the breakdown of inositol phospholipids elicited by the amine. They are indirectly involved in the histamine-mediated accumulation of cyclic AMP. All these biochemical responses mediated by H_1 receptors are calcium-dependent. H_2 receptors are coupled to an adenylate cyclase. In addition, a novel class of histamine receptors (H_3) are presynaptic autoreceptors and modulate the release of neuronal histamine.

In the Central Nervous System histamine has a dual cellular localization which presumably reflects multiple functions. Part of the amine is held in non-neuronal cells (probably mast cells) where it could be involved in vascular control or immune responses. On the other hand biochemical, electrophysiological and lesion studies have shown during the last decade that another pool of histamine is synthesized and stored in nerve terminals, emanating from a discrete set of neurons ascending from the posterior hypothalamus and possibly upper mesencephalon and projecting widely to the telencephalon.[1] Recently, the visualization of histamine neurons by immunohistochemical methods using antibodies raised against the amine itself or its synthesizing enzyme, L-histidine decarboxylase[2,3,4] have brought strong support to the previous data. Together with other monoamine systems, histamine neurons have been suggested to participate in the regulation of a variety of brain functions such as arousal, thermoregulation, and secretion of hormones like vasopressin or prolactin. A precise mapping of histaminergic neurons will be of great help to further elucidate histamine functions in brain, but evidence for a possible role of this amine in neuronal communication comes also from its interaction with specific receptors after its release upon depolarization of histaminergic nerve terminals.

Hence, the two classes of histamine receptors (namely H_1 and H_2) previously characterized in peripheral organs[5] were shown to be present in the mammalian brain.[6,7] The interaction of histamine with these specific receptors triggers a variety of intracellular biochemical processes eventually yielding to the final physiological response of the cell. This review will deal mainly with the direct identification of these receptors by radioligand binding studies and with the biochemical events identified as belonging specifically to these receptors.

Monique Garbarg, Dr. Sci.
Maitre de Recherches CNRS, Unité de Neurobiologie, Centre Paul Broca de l'INSERM, 2 ter rue d'Alésia 75014 PARIS
Jean-Charles Schwartz, Dr. Sci
Professor, Université René Descartes, Paris
Head, Unité de Neurobiologie Centre Paul Broca de l'INSERM, 2 ter rue d'Alésia 75014 PARIS

In addition, the presence of presynaptic autoreceptors modulating the release of the neuronal histamine and belonging to a novel class of histamine receptors (H_3) will be reported.

I. THE HISTAMINE H_1 RECEPTORS

1— BINDING STUDIES

Binding techniques which have been so fruitful for investigating the properties of a variety of CNS receptors have been applied successfully to histamine H_1 receptors in the brain. Hill et al.[8] first demonstrated that radiolabelled ^{3}H-mepyramine (a histamine H_1 receptor antagonist) could be used as a selective ligand of H_1 receptors in homogenates of smooth muscle of guinea pig ileum. It has been subsequently shown in several laboratories that ^{3}H-mepyramine labels H_1 receptors in particulate fractions of the brain of various animal species. ^{3}H-mepyramine binds to a single class of sites with an equilibrium dissociation constant (Kd) of about 1 nM, in good agreement with that obtained for the antagonism by mepyramine of the histamine-induced contraction of ileum, the reference biological system for an H_1 receptor mediated response.[5] Moreover, the pharmacological specificity of these binding sites, assessed by establishing the inhibitory potencies of a variety of histaminergic and non-histaminergic antagonists, leaves little doubt that they represent the recognition moiety of H_1 receptors.[9] Although selective lesions in the rat brain have failed to allow identification of the cells bearing the ^{3}H-mepyramine binding sites, other approaches have been more successful. A small fraction of the brain's total content is present on cerebral microvessels. On the other hand, the ontogenetic development and the synaptosomal localization of the H_1 receptors suggest a neuronal localization of ^{3}H-mepyramine binding sites. This view is strenghtened by autoradiographic studies which allow the visualization at the photon microscopic level of the receptor sites.[10] Radioautography of slices of the guinea pig brain showed a high density of H_1 receptors in the molecular layer of the cerebellum which was strongly reduced after destruction of neuronal cell-bodies by the neurotoxin, kainate. These data are consistent with the presence of H_1 receptors on dendrites of Purkinje cells. The association of H_1 receptors with neurons is also suggested by their presence mainly restricted to brain areas receiving histaminergic afferents.

Efforts to purify H_1 receptors are as yet in infancy. Only the first step, the solubilization, has been achieved by digitonin and it shows that the solubilized receptors are virtually identical with those obtained in the intact membranes.[11] This approach will offer new insights in the structure and function of the receptor molecules.

^{3}H-mepyramine can also be used to label cerebral H_1 receptors in the living mouse.[12] Thus, a few minutes following I.V. administration of ^{3}H-mepyramine in low doses, a saturable binding occurs *in vivo* which presents characteristics of regional heterogeneity and pharmacological specificity paralleling those observed in binding studies *in vitro*. A major interest of the *in vivo* test is that it shows that systemic administration of most H_1 receptor antihistamines in doses currently used in therapeutics to alleviate allergic symptoms results in the occupation of a major fraction of H_1 receptor in brain. This observation strongly suggests that the well-known central effects of H_1 antihistamines (like sedation, "mental clouding", increase in sleep duration) are indeed mediated by blockade of the actions of the endogenous histamine at H_1 receptors. This agrees well with the disposition of histaminergic neurons, similar to that of monoaminergic systems emanating from the brainstem, projecting diffusely to the entire telencephalon and also believed to control states of wakefulness. Interestingly, mequitazine and terfenadine, two H_1 antihistamines devoid of sedative properties do not occupy H_1 receptors in brain, probably because they do not easily cross the blood-brain barrier.[9]

Several antidepressants display significant H_1 antihistaminic potency but there is no correlation between their clinical efficacy and blockade of H_1 receptor. It is worthwhile to notice that H_1 receptor occupation at clinical dosage by these drugs seems well correlated with their sedative properties.[13]

2 — BIOCHEMICAL RESPONSES

Stimulation of cyclic nucleotide formation.
Kakiuchi and Rall[14] first demonstrated that histamine elevates the intracellular levels of cyclic AMP in slices of rabbit cerebellum. This *in vitro* model allowed the first characterization of histamine H_1 and H_2 receptors in the CNS. After a certain confusion due to a large extent to the use of histaminergic agents of limited specificity, it is now clear that brain tissues contain a histamine sensitive adenylate cyclase coupled to H_2 receptors, whereas, in slices, the histamine-induced accumulation of cyclic AMP involves not only this enzyme but also H_1 receptors possibly linked with a calcium translocation system.[6] Such an effect occurs to a various extent in different species and different brain regions. The guinea pig is the most sensitive species and has been studied extensively. Evidence was presented in the hippocampal slices that the response to histamine in concentrations above 10 μM is competitively antagonized by mepyramine with an affinity close to that expected for typical H_1 receptors and the apparent dissociation constants of a series of H_1 antihistamines are also close to their value on guinea pig ileum.[15] However, the presence of H_2 receptors is needed for H_1 stimulated cyclic AMP formation, suggesting an indirect effect. In cerebral cortex, the H_1 receptors also facilitate the cyclic AMP response induced by activation of adeno-

sine receptors.[16] The mechanism underlying this indirect effect is not yet clear but it appears that calcium ions play a role, since the effect mediated by H_1 receptors is strongly reduced in the absence of calcium and can be fully restored by addition of calcium ions.[9] The possible role of cyclic AMP as a second messenger of histaminergic neurotransmission is discussed below with H_2 receptor-mediated effects. In any case, the participation of H_1 receptors results in an enlargement of the response mediated by H_2 receptors.

The histamine H_1 receptors in brain are also likely to mediate the stimulation of cyclic GMP synthesis elicited by histamine but the evidence for such a role has been only provided until now with the bovine superior cervical ganglion and with murine neuroblastoma cells.[17,18] Although receptor-mediated stimulation of cyclic GMP synthesis has an absolute dependence on extracellular calcium ions, Snider et al.[19] failed to correlate activation of H_1 receptors with an increase of intracellular calcium ions measured by the bioluminescent protein aequorin in mouse neuroblastoma cells. The functional significance of the increase of cyclic GMP in association with the physiological response to the neurotransmitter is not yet clear.

Stimulation of glycogen breakdown. Glycogen constitutes a large energy reserve in various tissues and might be essential for sustaining glycolysis and meeting the high energy expenditure in the CNS.[20] Glycogen has been identified in both glial and neuronal elements in the brain and is likely to be under neuronal control. When brain slices are incubated in the presence of ^{3}H-glucose, they synthesize ^{3}H-glycogen which can be conveniently isolated and measured. Histamine exerts a powerful glycogenolytic effect on slices from mouse cerebral cortex.[21] From the relative potency of agonists and from the competitive antagonism by H_1 receptor antagonists and not by H_2 receptor antagonists, it can be safely concluded that only H_1 receptors mediate this response. Neither the cellular localization nor the functional role of this glycogenolytic response are yet established. It might, however, be hypothesized that histaminergic neurons control the energy supply of cerebral cells, a function shared with other monoaminergic neurons also projecting in a diffuse manner to telencephalic areas.

Prolonged exposure of the H_1 receptors linked to glycogenolysis and to cyclic GMP synthesis reduces their responsiveness to the stimulatory agents. This desensitization process might involve changes not only at the level of the H_1 receptors themselves but also at the level of events triggered by their activation by the amine. It has been recently shown that desensitization of muscarinic receptors in cultured neuroblastoma cells is accompanied by an inactivation of calcium channels to which they are coupled. It is tempting to speculate that a similar change might occur in the desensitization to the H_1 receptor-mediated responses to histamine which also seem to involve translocation of calcium ions.

Stimulation of inositol phospholipids breakdown. All the studies on H_1 receptors (like those on α-noradrenergic and cholinergic muscarinic receptors) suggest that they may use calcium as a second messenger. An early event associated with the activation of these receptors coupled to calcium mobilization might be changes in inositol phospholipid metabolism.[22] It has recently been shown that the products of cleavage might have a role as second messengers. *In vivo* studies first indicated that histamine injected intracerebrally (the amine does not penetrate the blood-brain barrier) stimulates the incorporation of ^{32}P into brain phospholipids and that the enhanced phospholipid labelling is selectively mediated by H_1 receptors. Characterization of the receptor-mediated breakdown of inositol phospholipids has recently been achieved by *in vitro* measurement of accumulation of ^{3}H-inositol-1-phosphate in the presence of lithium ions in slices from guinea pig and rat brain.[23] Although this response may be very complex, the good correlation between the magnitude of the response and the density of H_1 receptors labelled with ^{3}H-mepyramine in various regions of the guinea pig, together with the effect of agonists and the apparent dissociation constant of mepyramine strongly support that it is an H_1 receptor-mediated process. It is interesting to notice the requirement of calcium for this response as well as other H_1 receptor-mediated effects.

II. THE HISTAMINE H_2 RECEPTORS

1 — BINDING STUDIES

In spite of many attempts with the various available ligands, labelling of H_2 receptors remains a difficult problem.

^{3}H-cimetidine has first been tried as a ligand for H_2 receptors but it is clear that the observed binding of ^{3}H-cimetidine is not to the recognition site of H_2 receptors.[24] ^{3}H-ranitidine and ^{3}H-impromidine have also been tried unsuccessfully. ^{3}H-histamine has been tentatively used.[9] The tritiated amine labels sites with nanomolar affinity which cannot be simply ascribed to association with H_2 receptors, although the pharmacological specificity of these sites resembles that of H_2 receptors. They might correspond to a desensitized state of histamine receptors.

The early attempts with the potent H_2 receptor antagonist tiotidine ($Ki = 20$ nM) failed, probably due to impurities of the labelled tiotidine available at the time. Recently, specific binding of ^{3}H-tiotidine to histamine H_2 receptors in guinea pig cortex was reported.[25] The good correlation between the affinities of a series of H_2 receptor antagonists on the ^{3}H-tiotidine binding sites and on the histamine-sensitive adenylate cyclase is encouraging. Although some technical problems still remain with this ligand, the possibility of labelling the recognition moiety of H_2 receptors with ^{3}H-tiotidine certainly deserves attention until a better ligand with a higher affinity for H_2 receptors is available.

2 — BIOCHEMICAL RESPONSE

Stimulation of adenylate cyclase.

In cell-free preparations from guinea pig brain, a histamine-sensitive adenylate cyclase has been characterized, the enzyme being coupled to typical H_2 receptors strictly identified by the inhibition constant of antagonists and relative potencies of agonists.[26] In the brain-slice model, the participation of both H_1 and H_2 receptors in the overall response to histamine results in an enlargement of the limits of this response.

The presence of the H_2 receptors linked to an adenylate cyclase in the subcellular fractions containing synaptic membranes and their disappearance after destruction of neuronal cell-bodies by the neurotoxin kainate, render likely their association with neurons and, therefore, their possible involvement in histaminergic neurotransmission. Indeed, electrophysiological studies show that the iontophoretic application of cyclic AMP mimics that of histamine on brainstem neurons and that the histamine-induced depressions in hypothalamic neurons in culture is increased by inhibitors of cyclic nucleotide phosphodiesterase, the enzyme responsible for cyclic AMP breakdown. However, chronic interruption of histaminergic inputs increased the responsiveness of target-cells to iontophoretically-applied histamine without altering the cyclic AMP response to the amine. This absence of correlation raises the possibility that electrophysiological and biochemical responses are mediated by different receptors or elicited in different cells. In this respect, the participation of non-neuronal cells in the cyclic AMP response to histamine cannot be excluded since a histamine-induced accumulation of cyclic AMP has been evidenced in human astrocytoma cells and in a capillary-enriched fraction. Very recently, Haas[27] also suggested the involvement of cyclic AMP in a modulatory action of histamine observed in hippocampal slices, the potentiation of various excitatory signals elicited through activation of H_2 receptors.

Since they are present in the brain, histamine H_2 receptors might represent targets for psychotropic agents. The tricyclic and tetracyclic antidepressant drugs competitively antagonize histamine at the H_2 receptors as measured on the histamine-sensitive adenylate cyclase.[28] It has been proposed that this action might represent the molecular basis for their antidepressant activity. However, it became apparent that the potent antagonism of antidepressants at H_2 receptors occurs only when they are assayed on cell-free systems and does not occur when they are assayed on intact cell preparations, either slices or cultured cells.[13] This discrepancy is not yet understood but the latter preparations are more likely to represent what occurs *in vivo* and, therefore, do not support the idea that the clinical activity of antidepressants is related to interruption of histaminergic neurotransmission.

III. THE HISTAMINE AUTORECEPTORS (H_3)

It is well established that several neurotransmitters affect neuronal activity in the CNS through stimulation not only of post-synaptic receptors, but also of receptors located presynaptically which often display distinct pharmacological specificity and by which they may control their own release.[29]

The presence of receptors modulating neuronal histamine-release through a negative feed-back mechanism has been shown by studies using rat brain slices prelabeled with ^{3}H-histamine locally synthesized from ^{3}H-L-histidine and depolarized in a calcium-dependent process by K^+ ions or veratridine. On this model extracellularly-applied histamine inhibits both K^+– and veratridine-evoked release of ^{3}H-histamine in a concentration-dependent manner.[30] It is likely that this effect is a receptor-mediated process, since the inhibitory action of exogenous histamine is saturable and reversible. Moreover, it is antagonizable in an apparently competitive manner. A systematic study of a range of histamine-agonists and antagonists on the K^+-evoked release of ^{3}H-histamine allowed the pharmacological characterization of a new class of histamine receptors clearly distinct from H_1 and H_2 receptors. Exogenous histamine inhibits ^{3}H-histamine release evoked by K^+ with an EC_{50} value of 40nM, much lower than that observed for the stimulation of H_1 and H_2 receptors in various brain-slice preparations. Specific H_1 and H_2 receptor-agonists failed to mimic the inhibitory actions of histamine. Only the two $N\alpha$ and $N\alpha$, $N\alpha$-methyl derivatives, which display agonist properties at both H_1 and H_2 receptors, were effective, their relative potency to histamine being slightly higher than that on the two well-known classes of histamine receptors. While H_1 antihistamines are ineffective at concentrations at which they block H_1 receptors, several H_2 antihistamines antagonize in a concentration-dependent and surmountable manner the histamine-induced inhibition of release. However, it is clear that these latter effects cannot be attributed to blockade of H_2 receptors since the potency of the various compounds markedly differs from what they display at either peripheral or cerebral H_2 receptors. For instance, tiotidine is a very weak antagonist, whereas, burimamide is quite potent. The pA_2 value of 7.5 determined by Schild-plot analysis of the antagonist effect of burimamide is higher by two orders of magnitude than its value at H_2 receptors ($pA_2 = 5.1$). In addition, impromidine, a highly potent H_2 receptor-agonist, inhibits competitively the histamine effect with a pA_2 value of 7.5. Thus, from the relative potencies of histamine agonists, from the apparent dissociation constant of histamine antagonists as well as from the lack of effect of antagonists of other neurotransmitters, it can be concluded that the autoinhibition of histamine-release in brain is mediated by a novel class of histamine receptors which are proposed to be called H_3. The persistence of the H_3 receptor-mediated effect in slices from striatum after destruction of neuronal cell-bodies by kainate and in slices from cerebral cortex depolarized in the presence of tetrodotoxin (a drug which blocks the traffic of action potentials), suggests that interneurons are not mediating the inhibitory effect of histamine. The presence of these autoinhibitory receptors in all brain regions containing histamine-nerve terminals as well as in synaptosomes from cerebral cortex further supports the idea that they are localized presynaptically on histamine-synthesizing nerve terminals.[31] Although the *in vivo* situation clearly differs from the *in vitro* model, the various data are compatible with the view that these H_3 receptors are involved in the physiological control of histaminergic neurotransmission. For instance, antagonists like impromidine or burimamide not only reverse the inhibitory effect of exogenous histamine, but also exhibit a facilitatory action of ^3H histamine-release which can be interpreted as resulting from blockade of a feedback inhibition elicited by the endogenous amine. Thus, the released endogenous amine may trigger the brake by interacting with the presynaptic autoreceptors and modulating its own release.

The development of specific compounds able to stimulate or to block this new class of histamine receptors and possibly to be used as ligands for binding studies will be most useful for a better understanding of the functional role of these presynaptic autoreceptors at the histaminergic synapses.[32]

IN CONCLUSION, the biochemical studies of histamine receptors in the brain have allowed evidence of the presence of H_1 and H_2 histamine receptors as well as the presence of a new class of histamine receptors proposed to be called H_3 receptors. The biochemical events mediated by these receptors, in agreement with anatomical and electrophysiological knowledge, suggest for histaminergic neurons a role in the regulation of general levels of activity, of energy reserves, and of vascular controls in large areas of the brain.

REFERENCES

1. Schwartz JC, Pollard H, Quach TT. Histamine as a neurotransmitter in mammalian brain: neurochemical evidence. J Neurochem 35 (1): 26-33, Jul 1980.
2. Steinbusch HWM, Mulder AH. Localization of histaminergic neurons in the rat brain: an immunohistochemical study. Neurosci Letters Suppl 14: 356, 1983.
3. Pollard H, Pachot I, Legrain P, Buttin G, Schwartz JC. Development of a monoclonal antibody against L-histidine decarboxylase as a selective tool for the localization of histamine synthesizing cells. In: Frontiers in Histamine Research. Ganellin CR, Schwartz JC (Eds.). Pergamon Press 1985 pp. 103–118.
4. Watanabe T, Taguchi Y, Shiosaka S, Tanaka J, Kubota H, Terano Y, Tohyama M, Wada H. Distribution of the histaminergic neuron system in the central nervous system of rats: a fluorescent immunohistochemical analysis with histidine decarboxylase as a marker. Brain Res 295: 13-25, Mar 1984.
5. Ganellin CR. Chemistry and structure-activity relationship of drugs acting at histamine receptors. In: Pharmacology of histamine receptors. Ganellin CR, Parsons ME (Eds.). Wright PSG, 1982, pp. 10-102.
6. Schwartz JC. Minireview: histamine receptors in brain. Life Sci 25: 895-912, Sept 11, 1979.
7. Hough LB, Green JP. Histamine and its receptors in the nervous system. In: Handbook of Neurochemistry. Lajtha A (Ed.). Plenum Press, New York, 1984, vol. 6, pp. 145-211.
8. Hill SJ, Young JM, Marrian DH. Specific binding of ^3H-mepyramine to histamine H_1 receptors in intestinal smooth muscle. Nature 270: 361-361, Nov 24, 1977.
9. Schwartz JC, Barbin G, Duchemin AM, Garbarg M, Llorens C, Pollard H, Quach TT, Rose C. Histamine receptors in the brain and their possible functions. In: Pharmacology of Histamine Receptors. Ganellin CR, Parsons ME (Eds.). Wright PSG, pp. 351-391, 1982.
10. Palacios JM, Wamsley JK, Kuhar MJ. The distribution of histamine H_1-receptors in the rat brain: an autoradiographic study. Neurosciences 6 (1): 15-38, 1981.
11. Gavish M, Chang RSL, Snyder SH. Solubilization of histamine H_1, GABA and benzodiazepine receptors. Life Sci 25: 783-790, Aug 27, 1979.
12. Quach TT, Duchemin AM, Rose C, Schwartz JC. Labeling of histamine H_1 receptors in the brain of the living mouse. Neurosci Lett 17 (1-2): 49-54, 1980.
13. Schwartz JC, Garbarg M, Quach TT. Histamine receptors in brain as targets for tricyclic antidepressants. Trends Pharmacol Sci 2 (5): 122-125, 1981.
14. Kakiuchi S, Rall TW. The influence of chemical agents on the accumulation of adenosine 3'-5' phosphate in slices of rabbit cerebellum. Molec Pharmacol 4: 367-378, Jul 1968.
15. Palacios JM, Garbarg M, Barbin G, Schwartz JC. Pharmacological characterization of histamine receptors mediating the stimulation of cyclic AMP accumulation in slices from guinea pig hippocampus. Molec Pharmacol 14: 971-982, Nov 1978.
16. Daum PR, Hill SJ, Young JM. Histamine H_1-agonist potentiation of adenosine-stimulated cyclic AMP accumulation in slices of guinea pig cerebral cortex: comparison of response and binding parameters. Br J Pharmacol 77: 347-357, Oct 1982.
17. Richelson E. Histamine H_1 receptor-mediated guanosine 3',5'-monophosphate formation by cultured mouse neuroblastoma cells. Science 201: 69-71, Jul 7, 1978.
18. Study RE, Greengard P. Regulation by histamine of cyclic nucleotide levels in sympathetic ganglia. J Pharmacol Exp Ther 207: 767-778, Dec 1978.
19. Snider RM, McKinney M, Forray C, Richelson E. Neurotransmitter receptors mediate cyclic GMP formation by involvement of arachidonic acid and lipoxygenase. Proc Nat Acad Sci (USA) 81: 3905-3909, Jun 1984.
20. Yarowsky PJ, Ingvar DH. Symposium summary. Neuronal activity and energy metabolism. Fed Proc 40 (9): 2353-2362, Jul 1981.
21. Quach TT, Duchemin AM, Rose C, Schwartz JC. ^3H-glycogen hydrolysis elicited by histamine in mouse brain slices: selective involvement of H_1-receptors. Molec Pharmacol 17: 301-308, May 1980.
22. Michell RH. Inositol phospholipids and cell surface receptor function. Biochem Biophys Acta 415: 81-147, 1975.

23. Daum PR, Downes CP, Young JM. Histamine stimulation of inositol-1-phosphate accumulation in lithium-treated slices from regions of guinea pig brain. J Neurochem 43 (1): 25-32, 1984.
24. Warrander SE, Norris DB, Rising RJ, Wood TP. ^{3}H-cimetidine and the H_2-receptor. Life Sci 33 (12): 1119-1126, 1983.
25. Gajtkowski GA, Norris DB, Rising TJ, Wood TP. Specific binding of ^{3}H-tiotidine to histamine H_2-receptors in guinea pig cerebral cortex. Nature 304: 65-67, Jul 7-13, 1983.
26. Hegstrand LR, Kanof PD, Greengard P. Histamine-sensitive adenylate cyclase in mammalian brain. Nature 260: 163-165, Mar 11, 1976.
27. Haas HL. Histamine actions in the mammalian central nervous system. In: Frontiers in Histamine Research. Ganellin CR, Schwartz JC (Eds.). Pergamon Press, 1985 pp. 215–224.
28. Green JP. Histamine receptors in brain. In: Biochemical studies of CNS receptors. Handbook of psychopharmacology. Iversen LL, Iversen SD, Snyder SH. (Eds.). Plenum Publish Corp (New York) vol. 17, pp. 385-420, 1983.
29. Starke K. Presynaptic receptors. Annu Rev Pharmacol Toxicol 21: 7-30, 1981.
30. Arrang JM, Garbarg M, Schwartz JC. Auto-inhibition of brain histamine release mediated by a novel class (H_3) of histamine receptor. Nature 302: 832-837, Apr 28, 1983.
31. Arrang JM, Garbarg M, Schwartz JC. Autoregulation of histamine release in brain by presynaptic receptors. Neurosci 1985 15:553–562.
32. Schwartz JC, Garbarg M, Pollard H. Histaminergic transmission in the brain. Handbook of Physiology, Section 1, Vol IV. Mountcastle VB, Bloom FE, Geiger SR (Eds.). American Physiological Society (U.S.A.) pp 257–316, 1986. □

Chapter XI

H_1 and H_2 Receptors in the Skin: Role in Chronic Urticaria

Joel L. Cristol, M.D.

ABSTRACT

A general review of urticaria is given with emphasis upon the classification, etiology and causative mechanisms of urticaria. Treatment modalities are then introduced for the various types of urticaria. Finally, a comprehensive discussion is presented concerning the role of H_1 and H_2 antagonists in the treatment of urticaria and a comparison is made between the various H_1 and H_2 antagonists currently available for therapy.

In 1842, T.H. Burgess wrote in *The Management of Diseases of the Skin* "Urticaria is one of the few cutaneous eruptions which can be traced directly to its source." If this was true in 1842, unfortunately the secret has been lost. Today, urticaria remains one of the most puzzling mysteries of relationships between the immune system and the skin.[1]

Physicians must be aware of two classifications of urticaria, namely; ACUTE, consisting of a cutaneous eruption of transient, erythematous, papules or wheals, usually pruritic; and CHRONIC, consisting of episodes lasting longer than six weeks which may unfortunately persist for years. In approximately 80% of chronic urticaria patients, a specific cause is never identified.

The etiological factors in urticaria are many and varied, including: immunologic, anaphylactoid, miscellaneous (such as those associated with specific disease), idiopathic, physical, cholinergic, emotional, exercise, solar, mechanical pressure, vibration, trauma, cold, etc. Since urticaria usually cannot be considered as caused by a single entity in most cases, it is, therefore, most difficult to diagnose and treat. The cause is usually undetermined and the subsequent therapy must, especially, be directed toward controlling symptoms.

Acute urticaria is usually a manifestation of a Type I (IgE Mediated) Allergic reaction in which an interaction between an allergen and its specific IgE Antibody attached to the surface of mast cells cause a transmethyllation of membrane phospholipids followed by a movement of calcium ions into the mast cells, causing an eventual cascade of intracellular events, resulting in a release of chemical mediators including: histamine, ECF (Eosinophilic Chemotactic Factor of Anaphylaxis), NCF (Neutrophilic Chemotactic Factor of Anaphylaxis), SRS-A (Slow Reacting Substance of Anaphylaxsis) and leukotrienes C, D and E.

Other forms of urticaria are not mediated by immunologic pathways. A number of agents can act DIRECTLY upon the mast cells to release histamine. Such drugs as amphetamines, atropine, codeine and thiamine are examples. In addition, bacterial toxins, insect venoms, aspirin and indomethacin cause urticaria by blocking cyclooxygenase pathways in the metabolism of arachidonic acid.[1]

Typical causes of acute urticaria include foods, drugs, bites, stings, inhalants, contactants, and psychic or physical factors. Urticaria is often transient, of minor significance, and is usually a self-limiting disorder that

Associate Professor of Medicine, Chief Allergy Teaching Program, Chicago Medical School, North Chicago, Illinois

disappears in four to six weeks. The best advice for a doctor trying to find the cause of urticaria says Dr. L. Juhlin, is "to be curious and to continue to search for the cause."[2] In addition, since there are so many possible inciting agents or events, Dr. Kenneth Mathews states that "Taking a careful disease history, a general medical history, and performing a thorough medical examination are the key steps to finding the cause of urticaria."[3]

Since the episodes may recur, ideal treatment requires identification and removal of the offending agent if possible. Consequently, the preferred treatment then becomes AVOIDANCE of the causative agent and when avoidance is relatively easy to do as in the case of suspected foods, drugs, inhalants or contactants, then treatment is relatively simple. An explanation of the disease process and its triggering mechanism should be helpful for patients with cholinergic urticaria, dermatographism, and presssure or vibratory (trauma) urticaria. Environmental controls should be helpful in cold, solar, or heat urticaria.

Desensitization or immunotherapy has little role in the management of patients with urticaria with the only exceptions being patients with Hymenoptera sensitivity and the occasional case of prophylactic desensitization to penicillin, insulin or equine antisera.

Corticosteroids are often required for relief of hives and may be most useful for their anti-inflammatory effects.[4] Patients with chronic urticaria are usually treated with conventional antihistamines (H_1) but the response is good in no more than about 33% of patients.[5] The inability of conventional H_1 antihistamines to produce consistent suppression of urticarial wheals can be ascribed to several causes. Histmine released from skin mast cells in close proximity to skin blood vessels may achieve very high local concentration. Systemically administered antihistamines, although possessing a greater affinity for vascular histamine receptors than histamine itself may not achieve high enough local concentrations to compete successfully with histamine for blood vessel receptors.[6]

Since the primary mediator in the development of urticaria is histamine and the vasodilator and vascular permeability actions of histamine involve both H_1 and H_2 receptors, it seems rational to treat urticaria unresponsive to classical antihistamines with a combination of H_1 and H_2 antagonists. We now know that there are two types of histamine receptors, the first type (designated H_1) controls the increased vasodilation and smooth-muscle contraction caused by histamine and is inhibited by standard antihistamines (ex. hydroxyzine, chlorpheniramine maleate, and diphenhydramine hydrochloride). The second type (designated H_2) mediates the response not blocked by standard antihistamines (ex. gastric acid secretion, atrial contraction, and uterine contraction). This type of receptor is classically inhibited by the drug, cimetidine.[7,8]

The first evidence that human skin blood vessels might possess both classes of histamine receptors came from an observation that vascular flushing in the skin of human volunteers, who had received histamine intravenously could be suppressed by the administration of H_2 receptor antagonists.[9,10] Further evidence for the existence of H_2 receptors in skin blood vessels is that a synthetic histamine analogue with predominantly H_2 agonist activity injection into the skin will produce whealing, erythema, and pruritus.[11,12] A recent study showed that cimetidine caused a highly significant suppression of both the wheal and erythema response to histamine; the combination of cimetidine and chlorpheniramine caused a significantly greater suppression of histamine induced erythema than either drug alone;[13] another study showed that the combination of cimetidine and hydroxyzine caused a significantly greater reduction of histamine induced whealing than hydroxyzine alone.[14] The distribution of H_1 and H_2 receptors in human skin is now very well established, as is the fact that human skin blood vessels possess both H_1 and H_2 receptors which mediate vasodilation and increased vascular permeability.[15] Consequently, a combination of H_1 andH_2 therapy has been found to be more effective than H_1 alone in studies by Kaur, Greaves, and Eftekhari, 1981.,[16] Breathnach et al, 1973.[17]

The diverse roles of histamine in human physiology have been recognized since early in this century.[18] Yet the existence of the two histamine receptors and their important cellular regulatory functions were proven only recently.[19] The development by Black et al,[11] of the H_2 receptor antagonists has allowed them to be used along with H_1 in previously refractory cases of urticaria. This report was supported by human experimental data[20] and animal studies which suggested augmented suppression of histamine when used in combination.[21]

Hydroxyzine is currently the most potent available H_1 antipruritic and antihistaminic agent used in the treatment of urticaria.[22,23] When combined with cimetidine, the combination of H_1 and H_2 antihistmines produce a significant reduction in histamine-induced wheal size and a reduction in erythema. The results of this study were similar to the results obtained by Marks and Greaves.[20]

There are other reports documenting the use of cimetidine as an H_2 antagonist in conjunction with traditional H_1 antihistmines in the control of pruritus.[7,24-26]

When an H_2 blocker is added, the effect is approximately 10% greater; whereas doubling the H_1 dosage does not produce any reduction in the size of the wheals although increased soporific effects were apparent.[14] However, there still exists a controversy over combination therapy. Although the classical "Histamine-induced Itch" is mediated only through H_1 receptors,[27] in some studies, even if a combination of H_1 and H_2 receptor blockers are used, the therapy has not consistently proved more effective in relieving pruritus in patients refractory to conventional H_1 antihistamine alone.[7,28] Since it would appear that plasma histamine levels are only elevated in certain types of pruritus and urticaria, other vasoactive substances may be coincidentally operative in the urticarial reaction.

In a study by Monroe et al,[29] when individual patient responses were analyzed, 40 to 50% of the patients receiving a combination therapy showed a statistically significant improvement in itching and in the frequency, number, and size of their hives. The potential problem in the usage of an H_2 antagonist is the resulting inhibition of the negative feedback that histamine would exert on mediators released by the mast cells. Histamine itself, by interacting with an H_2 receptor on the mast cell, increases intracellular cyclic adenosine monophosphate levels and, thereby, inhibits the release of histamine.[8] Through interference with this mechanism, an H_2 antihistamine might potentially raise circulating histamine levels. *Consequently, an H_2 antihistamine should not be used by itself in treating urticaria.* The addition of an H_1 antihistamine to the H_2 antihistamine is intended to block all histamine receptors and, thus, counteract the effect of any extra circulating histamine.

Another theory on how an H_2 blocker works is that it may regulate gastric juice secretion, thus, suppressing urticariogenic chemical mediators and not by acting on the skin receptors directly. It is possible that the vasoactive substances liberated during the erosive process in the digestive tract are being transported by blood to the skin where they exert the inflammatory reaction.[30] If histamine played an exclusive role in urticaria, blocking H_1 and H_2 receptors would be expected to be uniformly effective, which is definitely not the case. Antihistamines blocking H_1 receptors fail frequently to control the rash and itching accompanying the urticarial wheals. Therefore, although a regimen of both H_1 and H_2 may be effective in many urticaria cases, there is evidence also that cimetidine (an H_2 blocker) is significant in affecting the "triple response."[31] However, the salutary effectiveness of blocking histamine receptors far outweighs possible deleterious results lowering the cellular level of cAMP and, thereby, promoting the liberation of histamine.[8] Finally, Rebhun[30] has postulated that cimetidine by blocking histamine which inhibits MIF (Macrophage Inhibitory Factor) production, may modulate the production of antibodies and antigen-induced cell proliferation affecting the chronic inflammatory cells seen in chronic urticaria. Since histamine exerts its effect on the skin by producing dilation of the blood vessels and increasing the vascular permeability, an H_2 blocker by regulating gastric juice secretion may decrease by some still unknown mechanism, the release of vasoactive mediators and ultimately the release of urticariogenic chemical mediators.

Finally, a new H_2 mediator antagonist has recently been introduced in this country. "Ranitidine" appears to be a more potent, more effective, and a safer H_2 receptor antagonist than cimetidine. Questions regarding side effects will be clarified by further long term clinical trials. If Ranitidine proves to be as effective as the initial studies suggest, it will be used for a number of clinical conditions that do not involve the gastrointestinal tract, as is the case with cimetidine. In dermatology, it may be used to treat chronic urticaria."[32]

REFERENCES

1. Berman BA, Ross RN, et al. Urticaria. Cutis 30:696,700-1,704, 1982.
2. Juhlin L. "Skin and Allergy News." 19:8, August 1983.
3. Mathews K. "Skin and Allergy News." 19:8, August 1983.
4. Beall GN. Urticaria, a review of laboratory and clinical observations. Medicine 43:131-151, 1964.
5. Champion RH, Roberts SO, Carpenter RG. Urticaria and angio-edema. A review of 554 patients. Br J Derm 81:588-97, 1969.
6. Dale HH. The action and uses of the antihistamine drugs as applied to dermatology. Br J Dermat 62:151-158, 1950.
7. Commens CA, Greaves MW. Cimetidine in chronic idiopathic urticaria: A randomized double-blind study. Br J Dermatol 99:675-79, 1978.
8. Lichtenstein LM and Gillespie E. Inhibition of histamine release by histamine controlled H_2 receptor. Nature 244:287-88, 1973.
9. Greaves MW, Marks R. Receptors for histamine in human skin blood vessels; A review. Br J Derm 97:225-228, 1977.
10. Burland WL, Duncan WA, Hesselbo T, et al. Pharmacological evaluation of cimetidine, a new H_2-receptor antagonist in healthy man. Br J Clin Pharmacol 2:481-86, 1975.
11. Black JW, Duncan WA, Durant CJ, et al. Identification and antagonism of histamine H_2-receptors. Nature 236:385-390, 1972.
12. Robertson J, Greaves MW. Responses of human skin blood vessels to synthetic histamine analogues. Br J Clin Pharmacol 5:319, 1978.
13. Moore-Robinson M, Warin RP. Some clinical aspects of cholinergic urticaria. Brit J Derm 80:794-799, 1968.
14. Harvey RP, Schocket AL. The effects of H_1 and H_2 blockade on cutaneous histamine response in man. J Allergy Clin Immunol 65:136-139, 1980.
15. Robertson E. and Greaves MW. Responses of human skin blood vessels to synthetic histamine analogues. Br J Clin Pharmacol 5:319, 1977.
16. Kaur S. Greaves M, Eftekhari N: Factitious urticaria (dermographism); treatment by cimetidine and chlorpheniramine in a randomized double-blind study. Br J Derm 104:185-190, 1981.
17. Breathnack SM, Allen R, Milford-Ward A, et al. Symptomatic dermographism natural history, clinical features, laboratory investigations, and response to therapy. Clinical Expt Derm (In press, 1983).
18. Code CF. Reflections on histamine, gastric secretion and the H_2 Receptor. N Engl J Med 296:1459-62, 1977.
19. Ash AS, Schild HO. Receptors mediating some actions of histamine. Brit J Pharmacol Chemo 27:427-39, 1966.
20. Marks R, Greaves MW. Vascular reactions to histamine and compound 48/80 in human skin: suppression by a histamine H_2-receptor blocking agent. Br J Clin Pharmacol 4:367-69, 1977.
21. Hutchcroft BJ, Moore EG, Orange RP. H_1 and H_2 antihistamines in allergic reactions (abstract). J Allergy Clin Immunol 61:192, 1978.

22. Baraf CS. Treatment of pruritus in allergic dermatoses; An evaluation of the relative efficacy of cyproheptadine and hydroxyzine. Curr Ther Res 19:32-38, 1976.
23. Cook TJ, MacQueen DM, Wittig HJ, et al. Degree and duration of skin test suppression and side effects with antihistamines. A double blind controlled study with five antihistamines. J Allergy Clin Immunol 51:71-77, 1973.
24. Harrison AR, Littenberg G, Goldstein L, Kaplowitz N. Pruritis, cimetidine and polycythemia. N Engl J Med 300:433-434, 1979.
25. Cook J, Shuster S. Lack of effect of H_2 blockade in chronic urticaria. Br J Dermatol, 101(Suppl 17):21-22, 1979.
26. Marks R. Treatment of chronic urticaria. Br J Derm 102:240, 1980.
27. Greaves MW, Davies MG. Histamine receptors in human skin; Indirect evidence. Br J Derm 107(suppl 23):101-105, 1982.
28. Cook J, Shuster S. Lack of effect of H_2 blockade in chronic urticaria. Br J Derm 101(Suppl 12):21-22, 1979.
29. Monroe EW, Cohen SH, Kalbfleisch J, Schulz CI, Combined H_1 and H_2 antihistamine therapy in chronic urticaria. Arch Derm 117:404-7, 1981.
30. Rebhun J. Hypothetical role of H_2 blockers in chronic urticaria. Annals Allergy 47:440-42, 1981.
31. Summers R, Sigler R, Shelhamer JH, Kaliner M. Effects of infused histamine on asthmatic and normal subjects: comparison of skin test responses. J Allergy Clin Immunol 67:456-64, 1981.
32. Tan O. Derm Capsule and Comment. p. 10, August, 1983. □

A special acknowledgement to Mrs. Sharon Glinski, Medical Librarian, Mrs. Jill Trzeciak, Medical Staff Secretary, and Mrs. Kathleen Laban, Medical Education Director, for their efforts in the preparation and presentation of this manuscript.

HISTAMINE RELEASE IN SURGERY

Chapter XII
Histamine Release in Anesthesia and Surgery

Jonathan Moss, M.D., Ph.D.

ABSTRACT

Histamine release can occur in response to anaphylactic or chemically mediated anaphylactoid reactions during general anesthesia. Narcotics and muscle relaxants have been demonstrated both in vitro and in vivo to cause significant histamine release. This histamine release appears to be directly related to changes in the cardiovascular system that are often seen during anesthesia. The use of combined H_1 and H_2 antagonists to attenuate the effects of anaphylactoid reactions in humans has been shown in several controlled trials. In addition, recent experience with chymopapain administration suggests that the use of H_1 and H_2 antagonists may be useful in the prophylaxis of immunologically mediated reactions.

Anesthesiologists and critical care physicians are acutely aware of anaphylactic and anaphylactoid reactions in their clinical practice. This is true for several reasons:

1. commonly used narcotics and muscle relaxants can induce a chemically-mediated release of histamine.
2. anesthesiologists often administer these drugs intravenously in a bolus fashion.
3. many anesthetic agents can moderate homeostatic sympathoadrenal mechanisms.

More recently, anesthesiologists have become aware of the relationship between immunologically-mediated anaphylactic reactions to drugs commonly administered in anesthesia and surgery. It is the purpose of this manuscript to review the literature which demonstrates that commonly used narcotics and neuromuscular blocking agents can cause dose-dependent increases in plasma histamine in humans, to demonstrate further that these increases in plasma histamine are temporally and quantitatively related to observed cardiovascular changes, and to review clinical strategies that can attenuate these cardiovascular changes in humans. We will also try to identify epidemiologic patterns of true immunologically-mediated reactions to anesthetic agents and chymopapain.

Numerous studies utilizing mast cell, basophil, and animal preparations have demonstrated that commonly used anesthetic agents can cause significant release of histamine.[1-5] A number of studies of rat mast studies demonstrated release with infusion of very high (10^{-2} to 10^{-4} M) concentrations of morphine or d-tubocurarine.[1] Numerous investigators have utilized organ baths or animal preparations in order to demonstrate that histamine could be released following the administration of a variety of anesthetic agents.[5] While these studies were extremely suggestive, the well-documented differences between human mast cells and cells from other species, as well as the variability and distribution of different types of mast cells within a given species, make extrapolation to humans very difficult.[6,7] As Dr. Beaven has alluded to elsewhere in this Symposium, the measurement of histamine in plasma is not trivial and the lack of sensitive, reliable methods to assay plasma histamine has ham-

Assistant Anesthesiologist, Massachusetts Eye and Ear Infirmary, 243 Charles Street, Boston, Massachusetts 02114; Associate Professor of Anesthesiology, Harvard Medical School

pered many human investigations.

Until recently, the most accurate predictor for whether a drug would be a potential histamine-releaser in man was the all-or-none indicator of the delayed-depressor response in the cat. Savarese[4] has attempted to quantify histamine release indirectly by measuring the "autonomic margin of safety" for a number of neuromuscular blocking agents. While no measurements of plasma histamine were made, the cardiovascular data were utilized to construct quantal dose response curves for presumed histamine release in animals. Potency to effect delayed-depressor response in cats appeared to correlate with the ability to produce flushing and hypotension in surgical patients. Recent studies with novel neuromuscular blocking agents, including BW444, document that the cat model may be relatively insensitive to compounds that marginally release histamine.[8,9] Thus, while it is possible to rule out drugs which are potent histamine releasers in humans, it may be difficult to extrapolate in marginal cases.[10]

In addition to the numerous *in vitro* studies and animal experiments, there are a plethora of case reports and clinical studies demonstrating that the administration of narcotics and neuromuscular blocking agents in usual doses can cause tachycardia, hypotension, and peripheral vasodilitation, signs that may be mimicked by the infusion of histamine.[11] Interpretation of individual case reports often is complicated because of the concomitant use of other drugs and the difficulty in distinguishing between direct and immunologically-mediated histamine release. Although immunologically-mediated release does occur, particularly following release of muscle relaxants, it appears to be a far less common event than does chemically-mediated release.[12] Immunologically-induced release by narcotics has rarely been documented.[13]

Studies by Professor Lorenz and Dr. Kaliner have demonstrated that infusion of very substantive amounts of histamine into humans can cause the same types of changes that are seen during anaphylactic or anaphylactoid reactions in anesthetized patients.[14] It is important to note, however, that the doses of drugs utilized in order to effect these cardiovascular changes may be very substantative. Thus, in the study by Kaliner et al.,[14] 210,000 ngs. of histamine were infused into a 70 kg. man over 30 minutes to result in elevation of 1 ng/ml in plasma histamine levels. Similar elevations can be achieved with ease following administration of clinically used doses of morphine or curare.[15,16] Thus, the overwhelming amount of catabolic enzyme present within humans and the rather short half-life of histamine makes infusion studies somewhat difficult to interpret. Extrapolation of infusion studies to endogenous release may not be quantitatively valid.

Lorenz et al[17,18] had previously demonstrated that administration of induction agents could cause elevations in plasma histamine which were coincident with significant cardiovascular changes in humans. We utilized a radioenzymatic assay based on the procedure described by Beaven in order to determine whether histamine release was significant following usual and customary doses of a variety of narcotics and muscle relaxants.[19,5] In our initial study, we administered d-tubocurarine to a series of 21 patients undergoing elective orthopedic procedures.[15] Each patient received the synthetic narcotic, fentanyl, followed two minutes later by thiopental. These patients were ventilated with oxygen and nitrous oxide. Four minutes after the administration of thiopental, d-tubocurarine was given intravenously as a rapid bolus in doses ranging from 0.25 to 0.75 mg/kg. Plasma histamine was measured before, two, and five minutes after the administration of the neuromuscular blocking agent. Blood pressure and heart rate were measured for each event. Our results indicated that following the administration of d-tubocurarine, significant changes in heart rate, blood pressure, and plasma histamine were observed. Hemodynamic changes and the changes in plasma histamine followed a similar time course (Fig. 1,2,3). While there is considerable variability from individual to individual, it is clear that with increasing doses of d-tubocurarine there is a tendency for plasma histamine at event four (which represents two minutes after curare administration) to be increasingly elevated and to return to normal by event five (five minutes after administration of curare). It thus appears that there is a quantal dose-response relationship, i.e. as the dose of d-tubocurarine is increased, there is increased likelihood that the patient will release histamine. We have recently described similar dose-response relationships (with similar interpatient variability for histamine release) following the administration of experimental neuromuscular blocking agents BW785 and BW444 in humans.[8,9] It is significant that these compounds have no ganglionic blockade. In contrast to d-tubocurarine, the bolus administration of ED95 doses of metocurine, the neuromuscular blocking agents atracurium or vercuronium, appeared to cause no histamine release.[20,21] The ability to generate dose-response relationships and the absence of prior sensitization suggests that a direct histamine release is occurring in these patients rather than an immunologically-mediated phenomenon.

While the effects of neuromuscular blocking agents are commonly seen only in the operating room or intensive care unit, the effects of narcotic-induced histamine release may be seen in many clinical settings. The classic description of morphine-induced histamine release emphasizes cutaneous manifestations. Despite intensive investigation by many distinguished physiologists and

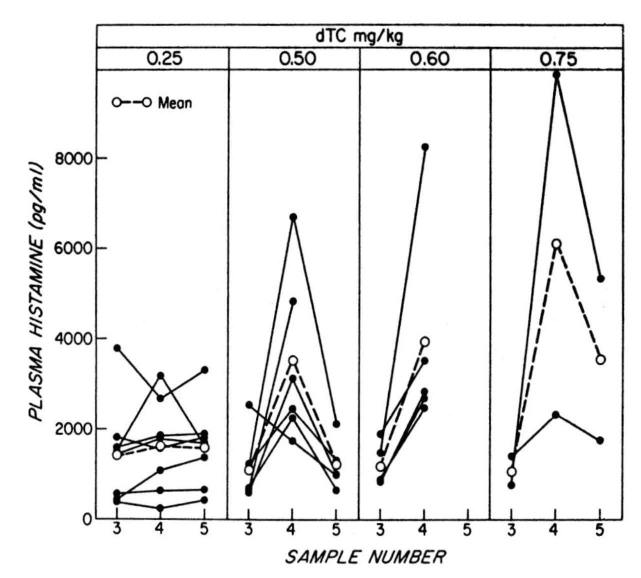

Figure 1. Plasma histamine following administration of indicated doses of d-tubocurarine to study patients. Dotted lines connect mean values. Plasma histamine was not measured in one patient in the 0.5 mg/kg group (event 5) and one patient in the 0.6 mg/kg group (events 3 and 4).

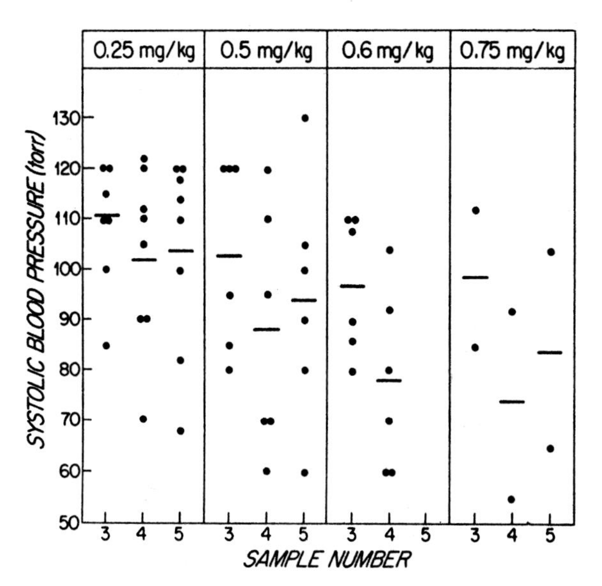

Figure 2. Systolic blood pressure following administration of doses of dTc to study patients. Horizontal bars indicate mean values.

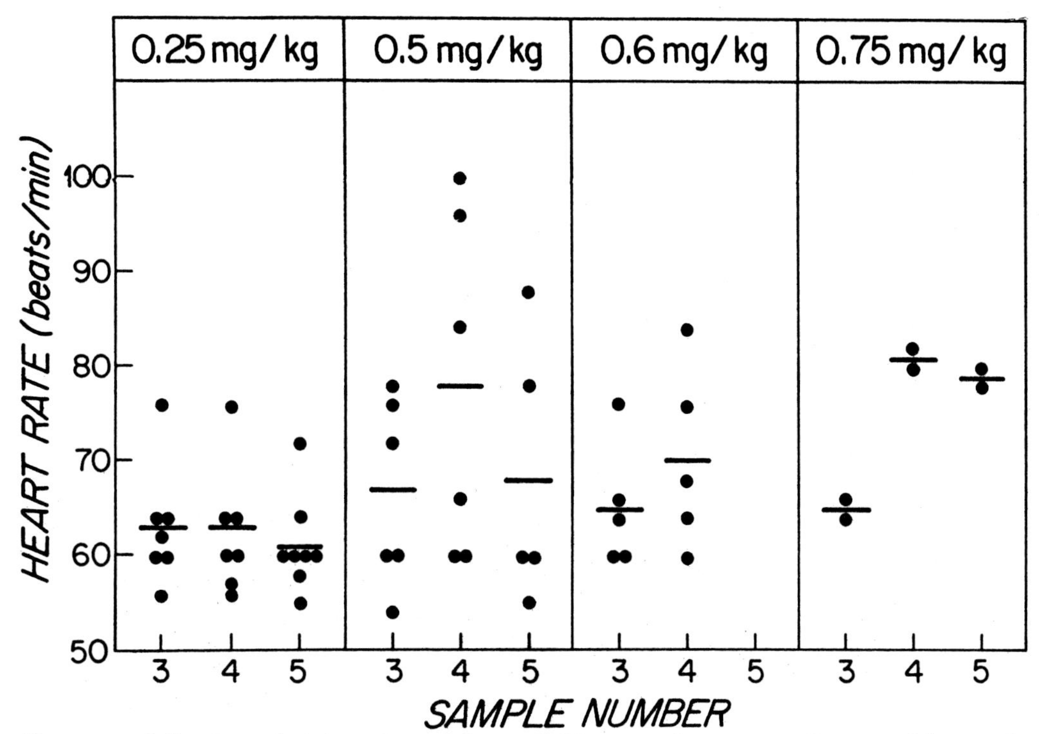

Figure 3. Heart rate following administration of doses of dTc to study patients. Horizontal bars indicate mean values. Heart rate was not recorded in one patient in the 0.5 mg/kg group (event 5) and one patient in the 0.6 mg/kg group (events 3 and 4).

(Figures 1, 2, and 3 reproduced by permission of authors and Anesthesiology. *Moss J, Rosow CE, Savarese JJ, et al: Role of histamine in the hypotensive action of d-tubocurarine in humans.* Anesthesiology *55:19-25, 1981).*

pharmacologists, it has only been recently demonstrated that the administration of intravenous morphine will cause an elevation in plasma histamine in humans.[16] In our laboratory, we demonstrated that the administration of intravenous morphine in doses of 1 mg/kg — which is the customary dose for cardiac surgical procedures — could elicit very significant histamine release. The variability from patient to patient was similar to that which was observed for neuromuscular blocking agents. Patients who received the synthetic narcotic, fentanyl, as their primary anesthetic agent in doses of 50 mcg/kg failed to show any elevation in plasma histamine. In addition to these studies, we have demonstrated that the narcotics, sufentanil, butorphanol, and methadone, release little or no histamine even in the substantive doses required for cardiac surgery.[22,23] A recent study by Flacke et al[24] demonstrated that meperidine may be a more significant histamine liberator than morphine. In their study, which was a double-blind study of patients receiving one of four different narcotics, they demonstrated that the proportion of patients who responded with histamine release varied with the potency of the narcotic. Thus, the very potent narcotics, sufentanil and fentanyl, demonstrated no histamine release, while meperidine appeared to demonstrate more release than did morphine. This suggests that there is a molar relationship for narcotics involving potency which may be important as a determinant of histamine release.

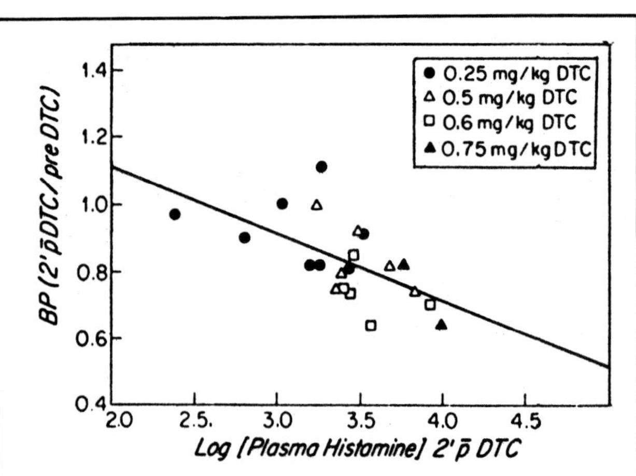

Figure 4. *Relationship between the decrease in blood pressure and plasma histamine concentration 2 min after the administration of indicated doses of d-tubocurarine (dTc) in 21 patients. The regression line for these data points is $y=0.2X-1.5$, with correlation coefficient of $r=-0.61 (P<0.005)$. The equation relating the three variables was:*

Systolic blood pressure 2 min after dTc / Systolic blood pressure before dTc = 1.37–0.27(dose dTc) –0.12 Log histamine.

(Reproduced by permission of the authors and Anesthesiology. *Moss J, Rosow CE, Savarese JJ, et al: Role of histamine in the hypotensive action of d-tubocurarine in man.* Anesthesiology 55:19-25, 1981.)

CARDIOVASCULAR SEQUELLAE OF HISTAMINE RELEASE

In other sections of this Symposium, there has been extensive discussion of the effects that histamine can exert on the human cardiovascular system. While the most sensitive effects appear to be the change in fibrillation threshold described by Levi and colleagues,[25,26] this has been difficult to measure in the clinical setting. Our experience, and that of other investigators, has been to attempt to correlate the amount of histamine released by various narcotics and muscle relaxants with the commonly observed and measured changes in blood pressure, cardiac index, heart rate, and systemic vascular resistance.[5] In the studies we performed with curare, while there was considerable variability between the amount of histamine released at any given drug dose in any given patient, it was possible to construct a significant regression line relating the change in blood pressure to the log of the plasma histamine concentration elicited by the administration of curare.[15] It thus appears that while individuals may have different threshold sensitivities, once the histamine is released there will be signicicant changes in blood pressure. (Fig. 4) In another series of elegant experiments, Dr. Philbin at our institution utilized a double-blind study of 40 patients undergoing elective coronary artery bypass surgery who were intensively monitored. In this study, it was shown that histamine release correlated with increased cardiac index and decreased blood pressure and systemic vascular resistance. In a similar study, we have demonstrated that the change in systemic vascular resistance correlates well with the log of plasma histamine concentration. (Fig. 5) The recent studies by Flacke et al[24] demonstrated similar changes. In addition, they and others have shown that the amount of epinephrine released in response to the histamine is quantifiable and represents linear relationship[24,27] (Fig. 6).

We have attempted to identify three strategies for attenuating the histamine-mediated hemodynamic effects of narcotics and muscle relaxants in man. These include alteration of the rate of administration, the use of antihistamines, and drug design.

Alteration of the rate of administration can be a very effective means of attenuating effects. Comparison of the alteration in hemodynamics and histamine release for the investigation of hemodynamics and histamine release for the investigational neuromuscular blocking drug, BW785, is demonstrated in the accompanying figure.[9] (Fig. 7) The dose-response relationship was determined when this drug was administered as a bolus or as a

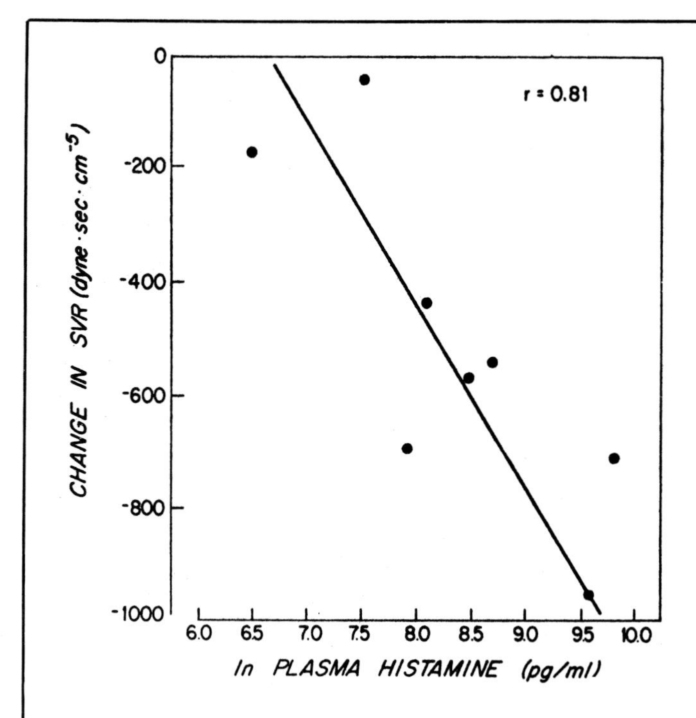

Figure 5. Correlation of plasma histamine (logarithmic transformation, see text) with peak change in systemic vascular resistance for patients given morphine. Data for fentanyl are not included since neither variable changed significantly in this group.
(Reproduced by permission of authors and Anesthesiology. *Philbin DM, Moss J, et al: The use of H_1 and H_2 histamine antagonists with morphine anesthesia: a double-blind study.* Anesthesiology *55:292-296, 1981).*

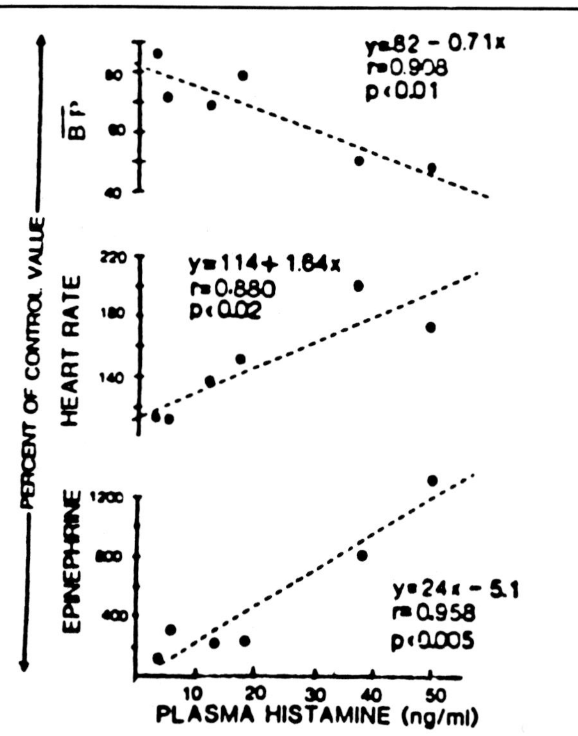

Figure 6. Correlation of hemodynamics, plasma epinephrine, and histamine levels. Patients who responded to the infusion of meperidine or morphine with histamine release were studied. Significant correlations between changes in blood pressure, heart rate, and epinephrine with histamine are given above.
(Reproduced by permission of authors and Anesthesiology. *Flacke JW, Van Etten A, and Flacke WE: Greatest histamine release from meperidine among four narcotics: Double-blind study in man.* Anesthesiology *59, 3A51, 1983).*

continuous infusion over a one-minute period. It is possible to demonstrate that there is a significant difference in the hemodynamic changes seen in the infusion versus the bolus administration. In other studies, we have been able to demonstrate that there is a significant difference between those drugs administered in a five second bolus and those administered in a 15 to 30 second slow bolus (J Moss, unpublished data). It thus appears that even small differences in the rate of administration of intravenous drugs can lead to a significant attenuation in histamine release and cardiovascular changes.

Several groups of investigators have performed studies demonstrating that the combined use of H_1 and H_2 antagonists can prevent the cardiovascular sequellae of anaphylactoid reactions that can accompany the administration of dextran, certain induction agents, and histamine itself.[14,28,29] Their experience in conjunction with data from human heart transplantation suggests that both H_1 and H_2 blockers must be administered in order to achieve significant attenuation of cardiovascular response.[30] Data published from our own laboratory demonstrated that the prophylactic administration of H_1 and H_2 receptor antagonists can attenuate morphine-induced hemodynamic changes. In a double-blind study, Philbin et al[31] randomly assigned patients to receive either a placebo, H_1 antagonist, H_2 antagonist, or a combination of H_1 and H_2 antagonists intravenously immediately before coronary artery bypass surgery.[31] Patients received morphine (1 mg/kg) at the rate of 5 mg/minute. Morphine-induced elevations in plasma histamine were the same in treatment groups, but those patients who received the H_1 and H_2 antagonists in combination were protected against the cardiovascular changes, particularly the changes in systemic vascular resistance (Fig. 8). Combination pretreatment with H_1 and H_2 antagonists completely eliminated the need for pressor support during induction, a major problem in the other three goups (Table 1). When the data were analyzed by analysis of covariance, it was demonstrated that there was no apparent interaction between the H_1 and H_2

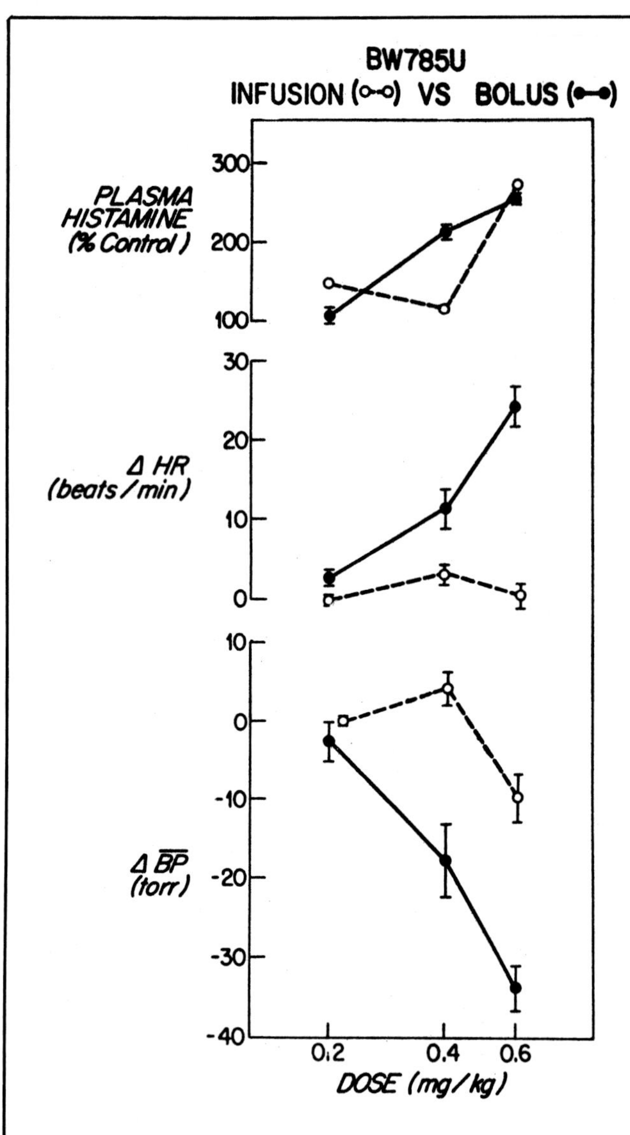

Figure 7. *Effect of method of administration on hemodynamics and plasma histamine. Patients received BW785U as a bolus or as an infusion over 1 min. The dose-response relationship for BP, HR, and histamine are significant (P<0.05). Slopes for bolus versus infusion are significantly different for plasma histamine (P<0.01). Data are given as mean +/– SEM.*
(Data are reproduced by permission of authors and Anesthesiology. *Rosow CE, Basta SJ, Savarese JJ, et al: BW785U: Correlation of cardiovascular effects with increases in plasma histamine.* Anesthesiology *55:S270, 1980).*

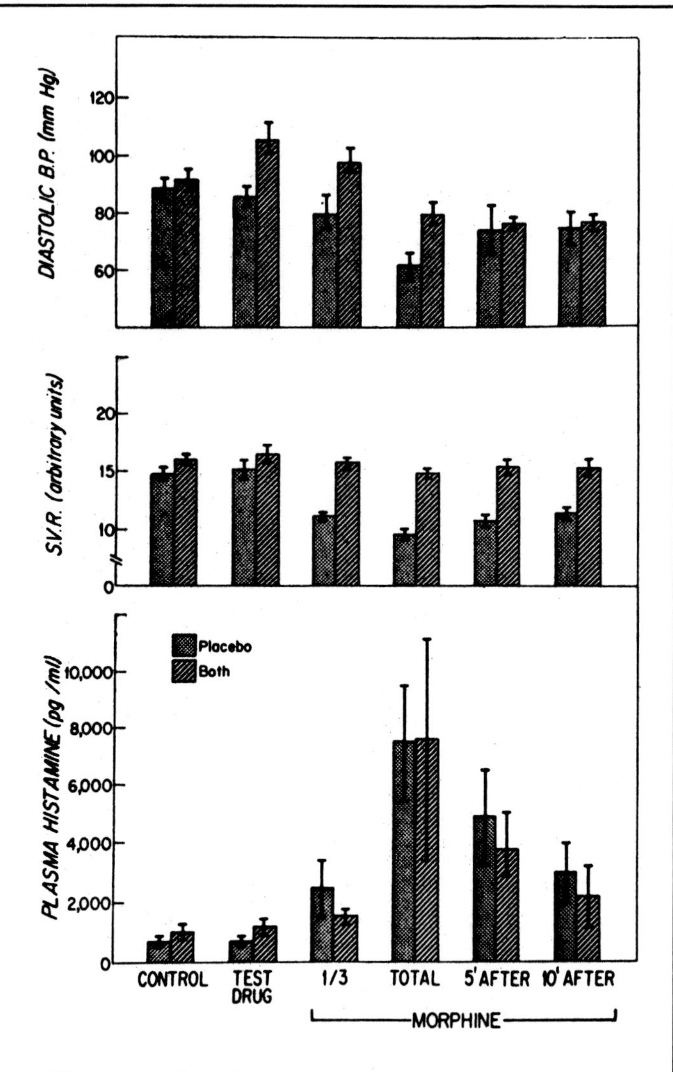

Figure 8. *The relationship between plasma histamine levels, SVR, and diastolic blood pressure for patients receiving placebo and patients receiving both cimetidine and diphenhydramine. The decreases in diastolic blood pressure and systemic vascular resistance are significantly different (P<0.05, P <0.01), although comparable histamine release is achieved. Data are given as mean +/– SD.*
(Data are reproduced by permission of authors and Anesthesiology. Philbin DM, Moss J, Akins CW, et al: The use of H_1 and H_2 histamine blockers with high dose morphine anesthesia: A double-blind study. Anesthesiology 55:292-296, 1981).

Table I

Group	Number of Patients Requiring Neosynephrine
Placebo	8
Cimetidine	6
Diphenhydramine	5
Cimetidine + diphenhydramine	0

Four groups of 10 cardiac surgical patients received either placebo, cimetidine (4 mg/kg), diphenhydramine (1 mg/kg), or a combination of cimetidine (4 mg/kg) and diphenhydramine (1 mg/kg) before administration of morphine (1 mg/kg). The number of patients requiring neosynephrine in each group suggests the extent to which H_1 and H_2 receptor antagonists provide cardiovascular protection.

Table II

Summary of Significant Comparison Among Treatments By Ancova*

	TREATMENT			
Variable	Slopes (P value)	C	D	C ×D (P value)
CI	0.19	0.02	0.62	0.23
Diastolic	0.51	0.18	0.001	0.95
BP	0.32	0.09	0.005	0.83
HR	0.67	0.08	0.18	0.98
SVR	0.07	0.0005	0.04	0.26

C = Cimetidine; D = Diphenhydramine

* *Analysis of covariance (ANCOVA). The data from Philbin et al. were analyzed by ANCOVA. The C designation represents patients receiving cimetidine; the D designation represents patients receiving diphenhydramine. The lack of significance in the C × D term (interaction) suggests that cimetidine and diphenhydramine confer protection independently and without interaction for any given cardiovascular variable. The significance level of cimetidine (C) and diphenhydramine (D) in providing protection for each variable is given in the "C" and "D" terms.*

P-values that are not significant indicate the model assumption of equal slopes holds.

receptors in the human cardiovascular system, i.e. they appear to mediate the cardiovascular responses independently (Table 2). These data are essentially in agreement with other work performed on plasma expanders and intravenous induction agents in which neither H_1 nor H_2 receptor blockade was effective but the combination worked. The importance of combined H_1 and H_2 receptor blockade has also been demonstrated for exogenously administered histamine.

Still another strategy utilized to attenuate clinically important histamine release involved minor alterations of molecular structure. This is particularly true in the development of new neuromuscular blocking agents. Thus, metocurine which is very similar to parent molecule d-tubocurarine, causes significantly less hypotension.[20,32,33] Recent clinical experience with atracurium and vecuronium, investigational neuromuscular blockers which may shortly be released for clinical usage in the United States, indicates that at a dose twice the ED95 for neuromuscular blockade there are no changes in the level

Table III

Incidence of Clinical Signs

Circulatory collapse	68%
Cardiac arrest	11%
Bronchospasm	23%
Widespread flush	55%
Oedema	25%

(Data reproduced by permission of Klinische Wochenschrift and authors. Laxenaire MC, Moneret-Vautrin DA, Boileau S, Moeller R: Adverse Reactions to intravenous agents in anaesthesia. Klinische Wochenschrift 60:1006–1009)

of plasma histamine in human volunteers.[20,21] Thus, it appears that more potent muscle relaxants and narcotics are less likely to release histamine at usual clinically administered doses. Given the relatively wide choice of compounds that are available as neuromuscular blocking agents and narcotics, it may be possible to select or design drugs that will be devoid of histamine release in those cases in which histamine can present a significant problem.

In addition to the studies of anaphylactoid reactions in anesthesia, there has been an increasing appreciation of the occurrence of immunologically-mediated reactions in anesthesia and surgery. Data from Australia and from France suggest that muscle relaxants are most often implicated as the cause of immunologic reactions to anesthetic agents.[12,34] This is particularly true of succinylcholine. These reactions occur more commonly in women than in men. While previous exposure could not be uniformly demonstrated, immunologic tests suggested an allergic origin. The analysis of the clinical symptoms of the reactions from Professor Laxenaire's work suggests that cardiovascular collapse rather than bronchospasm may be an important component of these true immunologically-mediated reactions (Table 3). They thus parallel what is seen in other studies of chemically-mediated anaphylactoid reactions.

In conjunction with anaphylaxis caused by anesthetic agents per se, chemonucleolysis with chymopapain may precipitate anaphylaxis in anesthetized patients. A large body of data regarding the epidemiology of anaphylaxis has become available since the clinical introduction of chymodiactin for the treatment of herniated nucleus pulposis.[35] The Phase III clinical trials of this compound in the United States suggested an anaphylaxis rate of approximately 1% following administration of the compound. There were 13 cases of anaphylaxis, and 2 deaths in the 1585 patients who received the enzyme.[36] The symptoms encountered were much the same as those described by Professor Laxenaire with cardiovascular collapse being most prominent. As with the muscle relaxants, there was a significant gender difference. In subsequent studies in which a large number of patients received chymopapain, the incidence rate has remained unchanged but there were no deaths in the first 17,000 cases reported.[37] One significant difference between the Phase III clinical trials and the Phase IV surveillance study, which could account for the dramatic fall in anticipated mortality, is the use of prophylactic antihistamines. Ninety-three percent of patients (in the Phase IV surveillance study) received H_1 and H_2 antagonists prior to the administration of chymopapain, while no patients received the combination of receptor antagonists during the Phase III clinical trials. The decreased mortality rate suggests that these reactions may be less severe. While physician awareness and case selection may be factors, the data suggest that pretreatment with H_1 and H_2 antagonists may be a factor in attenuating the severity of the reaction. Several case reports of anaphylaxis in intensively monitored patients suggest that the decrease in systemic vascular resistance may predominate over the negative inotropic effects of leukotrienes, etc.[40,41] The fact that incidence does not change only speaks to the fact that other vasoactive substances are released during true immunologically-mediated anaphylaxis.

The results of our investigations, as well as a review of the literature, suggest that both anaphylactic and anaphylactoid reactions can and do occur under anesthesia. These reactions can appear to be physiologically similar but can be separated out using immunologic techinques. Data from several studies suggest that pretreatment with H_1 and H_2 antagonists can significantly attenuate cardiovascular changes seen during either form of histamine release.

REFERENCES

1. Ellis HV 3rd, Johnson AR, Moran NC. Selective release of histamine from rat mast cells by several drugs. J Pharmacol Exp Ther 175(3): 627-631, 1970.
2. Feldberg W, Paton WDM: Release of histamine from skin and muscle in the cat by opium alkaloids and other histamine liberators. J Physiol 114, 490-509, 1951.
3. Paton WDM: The effects of muscle relaxants other than muscular relaxation. Anesthesiology 20:453-463, 1959.
4. Savarese JJ. The autonomic margins of safety of metocurine and d-tubocurarine in the cat. Anesthesiology 50:40-46, 1979.
5. Moss J, Rosow CE. Histamine release by narcotics and muscle relaxants in humans. Anesthesiology 59:330-339, 1983 (78 Ref.).
6. Owen DA, Harvey CA, Boyce MJ. Effects of histamine on the circulatory system. Klin Wochenschr 60:972-977, 1982.
7. Austen KF. Tissue mast cells in immediate hypersensitivity. Hos Pract 17:98-108, 1982.

8. Basta SJ, Moss J, Savarese JJ, Ali H, Sunder N, et al. Cardiovascular effects of BWA444U: correlation with plasma histamine levels. Anesthesiology 55:A198, 1981.
9. Savarese JJ, Basta SJ, Ali HH, Sunder N, Moss J. Neuromuscular and cardiovascular effects of BW 33A (Atracurium) in patients under halothane anesthesia. Anesthesiology 57:A262, 1982.
10. Moss J, Philbin DM, Rosow CE, Basta SJ, Gelb C, Savarese JJ. Histamine release by neuromuscular blocking agents in man. Klin Wochenschr 60:891-895, 1982.
11. Lim H, Churchill-Davison HC. Adverse effects of neuromuscular blocking drugs. Adverse Reactions to Anesthetic Drugs. (Monographs in Anaesthesiology, V8) Thornton JA. Amsterdam, Elsevier 1981.
12. Fisher MM, Munro I. Life-threatening anaphylactoid reactions to muscle relaxants. Anesth Analg 62:559-64, 1983.
13. Levy, JH, Rockoff MA. Anaphylaxis to meperidine. Anesth Analg 61:301-303, 1982.
14. Kaliner M, Shelhamer JH, Ottesen EA: Effects of infused histamine: correlation of plasma histamine levels and symptoms. J Allergy Clin Immunol 69:283-289, 1982.
15. Moss J, Rosow CE, Savarese JJ, Philbin DM, Kniffen KJ, et al. Role of histamine in the hypotensive action of d-tubocurarine in humans. Anesthesiology 55:19-25, 1981.
16. Rosow CE, Moss J, Philbin DM, Savarese JJ, et al. Histamine release during morphine and fentanyl anesthesia. Anesthesiology 56:93-96, 1982.
17. Lorenz W, Doenicke A. Histamine release in clinical conditions. Mt Sinai J Med (NY)45:357-386, 1978 (78 Ref.).
18. Lorenz W, Doenicke A, Meyer R, et al. Histamine release in man by propanidid and thiopentone: Pharmacological effects and clinical consequences. Br J Anaesth 44:355-369, 1972.
19. Shaff RE, Beaven MA. Increased sensitivity of the enzymatic isotope assay of histamine: measurement of histamine in plasma and serum. Anal Biochem 94:425-430, 1979.
20. Basta SJ, Ali HH, Savarese J, Sunder N, Moss J, et al: Relative histamine releasing properties of Atracurium (BW 33A), Metocurine and D-tubocurarine. Anesthesiology (In press).
21. Basta SJ, Savarese JJ, Ali HH, Sunder N, Moss JJ, et al. Vecuronium does not alter serum histamine within the clinical dose range. Anesthesiology 59:3,A273, 1983.
22. Rosow CE, Philbin DM, Keegan CR, Moss J. Hemodynamics and histamine release during induction with sufentanil or fentanyl. Anesthesiology 60:489-91 1984.
23. Rosow CE, Keegan CR, Moss J. Cutaneous signs of histamine release following butorphanol or morphine. Abstracts of Scientific Papers. American Society of Anesthesiologists Annual Meeting Las Vegas, 1982 Anesthesiology 57:3,A355, 1982.
24. Flacke JW, Van Etten A, Flacke WE. Greatest histamine release from meperidine among four narcotics: double-blind study in man. Anesthesiology 59:3,A51, 1983.
25. Levi R, Chenouda AA, Trzeciakowski JP, Guo ZG, Aaronson LM, Lee CH, Gay WA, Subramanian VA, McCabe JC, Alexander JC. Dysrhythmias caused by histamine release in guinea pig and human hearts. Klin Wochenschr 60:965-971, 1982.
26. Levi R, Owen DAA, Trzeciakowski J. Actions of histamine on the heart and vasculature in pharmacology of histamine receptors. Edited by Ganellin R, Parsons M. London, J Wright and Sons, 1982.
27. Fahmy NR, Sunder N, Soter NA. Role of histamine in the hemodynamic and plasma catecholamine responses to morphine. Clin Pharmacol Ther 33:5,615-620, 1983.
28. Owen DAA, Flynn SB, Gristwood RL, et al. The role of histamine in the cardiovascular system and in acute inflammatory processes: A review of current evidence. In: Symposium on Further Experience with H_2 Receptor Antagonists, Capri, Italy October 18-20 1979, Edited by Torsoli A, Luchelli PE, Brimblecombe RW. Excerpta Medica, Amsterdam, Oxford, Princeton 1980.
29. Lorenz W, Doenicke A, Schönig B, Mamorski J, Weber D, Hinterlang E, Schwarz B, Neugebauer E. H_1 and H_2-receptor antagonists for premedication in anesthesia and surgery: A critical view based on randomized clinical trials with haemaccel and various antiallergic drugs. Agents Actions 10:114-124, 1980.
30. Ginsburg R, Bristow MR, Stinson EB, Harrison DC. Histamine receptors in the human heart. Life Sci 26:2245-2249, 1980.
31. Philbin DM, Moss J, Akins CW, Rosow CE, Kono K, Schneider RC, Verlee TR, Savarese JJ. The use of H_1 and H_2 histamine antagonists with morphine anesthesia: A double blind study. Anesthesiology 55:292-296, 1981.
32. Antonio RP, Philbin DM, Savarese JJ. Comparative hemodynamic effects of tubocurarine and metocurine in the dog. Br J Anaesth 51:1007-1010, 1979.
33. Zaidan J, Philbin DM, Antonio RP, et al. Hemodynamic effects of metocurine in patients with coronary artery disease receiving propranolol. Anesth Analg 56:255-259, 1977.
34. Laxenaire MC, Monerat-Vautrin DA, Boileau S, Moeller R. Adverse reactions to intravenous agents in anesthesia in France. Klin Wochenschr 60:1006-1009, 1982.
35. Javid MJ, Nordby EJ, Ford LT, et al. Safety and efficacy of chymopapain (Chymodiactin) in herniated nucleus pulposus with sciatica. JAMA
36. Roizen MF. Illinois open trial. In: Chemonucleolysis. Anaphylaxis: recognition and treatment. Smith Laboratories Symposium, Sieber and MacIntyre, Chicago, Oct. 1982.
37. Moss J, Roizen M. Anesthesia for chemonucleolysis. Theory and practice. In: Intradiscal Therapy, A Modality of Treatment. Eds. Smith L, Nordby EJ, and Brown J. Charles B. Slack Co., 1984.
38. Moss J, Fahmy NR, Sunder N, Beaven MA. Hormonal and hemodynamic profile of an anaphylactic reaction in man. Circulation 63:210-213, 1981.
39. Beaupre PN, Roizen MF, Cahalan MK, Alpert RA, et al. Hemodynamic and two-dimensional transesophageal echocardiographic analysis of an anaphylactic reaction in a human. Anesthesiology 60:482-4, 1984.
40. Rosow CE, Basta SJ, Savarese JJ, et al. BW785U Correlation of cardiovascular effects with increases in plasma histamine. Anesthesiology 53:S270, 1980. □

ANTIHISTAMINES

Chapter XIII

Methods of Studying Antihistamines

John T. Connell, M.D.

ABSTRACT

A variety of ingenious methods have been devised to challenge and incite episodes of acute allergic rhinitis in susceptible individuals. These methods teach us much about basic mechanisms involved in the disease. There is some danger in using them for efficacy trials because antihistamines are only partially effective treatment for hay fever and the challenge administered could easily overcome the degree of protection. Additional studies may lead to a better understanding of the factors involved in challenges and hence, their usefulness in clinical testing.

The out-patient trial design is successful in demonstrating efficacy in 40 to 60 per cent of trials. The field trial is 70 to 90 percent accurate in its findings.

The clinical design of antihistamine trials has improved remarkably in the past 10 years. Because of the nature of the disadvantages discussed throughout this report, I would doubt that further improvements in design will occur in future years unless a substitute is found for subjective evaluations.

INTRODUCTION

Antihistamines, either alone or in combination with other agents, are perhaps the most commonly employed drugs in the world. They are used primarily in allergic disease and as drying agents in acute coryza. That they are efficacious to a degree is unquestioned but the exact degree of efficacy still eludes us. Some patients seem to derive excellent relief of symptoms but others notice little or no benefit. Why they are not completely effective may be due to several reasons. In some cases, misdiagnosis and use in inappropriate conditions may result in failure. Our deficiencies in understanding the pathophysiology and the role of mediators other than histamine may explain failure in other cases of allergic disease.

Of equal importance as the therapeutic effect are the side effects of antihistamines, the principle one being sedation. Estimates for the incidence of sedation range from those who claim a greater than 35 per cent incidence to those who say that significant sedation is less than three per cent and may in fact be limited to a small number of paitents who are genetically predisposed.

Clinical trials are required to demonstrate antihistaminic effectiveness. The clinical design of these trials and interpretation of results is poorly understood. Evaluations of clinical trials both for therapy and adverse reactions can be frustrating experiences. Different investigators often differ in their conclusions regarding an antihistamine and even the same investigator may have difficulty reproducing his results from experiment to experiment. In this essay, I will describe the various clinical methodologies, pointing out their usefulness, weaknesses, and strengths.

There are two well-defined types of antihistamine receptors, H1 and H2, and possibly a third H3 receptor in cerebral tissue. At the present, the H1 receptor appears to be primary for symptoms of allergic disease. The H2 receptor is located in various organs and plays a role in the G.I. tract and the myocardium. Because of its effect on cardiac output, it may occasionally play an

Nasal Diseases Study Center, Holy Name Hospital, Teaneck, New Jersey 07666

Reprint requests: John T. Cownell, M.D. 575 Jones Road, Englewood, N.J. 07631

important role in anaphylaxis. The H3 receptor, reputed to control histamine metabolism in the brain, may be significant in the sedation which sometimes accompanies antihistamine use.

LABORATORY PHARMACOLOGY

Animal studies are an important prerequisite for human clinical trials as they provide clues as to what may be expected in humans.

The first task in defining a new antihistamine is to determine its blocking characteristics. This may be done, for example, in the guinea pig ileum (H1 receptors defined by blocking the immediate contraction of the ileum when exposed to histamine) or the heart (blocking the chronotropic H2 receptor in the isolated guinea pig atria) utilizing appropriate blocking agents. Additional studies on animal tissues are performed to determine the blocking capacity of the compound for the various inflammatory mediators such as histamine, serotonin, and leukotrienes.

Most currently available antihistamines exhibit some anticholinergic activity. In fact, anticholinergic activity may be important therapeutically. The anticholinergic profile of a compound is studied by its blocking of the pilocarpine stimulation of salivary secretion and pupillary changes in rabbits.

Short term studies of tolerance to ever increasing doses and long term studies of prolonged administration define toxicity in the intact animal and in tissue sections of the animal. Metabolic and excretion studies show the mode of absorption, elimination, and detoxification of the substance.

Sedating characteristics may be determined by observation of the animals. Injection of radioactive tagged compound followed by radiographs demonstrate whether or not the compound gets into the brain and its potential for causing sedation.

TRIALS IN MAN

Trial Design for Studying Toxicity

Many symptoms have been reported coincidentally with antihistamine therapy. Most, such as dizziness, abdominal distress, and rashes, are extremely rare. Sedation of varying degrees is the most prominent side effect.

Sedation may be studied by crude simple procedures such as a questionnaire or evaluated by more sophisticated techniques. One of the more sophisticated techniques is critical flicker fusion. Critical flicker fusion evaluates the ability of a patient to differentiate distinct pulses from a light source. The rate of pulsation may be varied and when the pulsations are rapid the patient sees only a constant light. The test measures the neurotransmission and assimilation of the stimuli of the light source. A variety of performance tests which again measure alertness and neurotransmission of sensory stimuli can be done. These include driving through an obstacle course, simulated driving, mechanical puzzles, and word tests. Electroencephalography provides information about sleep latency and depth. A sedation profile of an antihistamine may be obtained by using a combination of these tests.

Although these tests define alertness or drowsiness in some fashion, we are still perplexed by the clinical findings that some patients with drowsiness may function rather normally under stress while others with even less drowsiness are functionally impaired.

METHODS OF DETERMINING ANTIHISTAMINE EFFICACY

Disease State For Studying Efficacy

Antihistamines are useful in treating a number of allergic symptoms including those which occur in rhinitis, asthma, and urticaria. It is of utmost importance that the clinical condition respond to antihistamines if efficacy is to be truly measured. In each condition mentioned, the differential diagnosis includes a number of diseases in which antihistamines are not effective. For instance, asthma associated with infection, nasal polyps, or exertion rarely responds to antihistamines and in fact antihistamines may be contraindicated in infectious asthma. Similarly, urticaria due to genetic defects in the complement system is unresponsive. Rhinitis due to nasal mastocytosis, nonallergic eosinophilic disease of the nose, nasal polyps, and deviated septum, conditions sometimes confused with allergic rhinitis, are all unresponsive to antihistamines. Patients with these conditions should not be enrolled in studies designed to show the efficacy of these drugs.

The ideal disease state for studies of efficacy are those that are common, easily diagnosed with little chance of confusion, and those whose pathophysiology has at least partly been shown to be caused by the release of histamine. IgE mediated conditions are the most likely to respond. Most cases of asthma, urticaria, and perennial rhinitis fail to meet some or all of the criteria. The disease state that meets these criteria best is seasonal allergic rhinitis. Seasonal allergic rhinitis occurs in a high percentage of the population during specific seasons, skin or blood tests are available to confirm the presence of specific antibody in patients, and histamine is a known mediator that plays a role in the pathophysiology. Therefore, most clinical trials should be done in seasonal allergic rhinitis. Efficacy is more difficult to demonstrate in studies done in asthma, poorly defined perennial rhinitis, and urticaria, because the underlying mechanism may be difficult to ascertain. The methods described below are primarily for the study of antihistamines in allergic rhinitis.

GENERAL FEATURES OF THE PATHOPHYSIOLOGY OF ALLERGIC RHINITIS AFFECTING OBSERVATIONS OF EFFICACY

The complete picture of the pathophysiology of allergic rhinitis is still unknown. Histamine is one of the major mediators involved in the reaction. On the other hand, the role of leukotrienes, eosinophil chemotactic factor, major basic protein from eosinophils, platelet activating factor, various polymorphonuclear mediators and chemotactic factors, and mediators released by lymphocytes, still have to be defined.

During inspiration, turbulent air flow causes particulate matter in the inhaled air to be trapped on the mucus blanket. Antigenic substances are solubolized. In one theory, the antigens bind to IgE attached to the surface of mucosal mast cells (most likely of the basophilic series). These cells are located on the surface of the epithelium or between the epithelial cells and should be differentiated from the tissue mast cells lying deeper in the mucosa. Histamine is released, initiating sneezing and rhinorrhea via a reflex neurogenic arc. Solubolized antigen penetrates the epithelial surface reaching mast cells deeper in the tunica propria. Additional mediators are released by this reaction thereby extending the pathology.

Patients who have not been exposed to antigens for some time are relatively resistant when exposed again. However, repeated exposure over hours or days reduces resistance so that eventually patients respond with symptoms to very minimal amounts of antigen. This alteration in reactivity is called the priming effect.[1] One explanation for the priming effect is that the basement membrane underlying the epithelial cells is disrupted and made more permeable so that antigen more easily gains access to the cells and structures in the tunica propria. Eosinophils which break down in the tissues may release major basic protein, a substance which could cause degeneration of the basement membrane and hence promote greater and more rapid absorption of solubilized surface antigen. Another possible explanation is that basophils are attracted to the epithelium by initial exposures to antigen, enhancing the reaction to future exposure.

Delayed nasal reactions occurring four to eight hours after exposure have been described. As yet these are difficult to evaluate since they may be true delayed reactions or they may be an additional acute episode due to undetected exposures to other environmental antigens.

An understanding of these events is helpful in assessing efficacy or lack of efficacy of antihistamines in clinical trials.

Criteria for Selecting Subjects

The major criteria for accepting subjects for efficacy trials in allergic rhinitis are the patient's general health and the certainty of the diagnosis. It is obvious that the patient should be in good health. He should not have nasal infection or other nasal conditions which would interfere with the evaluations. Intranasal steroids should be prohibited for at least two weeks and steroid injections for at least six weeks prior to the trials. Twenty-four hours off antihistamine therapy should be sufficient for washout of the clinical effects of antihistamines even though traces of the drug may still be in the blood. Decongestants have little or no effect on the symptoms of allergic rhinitis and may be continued up to 12 hours before the trial. A history of previous positive or negative responses to antihistamines might be important except that these responses are difficult to evaluate. In most patients, a careful history will show that on some days an antihistamine works and on other days, it seems to have little effect. In most cases prior failure of antihistamines suggests a misdiagnosis. The current use of immunotherapy is permissible providing that the patient is still symptomatic and injections are not given for a few days prior to onset of the trial or during the trial. There is little likelihood that one injection of antigen will cause improvement and affect evaluations but an injection could cause a temporary exacerbation of symptoms for one to several days. The patient must have the ability and most important the desire to comply with elements of the protocol. The selection of subjects can be crucial to the outcome.

I do not find that severity of symptoms at the time of enrollment is a significant factor as long as the subject does have some symptoms. In fact, patients with fewer symptoms often have a better response to antihistamines than patients with severe disease. In general, patients with severe symptoms may improve when taking placebo because they were enrolled at the height of their disease while patients with few symptoms at enrollment often get worse on placebo.

Efficacy is determined by changes in symptoms. Only the subject can appreciate and evaluate these changes so that the type of subjects selected is important. The source of subjects can vary from private patients of the investigator, to unpaid volunteers who merely want to be helpful, to subjects obtained through various types of advertising and who receive some type of compensation for their services. Private patients and unpaid volunteers will possibly be the most compliant. However, private patients really come to the physician because they are sick and they expect relief. Therefore, if they are treated with placebo, they are the ones most likely to drop out. This type of subject has an additional disadvantage in that some are prone to want to improve thinking that improvement will please the physician or investigator, a reason that can destroy a study. Possibly the best subjects are those obtained through sources such as advertisements. They are emotionally neutral towards the investigator and more likely to report realistically. However, a few are involved only for the money and these few may fail to comply with the protocol and deceive the investigator. It is most important that the subject understand that accurate reporting is required and that a good result for him is not necessarily equated with clinical improvement. In the final analysis, efficacy can only be demonstrated when the placebo group does worse than those treated with drug.

The subject should have a history of at least two years of seasonal symptoms to fulfill the seasonal requirement. Symptoms should include most of the following: rhinorrhea, sneezing, nasal itching, itching of the throat, eyes or ears. Nasal itching occurs in almost every patient with allergic rhinitis but is most often absent in rhinitis which is not IgE mediated. Eye symptoms in addition to nasal symptoms is an important aid in diagnosis since nasal symptoms alone are more likely in non-allergic disease. Post nasal drip is common and one of the first symptoms to occur and the last to disappear in a patient with allergic rhinitis. Unfortunately, it is common in almost every other form of rhinitis and therefore not a good diagnostic symptom. A history of definite allergic rhinitis in another family member is of definite help in making the diagnosis. Less reliable is a family history of rhinitis, asthma, or urticaria of unknown etiology since these diseases may not be IgE mediated and therefore not represent a true family history of allergy.

Identification of specific IgE antibodies insures that the subject is allergic. This may be done by skin testing or the finding of a positive RAST (radioallergoadsorbent test) for the antigens present in the environment during the trial. A positive RAST is almost always indicative of a positive skin test. If the RAST is negative, the patient should be skin tested to demonstrate the antibody. RAST testing may be the preferred test for new subjects previously unknown to the investigator because it is noninvasive and cannot cause a serious systemic reaction. Generally, higher levels of antibody correlate with more severe symptoms. However, for entrance criteria, the level of antibody is not critical because some patients with low titers or relatively insensitive skin tests may have severe allergic rhinitis whereas others with high antibody levels may display few or no symptoms.

Allergic rhinitis cannot be diagnosed by nasal examination alone, Congested pale mucosa and clear secretion are helpful compatible findings but even when a patient is experiencing severe hay fever, the mucosa may appear normal or red in 50 per cent of subjects. Only about 70 per cent of subjects have nasal congestion so that this criterion is not diagnostic. Nasal examination is more important in the exclusion of subjects. Patients who have an anatomical defect which might interfere with the outcome should be excluded as should patients with nasal polyps. Nasal polyps do not respond to antihistamines and they are frequently found in non-IgE mediated disease. Nasal eosinophilia is only helpful providing all other diagnostic criteria are met. Nasal eosinophilia in the absence of a seasonal history and a positive antibody test probably indicates non-allergic disease.

In allergic rhinitis, sex or age is not important except that a subject must be capable of complying. Care should be taken that in studies done in children, the subjective reporting is that of the child and not the parent's idea of what he thinks the child's symptoms should be.

Weight does not seem to be an important factor in antihistamine trials, although it is with some pharmaceutical agents.

Smoking is frequently mentioned as a criterion. It would be best if patients were not smokers but realistically 50 per cent of patients with allergic rhinitis do smoke and smoking does not appear to have an effect on efficacy studies. An attempt to prohibit smoking during a study probably does more harm than good. It may cause emotional tension and unbalance neurogenic mechanisms that interfere with the response to disease or treatment. However, if the study site is an enclosed area such as a room and a number of subjects are in the room, smoking by one may affect the results of the others. In this case, I find it advantageous to provide a separate area where smokers may go when they wish to smoke.

It is important to consider the natural history of allergic rhinitis in designing studies for assessing effectiveness. As an example, symptoms of allergic rhinitis are usually worse in the morning as compared to the afternoon and evening. Thus, a patient enrolled in the morning will frequently show improvement on any type of treatment. Patients are usually worse outdoors than they are indoors. Multiple antigen exposures are important in some patients even though they have seasonal disease. This is so because of the priming effect previously described. Thus, in a study conducted during the ragweed season, a patient allergic to animal dander and exposed to the animals will have a much stronger response to both the animal and the seasonal antigen. These ragweed sensitive patients will be influenced by exposure to the animals as compared to others in the study who have no animal sensitivity. The natural history of allergic rhinitis through a season is such that exposure to the antigen even in large amounts early in the season causes fewer symptoms than a like exposure later in the season, again because of increased nasal reactivity due to the priming effect. Air conditioning and air filtration have an obvious effect in reducing symptoms through reduction of antigen exposure and can affect the results of a study.

The major symptoms of hay fever which can be measured subjectively occur in the nose, eyes, and pharynx, but rarely the ears. In the nose, rhinorrhea, sniffling, sneezing, nose blowing, and itching are the symptoms that respond best to antihistamine therapy. Occular itch appears to be a more responsive symptom than changes in lacrimation or watery eyes. Pharyngeal itch responds moderately to anithistamines but postnasal drip does not. Symptoms due to eustachian tube obstruction do not respond well and are poor measures of antihistamine efficacy.

DESIGNS FOR EVALUATING SYMPTOMS

The very essence of any clinical trial is to determine how the patient feels as accurately as possible. The patient's perception of disease is purely subjective and must be translated into an evaluation useful in clinical studies. When this is properly done it is quite accurate. Therefore, the HOW, WHEN, and by WHAT METHOD symptoms are reported is basic and critical to any study, HOW is the translation of severity to a scale and the manner in which the question is posed. WHEN defines the periodicity and timing of reporting. BY WHAT METHOD is the mode of tracking evaluations.

The patient is often criticized because his evaluations do not agree with the treatment he received. More often, the fault lies with the study design which may require the patient to do the impossible when evaluating symptoms. What we wish to know about a symptom during a specified interval was HOW severe was it and its duration, a confusing and complicated combination to evaluate. Usually the study design does not specify how this should be done and the patient must make his own judgement of what severity and duration are. Or, a patient may be asked to compare how he is at the time of the report compared to another time period. This is even more difficult since it means two sets of evaluations from memory and then a judgement comparing the two.

Accuracy of evaluations varies with the duration of the periods of observation, shorter periods being more accurate than longer ones. Because it is difficult to remember and assess the duration and severity of each symptom, reports should be made as soon as the observation period ends. A report made one day later or even hours later is probably quite useless. My subjects are instructed to skip reports that are not done on time. No information is better than the possibility of misleading data. The simplest and most accurate assessment is "how do you feel right now" (at the time the report is being made). Duration is sacrificed with this method unless assessments are made at frequent intervals during a day (see Field Trial Method). Frequency and complexity of evaluations and compliance go hand in hand; the more evaluations requested and the more complicated they are, the lower the compliance. Obviously, compromises must be made to secure the optimum amount of data.

Scales for reporting symptoms can markedly affect the outcome. Scales may vary from the simplest 0 = none, 1 = slight, 2 = moderate, and 3 = severe, to the most complicated analog type of reporting. When using an analog scale the patient is asked to judge severity by marking a 100 mm line on which one end is marked "none" and the other end "severe." The difficulty with the simple method is that the majority of symptomatic subjects will check one or two pretreatment which leaves very little room for change post treatment. Thus, the range is too restricted and it is difficult to show statistical differences among treatments. The analog scale is excellent theoretically but symptoms are subjective and reported emotionally. The blank 100 mm line with its infinite possibilities and no guidelines may frustrate the patient so that the mark he makes has little relationship to his symptoms.

The ideal scale is a range of five to ten choices which permits the patient some latitude without frustration. I employ a six point scale 0 = none, 1 = just perceptible, 2 = slight or definitely present, 3 = moderate, 4 = severe, and 5 = very severe. In double-blind studies, this scale almost always provides relevant statistical information.

The physical method used to record symptoms may influence the outcome of a trial. The simplest method is a single page on which symptoms are listed and columns supplied for as many days as desired. The patient may report once a day or several times each day. The disadvantages are that the patient can see his previous reports and be influenced by them and even more important may fail to report daily but may report a number of days at one time. In order to circumvent the latter problem, the patient may be asked to mail in a daily report or telephone in the results each day. Instead of a report card, an interviewer may query the patient by phone. The interviewer has a boring task repetitively asking the same question and great care must be taken to make sure that the question is asked in the same way each time. With each additional step in complexity, compliance is reduced.

Physician assessment of symptoms made during periodic visits is a measure often used in the belief that the physician will provide objectivity. In reality, the physician's assessment is a subjective evaluation of the patient's subjective evaluation and therefore probably less accurate. Furthermore, the physician may only see the patient for a few moments after days or a week of treatment, on a day which may be a good one or a bad one for the patient's disease. Thus, the physician evaluation is prone to unavoidable error. Another danger with a physician (or other study personnel) interview is that the interviewer may imply or suggest that the patient's baseline for evaluation is incorrect, thereby confusing the patient. His subsequent scoring may be adversely affected by this advice.

The assessment of symptom severity, simple as it seems, is a difficult task and as yet there are no exacting or standard methods.

In another effort to eliminate subjectivity, nasal airway resistance (an objective measurement of congestion), is substituted for symptom evaluation, NAR measurements are excellent for assessing congestion but are not useful for evaluation of antihistamines because antihistamines do not affect congestion. Furthermore, the degree of nasal congestion frequently bears no relationship to the other major symptoms of hay fever. Congestion is only one symptom of allergic rhinitis, and is absent in 30 per cent of patients with severe hay fever. The NAR measurement is an ancillary device for assessing hay fever but is NOT a substitute for symptoms evaluations.

DESIGN OF STUDIES

Four general methods are used for studying antihistamine efficacy. For the purposes of this report they will be called the out-patient method, field trials, challenge trials, and skin test wheal studies. In the out-patient method, subjects are given the treatments to take at home while exposed to the antigen in their usual environment. In the field trial, all subjects are observed at the same time for limited periods while in the same location. The challenge techniques utilize quantitated or semi-quantitated amounts of antigen administered to the shock tissue. In the skin test method, antigen is injected into the skin and the reaction observed and measured. Each method has its own advantages and defects.

Regardless of the techniques used, it is desirable to use a positive control (known active drug) and a placebo control. Needless to say, it is imperative that the treatments be double-blinded since all of the assays are subjective. These controls help to determine the accuracy of the results and assess the proficiency of each laboratory where the study is conducted.

An informed consent is a prerequisite for any clinical study. The Food and Drug Administration (FDA) guidelines include about 13 elements which should be included in the consent. The FDA has also described guidelines for institutional review of the protocol for human testing and can refuse to accept data from a study which has not been properly reviewed.

CHALLENGE METHODS

Antigen applied to the nasal mucosa causes an attack of allergic rhinitis. Antigen challenge can be done in a number of ways. When the antigen is a pollen, pollen grains themselves may be administered. Because of the great difficulty in quantitating the number of microscopic pollen grains administered, most study designs employ administration of aqueous extracts of the pollen.

In one method, patients inhale the natural pollen grains from a specially designed reservoir.[2] The number of pollen grains inhaled and the rate of pollen administration can be controlled. The original method as described was tedious and required experience as the estimation of pollen administered was done by sampling the airstream going to the patient and counting the sample visually using a microscope after the inhalation was completed. The technique has been improved in that the airstream going to the patient now passes through a modified particle counter. Thus, as the subject breathes, a digital counter continuously displays the number of grains inhaled. Since the patient inhales the pollen, the laws of physics pertaining to the action of particles in an airstream govern the distribution of pollen on the mucosa. These forces cause the inhaled pollen to be distributed on the mucosa as it is during natural exposure.

Pollen grains are administered to one nostril at a predetermined rate for about one hour. The patient scores his symptoms of hay fever once every three mintues. Symptoms may begin in a few minutes or at any time during the hour of challenge. An acute attack of hay fever has been produced with as few as seven pollen grains administered over three minutes while as many as 6000 pollen grains were administered to another patient and did not produce symptoms, illustrating the wide variation which may be seen. The technique has the added advantage that the challenge can be directly equated to environmental exposure. For reference, the number of pollen grains inhaled during seasonal exposure may vary from about one per minute on a mild pollinating day to 70 per minute on a severe pollinating day. The episode of hay fever resembles in every way that which occurs during natural exposure. The time of onset and severity of symptoms are dependent primarily on the reactivity of the nasal mucosa on the day of challenge. The reactivity of the mucosa depends to a great extent on exposure to any significant antigens during the preceeding days (priming effect). Thus, in a patient who has not been exposed for weeks, even a large initial challenge will produce few symptoms. In this event, challenges may have to be done on several consecutive days to increase nasal reactivity prior to the actual drug trial. Once symptoms begin, they usually increase in severity even though the challenge is maintained at the same rate. Symptoms increase or decrease in intensity if the challenging dose is increased or stopped. Symptoms will usually subside within minutes after the antigen challenge ceases.

Antihistamine efficacy may be determined by administering the drug at a predetermined time prior to the beginning of the challenge and comparing this result to a placebo treatment given prior to challenge. The degree of protection may be gauged by varying the amount or rate of administration of antigen, the total dose given, the time of onset of symptoms, and number and severity of symptoms.

In another method[3], pollen grains mixed with lactose are placed in capsules. Each capsule may contain ten to 5000 pollen grains. The capsules are inserted in a Spinhaler device and the entire contents of a capsule inhaled. Challenges are started by administering the contents of the capsule containing the lowest appropriate dose of pollen followed by an observation period. If symptoms do not occur, the next stronger dose is administered. The process continues until symptoms occur.

Another challenge method utilizes paper discs about 3 mm in diameter which have been soaked in various dilutions of antigen. The discs are then placed under direct vision on the mucosa of the turbinate. Challenge is usually begun with discs saturated with the weakest concentration of antigen so that the non-reactive concentration may be determined. If symptoms do not occur in ten minutes, a disc of 10× greater strength is placed and the reaction observed. Discs of increasing strength are placed until recognizable symptoms occur.

Aqueous extracts of pollen have been employed for challenge as drops, sprays, or as a mist placed on the nasal mucosa under direct vision or blown into the nose with some type of metering device. Weakest concentrations are administered first and if a reaction does not occur in a specified period of time, stronger concentrations are used.

Whether the antigen is administered as grains per capsule, drops, sprays, or mists, the protective effect of antihistamines is assessed by comparing the effects of titrations of antigen and the symptoms they cause after drug administration as compared to a placebo treatment.

Advantages and Disadvantages of the Challenge Methods

The challenge method of administering and counting pollen grains (as described by Connell) is the challenge which compares most favorably to the naturally occurring disease and the dose of pollen causing the attack can be directly compared to environmental exposures. The procedure itself does not require nasal instrumentation and therefore, symptoms due to manipulation are not incited in patients with hyperactive nasal mucosa. The physical properties of the pollen grains do not cause stimulation as one million pollen grains were inhaled by non-allergic patients and no symptoms occurred. Another advantage is that thresholds of exposure may be determined.

Major disadvantages are that the method is tedious in that pollen is administered every two or three minutes for an hour and only two to three patients can be done simultaneously. The pollen reservoir is a specially designed instrument and not available commercially. The particle counter used to count the pollen grains is expensive and those commercially available must be altered for experiments of this type. Some facility with the system must be gained by experience as it is possible to administer thousands of pollen grains during one inhalation if the procedure is not done properly.

Administration of pollen grains in capsules has the distinct advantage of simplicity. A possible disadvantage is the accuracy in producing capsules containing the proper number of grains. When one considers that there are approximately 33 million ragweed pollen grains in one mg of pollen, one recognizes the difficulty in making a dilution of pollen grains and lactose so that each capsule contains ten or 100, etc., pollen grains. It has also been shown that in carefully prepared pollen grain-lactose mixtures the amount of pollen delivered was less than anticipated because electrostatic forces on the pollen grains caused them to adhere to the walls of the containers.

Challenges utilizing pollen grains in capsules or solutions of antigens have several advantages. The challenge procedure is relatively easy and requires minimal training. Equipment is simple and inexpensive. Little time is required for each subject as the challenge with an individual concentration of antigen requires only a few seconds of investigator effort.

A major defect when using extracts of antigen is the quantitation of antigen and the possible non-allergenic stimulation of the nose by the delivery procedure. This may be particularly troublesome with antigen soaked discs. Placement of the disc requires exposure of the turbinate with a speculum and the placement of a disc on the mucosa. Such manipulation can cause rhinorrhea and sneezing in an already allergically stimulated nose or in a non-allergic hyperreactive nose. It is well-recognized that any aqueous solution administered intranasally by drops or sprays may cause acute nasal symptoms such as sneezing and rhinorrhea in many patients due to the physical characteristics of the solutions. These reactions can be confused with the expected symptoms associated with antigen challenge.

The amount of antigen required to produce an attack may be inexact when using pollen capsules or aqueous extract because the quantitative variation between successive challenges may be as much as ten-fold. Since repetitive doses are used one cannot be certain whether the attack is a result of the cumulative dose or the last dose administered. An additional area of difficulty is that with aqueous solutions, the amount delivered from the administering device may not be the amount that lands on and adheres to the mucosa. The quantitation of the aqueous delivery systems is difficult to control and even when delivery is well executed, many patients report swallowing some of the material. The amount of antigen in aqueous solutions cannot be compared directly to the number of pollen grains inhaled during natural exposure.

One problem associated with all challenge techniques is that the reactivity of the nasal mucosa is usually in a state of flux varying from day to day due to exposure to extraneous antigens in the environment. Challenges comparing drugs to placebo for efficacy in the same patient should ideally be done on consecutive days to reduce the effect of nasal variability. At times, due to the information desired or the design of the protocol, the challenges have to be done with many days or even weeks intervening. When this happens, the possibility of alterations in nasal reactivity due to extraneous environmental antigen exposures must be considered.

A major advantage of extracts over materials, which must be recognized visually or have a large size such as pollen grains, is that many more antigens are available in extract form. For instance it would be impossible to titrate the test with animal danders using the challenge methods used for pollen grains.

Challenges have many distinct advantages. They may be done at the investigator's convenience. Exposure to a single antigen is possible and within the limits of the technique, the amount of antigen delivered is known. Many of the variables present in clinical trials can be controlled or at least recognized in challenge studies.

Although a great deal of important and pertinent basic information has been learned from challenge studies, use of the methods in therapeutic trials is still in its infancy. Antihistamines do not abolish the allergic reaction but only blunt it. One major problem in interpretation of results is that the amount of antigen required to produce symptoms may be very close to the amount which cannot be controlled by antihistamine therapy. It is possible that the method using a continuous pollen grain challenge over one hour will be fine tuned enough to illicit the endpoint since the dose of pollen administered increases in small increments.

OUTPATIENT TRIALS

In outpatient trials a physician's office or clinic is used as the processing area. Patients are screened, enrolled, and taught about their treatments and a symptom evaluation system. They are then sent off to their usual environment for a period of days or a week to take the treatment and assess their condition. At the return visit they are examined and the observer attempts to assess how they have done.

An advantage of outpatient trials is their simplicity. No special locations or equipment are required. Disadvantages are numerous. The enrollment criteria usually include specifications for at least a certain degree of symptom severity. Since hay fever may vary in intensity over days, it is possible that a patient could be rejected on one day when he has few symptoms and doesn't meet the severity criterion and yet, be accepted on another when symptoms are worse. If accepted when at his worst, the patient will most often show improvement on his good days even when taking placebo. Enrollment for a study is often done over a period of weeks so that some patients may be enlisted early in a season while others enrolled later after having experienced hay fever for some time. The time of entry can be critical.

One major area of concern is compliance while away from the study site. Patients may not report on the prescribed schedule as previously described, they may not take the study treatment as directed or they may even substitute their own favorite treatment. The patient's usual environment and its antigenic content can vary markedly from that of other patients. For some, the environment may be cleaned by air conditioners or air filtration systems which reduce antigen exposure. Other subjects may live in relatively dirty antigenic surroundings. The antigenic content of the environment could significantly affect the results.

A large number of patients, usually in the hundreds, are required to show efficacy because of the marked variations previously described. Single investigators usually cannot secure enough subjects and multicenter trials must be employed in which different doctors in different parts of the country collect data. All of the disadvantages mentioned are compounded by this technique and a new one is added, the inter investigator differences.

Because of the difficulties described out-patient trials are only successful in approximately 50 percent of the studies. Reproducibility of results is often difficult to achieve in the same laboratory or among different investigators.

FIELD TRIALS

The field trial[4] was designed in an attempt to circumvent some of the disadvantages of the outpatient method. The location of a field trial is at some site where outdoor facilities are available to accomodate a large number of subjects for eight to 12 hours each day. As an example, I usually rent a conference room in a motel which is equipped as the laboratory. The grounds immediately outside this room consist of a large lawn. Patients stay in this outdoor area so it is equipped with canopies and picnic tables for their comfort. All patients arrive each morning at 9 am and stay until 5 pm.

Each patient assesses his condition by completing a 17 symptom report each hour. This can be done with appropriately printed forms. In the past I used special computer cards that the patient completed to evaluate symptoms but am now using computers with touch-screens. Questions and a choice of answers are displayed on the screen. Areas of the screen are sensitive to touch so that the patient merely records his answer by touching the appropriate section of the screen. Patients are asked to evaluate each symptom as to how they feel at the time. Patients are not permitted to see previous evaluations as they complete their current one. The data collected during the first two to four hours is baseline data serving to define each patient's severity of symptoms for that day. At the treatment hour, the computer is programmed to analyze all of the baseline data and pair the patients according to severity of hay fever. Treatments are administered so that of a pair of patients who have equal severity of symptoms, one will receive the placebo and one the active treatment. Reports are then continued hourly until the patient leaves that day. Reports are continued at home that evening on specially prepared forms. The same subjects return the next day and continue assessments for another eight hours under observation at the study site. Treatments are administered during the period according to the protocol. Patients are all fed at the same time and the food is the same for all. Since the studies are done during pollen seasons, the outdoor air is monitored with pollen counters hourly. There is no question of compliance utilizing this technique since treatment administration is observed and patients complete reports at exact times. We have studied as many as 70 patients in a single day in this manner.

A combination of the field trial and the out-patient trial is possibly the ultimate in studies. As an example, the first two days of the study are conducted at the study site as described. The subjects then continue treatment and symptom reports at home for a number of days. The study may then be completed with a final day at the study site. Of course any variation of the combination is possible.

There are disadvantages of the field trial. The investigator or assistants are required full time. If computers are utilized, their expense and the expertise using them must be considered. Inclement weather (usually infrequent) may force cancellation of study days. And of utmost importance is organization. The study is run by a clock which is unforgiving and personnel and equipment must be available as scheduled.

I find that field trials produce definitive results in 70 to 90 percent of trials when effective drugs are studied. The number of subjects required is small because many variables associated with hay fever are equalized by study design. Antihistamine efficacy may be demonstrated with as few as 30 to 40 patients per treatment group.

SKIN TESTS

Skin tests may be used to assess the efficacy of antihistamines. As a baseline, skin tests are performed with dilutions of histamine or an appropriate antigen and measured to determine the subject's reactivity. The materials used for testing must be made at frequent intervals since dilute solutions rapidly lose their potency. Very dilute solutions can become inactive in hours or a day. Skin tests are repeated at the desired intervals after administration of the treatments being investigated. Measurements of the reactions are again made and compared to baseline determinations. The degree of suppression of skin reactivity is a measure of the protective effect of the treatment. However, the reactivity of the skin does not always correlate with nasal protection for a number of reasons (see section describing nasal hyperreactivity). One advantage of the method is that the skin reactivity is relatively constant whereas the nasal sensitivity may change markedly depending on the degree and duration of exposure to environmental antigens.

RESULTS OF ANTIHISTAMINE TRIALS

Reports of antihistamine trials in the early literature often showed 75 to 100 percent relief of symptoms in 85 to 100 percent of patients. These trials were of the out patient variety, were not double-blinded and symptom evaluation procedures were less exacting. In the present era these results appear far too optimistic. Symptom relief with currently designed out-patient or field trials using a 4 mg. dose of chlorpheniramine given q.i.d. generally produce a 40 to 60 percent reduction in symptoms with few patients demonstrating complete relief.

As a general rule my field trials employing antihistamines commonly prescribed over the past two decades produce slightly greater improvement in the "wet symptom complex" (rhinorrhea, nose blowing, sniffles) than of the "itching complex" (itching of nose, eyes, and palate). These findings suggest that part of the favorable therapeutic response is due to an anticholinergic effect and that the total response to the older antihistamines is a combination of anticholinergic and antihistaminic effects.

In almost all studies a "placebo effect" or spontaneous improvement of some degree is observed. The placebo response generally varies from ten to 25 percent improvement but can be as high as 30 to 40 percent. As might be anticipated, in some studies the placebo effect is so great that it destroys the demonstration of efficacy of the drug being studied. The placebo effect has often been attributed to psychological factors in that the subject, having received a treatment, improves merely because of the treatment. I believe that a major portion of the placebo effect is caused by study design. For instance, in out-patient trials, the subjects usually have to have symptoms of a certain degree of severity to enroll. Unfortunately, this means that for many, on enrollment day they are as bad as they will get so that on a hay fever day of lesser severity, they will show improvement even though they get a placebo. Similarly, in field trials, the baseline is derived from symptoms experienced during the morning hours which is generally the time of highest pollen counts and greatest symptoms. Once again, improvement would be expected during subsequent hours of the day even though placebo was administered.

Alterations in study design could reduce the placebo effect. For instance, if one were to use afternoon symptom evaluations which are less severe as a baseline, placebo treated patients would be worse on the following morning and drug treated patients would show improvement but not as much as they currently do. Or, if patients enrolled in out patient trials were accepted with no minimum symptom score, some would obviously get worse during the course of the trial. Proper instruction of the patient is critical in reducing the placebo effect. Patients instinctively feel that a treatment should cause improvement, they want to get better, and they associate improvement with pleasing the doctor. Therefore, to counteract these tendencies, patients must be indoctrinated with the concept that they might get a placebo, that the placebo may have little effect on their symptoms, and they must report what they feel and not anticipate improvement. The indoctrination must be an active process before treatment and must be reinforced throughout the course of the study. It is not enough to assume that just because the patient has read about the placebo in the consent form, he understands its purpose.

SUMMARY

A variety of ingenious methods have been devised to challenge and incite episodes of acute allergic rhinitis in susceptible individuals. These methods teach us much about basic mechanisms involved in the disease. There is some danger in using them for efficacy trials because antihistamines are only partially effective treatment for hay fever and the challenge administered could easily overcome the degree of protection. Additional studies may lead to a better understanding of the factors involved in challenges and hence, their usefulness in clinical testing.

The out-patient trial design is successful in demonstrating efficacy in 40 to 60 per cent of trials. The field trial is 70 to 90 percent accurate in its findings.

The clinical design of antihistamine trials has improved remarkably in the past 10 years. Because of the nature of the disadvantages discussed throughout this report, I would doubt that further improvements in design will occur in future years unless a substitute is found for subjective evaluations.

REFERENCES

1. Connell JT. Quantitative intranasal pollen challenges. III. The priming effect in allergic rhinitis. J Allerg, 43:33–44, 1969.
2. Connell JT. Quantitative intranasal pollen challenges. I. Apparatus design and techniques. J Allerg, 39:358, 1967.
3. Naclerio RM, Meier HL, Kagey-Sobotka A. Mediator release after nasal airway challenge with allergen. Am Rev Respir Dis 128:597–602, 1983.
4. Connell JT. A novel method to assess antihistamine and decongestant efficacy. Ann Allergy 42:278–285, 1979. □

Chapter XIV

H-1 Blockers—Classical Antihistamines

James W. Cooper, Jr., Ph.D.

ABSTRACT

The H_1-blocking antihistamines pharmacology, pharmacokinetics, uses, toxicity and special precautions are presented. Newer agents may offer advantages of longer half-life and lower levels of sedation and motor impairment. Therapeutic considerations are listed with attention to sustained therapeutic efficacy.

Antihistamines, or classical H-1 blockers, were brought into clinical medicine in the early '40's with the introduction of pyrilamine maleate.[1] Over the past 40 years twenty separate chemical entities under scores of proprietary names have been introduced.[2-4] Classical antihistamines, or H-1 receptor antagonists, competitively inhibit most of the pharmacologic actions of histamine. Their pharmacologic effects are summarized in Table 1. Very little is known about the pharmacokinetics of antihistamines. Antihistamines appear to be well absorbed orally, have protein binding that varies from 72% with chlorpheniramine to 98% with diphenhydramine. Metabolism appears to be primarily hepatic with little renal effect. The elimination half-life is reported to be from five hours with triprolidine up to 15–25 hours with chlor- and brompheniramine.[2,3,7] Newer agents have even longer half-lives ranging from 16–23 hours with terfenadine, 38 hours, with mequitazine and 104 hours with astemizole.[5] In terms of pharmacodynamic distribution of the antihistamines, the highest concentrations appear to be found in the lungs and lower concentrations in spleen, kidneys, brain, muscle and skin. Small amounts of the drug appear to be distributed into breast milk. Onset of action varies from 15 to 60 minutes by the oral route. parenterally from 15 to 30 minutes, and rectally from 30 to 45 minutes. Peak effect is usually seen within three to 12 hours with nonsustained release formulations and in eight to 12 hours up to 24 or more hours with prolonged release dosage forms.[1-3]

Uses of antihistamines may be found in Table 2 along with a relative indication of the efficacy for that usage. The key concept with the use of antihistamines is that they are *not curative;* antihistamines are adjunctive and palliative in pharmacotherapy.

The different chemical classes of antihistamines with representative members and side effect differences are indicated in Table 3.

Professor and Head, Department of Pharmacy Practice,
University of Georgia College of Pharmacy
Athens, GA 30602

Special Precautions

Sedation is especially common among all classes of H_1-blockers with a great deal of interindividual variation. Table 3 indicates differences in tendency to sedate between classes. Concurrent use of alcohol and other CNS depressants such as anxiolytics, sedatives, hypnotics, antidepressants and antipsychotics can greatly increase sedation and motor impairment tendency. Decreased dose, temporary discontinuance or stopping of other CNS depressants, switching to another

Table I	
[1-5]Pharmacologic Actions of Antihistamines	
Antihistaminic	Antihistamines are effective in treatment of allergic manifestations by competing for H-1 receptor sites on effector cells, preventing the effects of histamine on the target cell.
Anticholinergic	The anticholinergic effects of most antihistamines also provide a drying effect on the nasal mucosa and pulmonary tree and decreased gastrointestinal motility.
Antidyskinetic	Diphenhydramine is effective in cholinergic excess-associated parkinsonism and in drug-induced dyskinesias by central antagonism of the actions of acetyl choline.
Antiemetic effects	May be related to central antimuscarinic actions, decreased vestibular stimulation and labyrinthine function with possible effect on the chemoreceptor trigger zone.
Antitussive	Diphenhydramine directly suppresses cough reflex center in the medulla.
Sedation/hypnosis	Antihistamines may cause sedation by inhibiting histamine N-methyl-transferase, blocking central histaminergic and serotonergic receptors, anticholinergic and alpha adrenergic blocking activity.[5]
Local anesthetic	Antihistamines bear a structural relationship to local anesthetics and have similar, though lesser, activity as local anesthetics.

Comment: H_1-blockers suppress salivary, lacriminal and other exocrine secretions, but not gastric secretions. In addition, neither H_1- nor H_2-blockers inhibit histamine release.[1]

antihistamine class or use of caffeine as a stimulant may lessen the sedation tendency. Sedation usually is transitory (from day to weeks) due to the development of tolerance, which also limits the use of antihistamines as sedatives or hypnotics to intermittent use several days at a time. Newer antihistamines, terfenadine and astemizole have been shown to have less sedative tendency. More importantly, these newer agents do not appear to impair driving performance when compared to other antihistamines.[6] This impairment makes it imperative for clinicians to warn patients using antihistamines that they should take special precautions or *not drive* vehicles or operate hazardous machinery. Recent litigation has found that failure to warn is expensive on personal injury and medicolegal bases.

Other CNS side effects of antihistamines include dizziness, hypotension and confusional states, especially with geriatric patients. In addition to general motor incoordination and performance impairment, lassitude and muscle weakness are commonly evident on careful history-taking. Patients with cerebral cortex lesions or seizure disorders may have epileptiform seizures especially with the phenothiazine class.

The organ system affected with the next most frequent side effects is the gastrointestinal tract. Patients should be told to increase their fiber intake to anticipate and prevent antihistamine exacerbation of patients most frequent functional complaint—constipation. Anexoria, epigastric distress, nausea and vomiting can occur, most commonly with the ethylenediamine class (see Table 3), and may be avoided by drug administration with meals, milk or antacid.

Anticholinergic effects of dry mouth urinary retention (especially in geriatric males), vertigo, blurred to double vision, impotence and tremors may all be seen with varying incidence and severity.

The safe use of antihistamines in pregnancy has not been established. Decreased lactation and nursing infant sedation may be problems when antihistamines are used by the nursing mother.

A final *caveat* is that antihistamines should be stopped at least four to seven days before skin testing to prevent masking of dermal reactivity to allergens. A complete listing of special considerations for antihistamine use may be found in references.[1-4]

There are therapeutic considerations in use of these agents.

Therapeutic Considerations

Several therapeutic points should be emphasized in the chronic use of antihistamines in various conditions.:

1. While hydroxyzine may be the preferred antihistamine for long term use in allergic phenomena,

Table II

Classical Antihistamine Uses

Use	Relative Efficacy	Comments
Rhinitis or nasal allergies	Hay fever (seasonal rhinitis) and perennial non-seasonal allergic rhinitis, appear to be more improved than vasomotor rhinitis.	Chronic nasal congestion and headache may be refractory to antihistamines unless the chemical class is changed every one to three weeks. Seasonal rhinitis treatment efficacy may be improved when therapy is initiated at the beginning of the hay fever season or when pollen counts are low. Oral decongestants or antihistamine–decongestant combinations may be indicated in the nonhypertensive individual. Antihistamines should be used with caution in patients with both hay fever and asthma due to anticholinergic and drying effects which may cause thickening of bronchial secretions, leading to increased airway obstruction in the asthmatic. Antihistamine combinations given concurrently are no more effective than one antihistamine by itself. It is preferable to alternate antihistamine class rather than giving two antihistamines at the same time. Hydroxyzine may be the preferred antihistamine in chronic rhinitis.[7]
Puritis or allergic dermatoses	Variable efficacy depending on the causative agent and symptoms. Removal of the allergen is essential. Best results seen when antihistamine class varied at one to three week intervals.	While itching and hives accompanying conditions may be temporarily relieved, edema is usually resistant and serum sickness type reactions not benefited. Symptomatic relief of itching with a contact dermatitis, pruritis ani or vulvae and insect bites may be important. Hydroxyzine has been shown to suppress the flare and wheal reactions for the longest period to date, but has not been compared with newer agents with longer half-lives (e.g. astemizole).
Angioedema, urticaria	Antihistamines may provide symptomatic relief of pruritis associated with these reactions and in dermatographism. Cyproheptadine is useful for cold urticaria.	Combinations of antihistamines and decongestants may be the only method to effectively control chronic urticaria. Changing chemical classes every one to three weeks may be needed to restore therapeutic response.
Anaphylactic reactions	Antihistamines are useful only as adjunct to epinephrine therapy.	Allergic bronchoconstriction is medicated less by histamine than by other autacoids such as SRS-A.
Transfusion reactions	Useful only for mild transfusion reactions not caused by ABO incompatabilities.	Antihistamines should not be added to blood being transfused. Antihistamines should be given prophylactically to patients with a history of transfusion reaction but not routinely to patients receiving blood.
Desensitization Procedures and allergic reactions to radiographic contrast media	Antihistamines may be helpful in desensitization and prevent mild reactions to contrast media.	Prophylactic antihistamine use may mask early signs of a severe allergic reaction.

Table II—*Continued*

Use	Relative Efficacy	Comments
Parkinsonism or extrapyramidal reactions (drug-induced)	Diphenhydramine is useful for symptomatic treatment of Parkinsonism and drug induced extrapyramidal reactions in elderly patients unable to tolerate more potent anticholinergics (e.g. Cogentin, Artane, Kemadrin) or in other age groups with mild Parkinsonism or in combination with centrally acting antimuscarinic agents.	The drying of skin, inhibition of micturation and constipating effects of these drugs must be considered, especially in the elderly.
Nausea or vomiting	For prophylaxis or treatment dimenhydrinate and its component diphenhydramine are indicated for the prevention and treatment of nausea and vomiting of motion sickness. Promethazine is most effective in controlling nausea and vomiting not related to the vestibular system.	Some antihistamines, such as buclizine, cyclizine, meclizine and promethazine are also useful in the symptomatic treatment of vertigo associated with vestibular system diseases such as Meniere's Disease or non-specific labyrinthitis.
Cough Suppressant	Diphenhydramine is currently indicated as a non-narcotic cough suppressant.	FDA OTC review panel has classified diphenhydramine as lacking sufficient evidence of effectiveness as a cough suppressant.
Sedation or Hypnosis	Diphenhydramine, doxylamine and pyrilamine have been used as daytime sedative and sleep aids.	Diphenhydramine or hydroxyzine (50 mg) are about as effective as 60 mg pentobarbital on short-term use.[9] Tolerance to sedative effect develops rapidly with daily use. All except newer antihistamines[5] have some degree of sedation with great individual variation.
Local Anesthesia	Parenteral diphenhydramine has been used in patients hypersensitive to amide or ester-type local anesthetics. Other antihistamines have been used topically.	While most antihistamines have local anesthetic activity their local hypersensitivity and irritant effects prevent this use.
Other Uses	Cyproheptadine has been used in Cushing's Disease and as an appetite stimulant. In addition cyproheptadine has been shown to partially block the harmful effects of the anti-tumor drug danorubicin, and restore female orgasmic response inhibited by tricyclic antidepressants.[8]	Unapproved uses.

Table II—*Continued*

Use	Relative Efficacy	Comments
Otitis media	Antihistamines usually combined with decongestants, are frequently used on the basis that this combination prevents eustachian tube obstruction.	An unproven use but nevertheless commonly utilized adjunct in otitis media.
Coryza	While decreasing symptoms of nasal congestion and postnasal drip the duration of viral illness is unaffected.	Common use by prescription and OTC use patterns.

Table III

Antihistamine Classes

Chemical Class	Generic Name	Trade Name	Comments
Ethanolamine	bromodiphenhydramine HCl	Ambrodyl	Frequent sedation and anticholinergic effect
	carbinoxamine maleate	Clistin	Lowest sedation effect of class
	clemastine fumarate	Tavist	Frequent drowsiness
	diphenhydramine HCl	Benadryl	Frequent drowsiness and anticholinergic effect
	doxylamine succinate	Decapryn	Frequent drowsiness
Aklylamine	brompheniramine maleate	Dimetane	This class has less sedation than other classes. Paradoxical stimulation seen, especially in very young patients.
	chlorpheniramine maleate	Chlor-Trimeton	
	dexchlorpheniramine maleate	Polaramine	
	dimethindene maleate	Forhistal	
	triprolidine HCl	Actidil	
Ethylenediamine	tripelennamine citrate	PBZ	Moderate sedation and dizziness, GI effects more common. (e.g. nausea, vomiting epigastric distress.)
	pyrilamine	usually in combination products	
	methapyriline	Histadryl	
Phenothiazine	methdilazine	Tacaryl	Primarily used as antipruritic, least sedating phenothiazine.
	promethazine HCl	Phenergan	Most sedating phenothiazine, also extrapyramidal effects plus photosensitization.
	trimeprazine tartrate	Temaril	Used primarily as antipruritic.
Piprazine	hydroxyzine HCl	Atarax	May be preferred in chronic therapy, but Anticholinergic effects and drowsiness common.
	hydroxyzine pamoate	Vistaril	
Miscellaneous	azatadine maleate	Optimine	Less sedation than many other drugs.
	cyproheptadine	Periactin	Weight gain and pronounced sedation common (especially usefully in cold urticaria).
	terfenadine	Seldane	Less sedation and motor impairment than other classes, but slightly less effective than other antihistamines.[10]

several newer agents with long term effect and less sedation should be evaluated.[5] Tolerance to sedation and therapeutic effect may develop over days to two weeks. The latter effect may be avoided by periodically (every one to three weeks) changing the chemical class of antihistamine used (see Table 3).

2. Using more than one antihistamine at a time has no basis in therapeutics.
3. If events that would *worsen* allergic conditions are anticipated, a dose of antihistamine should be taken one to three hours before the event.
4. Patient compliance and medication errors should be assessed by calling the pharmacist and checking refill dates by prescription number to ensure timely refills as well as appropriate use. Encourage the pharmacist to reinforce your counseling on appropriate use of the drugs, warn about sedation and recognize and report to you drug-related adverse effects as well as misuse.
5. Chronic problems may require long term, regular not *prn* usage of antihistamine and/or decongestants.
6. Treat specific symptoms with single drugs when possible or use effective combinations of single ingredients when indicated (see Table 3).

In summary this chapter has reviewed the pharmacologic effects, uses, precautions and therapeutic considerations in the utilization of antihistamines.

REFERENCES

1. Goodman AG *et al.* (eds.) The Pharmacologic Basis of Therapeutics 6th ed. MacMillan New York 622–632, 1980.
2. USPDI 5th ed. 1985 Mack Printing Co., Easton PA 194–204, 1985.
3. Facts and Comparisons JP Lippincott, St. Louis MO 612–629, 1981.
4. Drug Information 1985 American Hospital Formulary Service, American Society of Hospital Pharmacists, 2–16, 1985.
5. Normal PS. New Developments in Treating Allergic Rhinitis *Drug Therapy* 117–126, 1984.
6. Betts T, Markman D, Debenham S, Mortiboy D, McKevitt T. Effects of Two Antihistamine Drugs on Actual Driving Performance *Br Med J* 288:281–282, 1984.
7. Hendeles L, Weinberger M, Wong L. Medical Management of Noninfectious Rhinitis *Am J Hosp Pharm* 37:1496–1504, 1980.
8. Wilbur RM. Cyproleptadine Findings. *Drug Topics* 22:60, 1984.
9. Katcher BS *et al.* (eds.) Anxiety and Insomnia, in Applied Therapeutics, Applied Therapeutics Inc., 43, 1983.
10. Connell JT, Pharmacology and Efficacy of Terfenadine a New H_1-receptor Antagonist. *Pharmacotherapy* 5:201–208, 1985. □

Chapter XV

H_2-Receptor Antagonists: Development and Application

Saul Feldman, M.D.

ABSTRACT

The advent of H_2-receptor antagonists has dramatically advanced the understanding and treatment of peptic ulcer disease. Ranitidine and cimetidine have been shown to be safe and effective in healing duodenal and gastric ulcers and in prevention of duodenal ulcer relapse. Due to differences in chemical structure, ranitidine is more potent and has a longer duration of action and fewer side effects than cimetidine. The current trend in therapy is toward less frequent dosing patterns with more attention toward controlling nocturnal acid secretion. Possibilities for other therapeutic uses of H_2-receptor antagonists are suggested.

Peptic ulcer disease is a prevalent disorder. It is estimated that four million people suffer from active peptic ulcers in the United States alone, and that about 10 percent of Americans will develop this disease at some time during their life[1]. The treatment of peptic ulcer disease has been revolutionized since 1976 with the availability of compounds which specifically antagonize histamine-induced release of acid from parietal cells.

Associate Clinical Professor of Gastroenterology, Yale University Medical Center

Presented at the National Symposium on H_1 and H_2 Histamine Receptors Sponsored by Brown University and Rhode Island Hospital on December 7, 1983

Histamine has been recognized for several decades as a powerful stimulant of gastric acid secretion. The antihistamines developed in the 1940's, however, are totally ineffective in blocking the actions of histamine on the gastric parietal cell. Research into the mechanisms of the biological actions of histamine and antihistamines led to the concept that there is more than one type of histamine receptor.

In the mid-1960's, research efforts, led by Dr. James W. Black at the Smith Kline and French Laboratories in England, were directed toward developing compounds which would specifically block the histamine receptors resistant to the conventional antihistamines[2]. Black and his group developed a series of compounds which were progressive modifications of the structure of histamine. Their efforts over the next decade resulted in several compounds and substantiated the hypothesis of two separate and distinct histamine receptor populations. In 1972 they introduced burimamide and demonstrated that it is highly specific in blocking non-H_1 tissue systems *in vitro* and *in vivo*[3]. Studies on the human pharmacology of burimamide were disappointing, however, as it was neither potent enough nor absorbed well enough to justify development as a useful therapeutic agent. The discovery of burimamide was a significant advance, nevertheless, and enabled Black's group to define and characterize H_2-receptors as those histamine receptors which are specifically blocked by burimamide.

The next step forward came with the development of metiamide, which is four to six times more potent than burimamide in the inhibition of gastric acid secretion *in vivo*[2]. Metiamide proved to be effective in the treatment of duodenal ulcer disease but was soon found to be associated with a reversible granulocytopenia in some patients[2,4].

Further modifications of the histamine-like molecule resulted in the development of cimetidine, a highly effective and well-tolerated H_2-antagonist which has been hailed as the most important discovery in drug research in the last two decades[4].

The effectiveness and safety of cimetidine have been widely studied since clinical trials began in 1974. Cimetidine was approved for clinical use in the United Kingdom in 1976 and in the United States the following year. It has been used by an estimated 30 million patients throughout the world for the treatment of acid-peptic disorders. This extensive use accounts for much of our present day knowledge of H_2-receptors.

An oral dose of 300 mg cimetidine inhibits basal gastric acid secretion by 90% for four hours and nocturnal acid secretion by 90% for seven hours[5]. Cimetidine is capable of diminishing gastric acid secretion in response to stimuli including food, gastrin, and acetylcholine, possibly by blocking a powerful potentiating effect on histamine[5].

Cimetidine has been proven effective and is currently indicated for use in the short-term treatment of active duodenal ulcer and benign gastric ulcer, for prophylactic use in lower dosages for prevention of duodenal ulcer recurrence, and in the treatment of pathological hypersecretory conditions, such as Zollinger-Ellison syndrome, systemic mastocytosis, and multiple endocrine adenomas[6].

Treatment of duodenal ulcer with cimetidine 300 mg four times daily for six weeks resulted in complete healing for 76% of the patients evaluated by endoscopy in a U.S. multicenter study[7]. The same therapeutic regime has been shown to be effective in healing gastric ulcers over an eight week treatment period[8].

Despite the success of short-term therapy with H_2-antagonists in the healing of ulcers, such treatment does not cure ulcer disease. After cessation of cimetidine therapy, relapse occurs in up to 70% of the patients within three months and in up to 90% of the patients within one year of treatment[5].

Maintenance therapy with cimetidine 400 mg once or twice daily for up to one year has been shown to be effective in preventing ulcer recurrence. Relapse rates during one year of maintenance therapy have been reported for 13–45% of patients on cimetidine 400 mg at bedtime compared with 53–90% of patients on placebo[5].

Treatment of hypersecretory conditions, such as Zollinger-Ellison syndrome requires larger doses than the usual 1.2 g per day. Up to 2.4 g per day is recommended for treatment of Zollinger-Ellison syndrome, but most patients with this disorder require even larger doses or additional therapy to control gastric secretion[9]. Use of these higher dosages of cimetidine has been associated with undesirable effects, such as gynecomastia and impotence in males[10]. These effects have been attributed to the weak anti-androgen effect of cimetidine[11].

Table I

Drugs Which Interact With Cimetidine*

Drugs
Warfarin
Benzodiazepines
Diazepam
Chlordiazepoxide
Beta-blockers
Propranolol
Metoprolol
Theophylline
Lidocaine
Anticonvulsants
Phenytoin
Phenobarbital
Carbamazepine
Sodium Valproate
Tricyclic Antidepressants
Imipramine
Nortriptyline
Aminopyrine
Metronidazole
Quinidine
Ethanol

* *Adapted from Powell and Donn, 1983*

The extensive use of cimetidine has unveiled other untoward effects as well. The most common side effects are symptoms of central nervous system dysfunction, especially in the elderly, patients receiving high doses, or patients with hepatic or renal disorder[12]. Additional adverse reactions include gastrointestinal disturbances, headache, rash, and other relatively minor complaints. The incidence of any of these adverse events is very low.

One of the more disturbing side-effects of cimetidine is that it interferes with the metabolism of at least 15 other drugs[13], some of which are listed in Table I. Within two years of its release, cimetidine was shown to promote an increased prothrombin time in patients receiving warfarin[14]. It is now known that cimetidine binds to hepatic mixed-function oxidase microsomal enzymes and can reduce the clearance of certain drugs by 20–60%[13]. These interactions have been attributed to the binding of the imidazole ring of cimetidine to the cytochrome P-450 enzyme.

In short, cimetidine is the first H_2-receptor antagonist widely available for clinical use, and it has been extensively studied. Its effectiveness in the control of gastric acid secretion is well-established. Overall, cimetidine has been shown to be a safe drug, provided that the dosages do not exceed recommended limits and that the patient is not taking concomitant interacting medication. Optimal treatment for any chronic disorder, however, would require a more limited interaction with other medications which the patient might require as well as a dosing schedule less rigorous than an four-times daily regimen.

While cimetidine was being marketed and studied world-wide, another H_2-receptor antagonist ranitidine, was developed. Ranitidine (Zantac®) differs from cimetidine in that the imidazol nucleus and side chain cyano moiety was replaced with a furan ring and a side chain methyl-nitro group[15]. These substitutions succeeded in producing a compound which is eight times more potent than cimetidine in inhibiting histamine-induced gastric acid secretion[16] and which has poor affinity for the cytochrome P-450 enzyme system, thus eliminating potential interaction with the hepatic drug-metabolizing system.

Several recent studies have indicated that ranitidine 300 mg per day is either equivalent or superior to cimetidine 1000 mg per day in the treatment and prevention of duodenal and gastric ulcer[15,17]. In a multicenter, double-blind study involving 484 patients with recently healed duodenal ulcers, ranitidine 150 mg HS was superior to cimetidine 400 mg HS in preventing ulcer recurrence throughout a full year of maintenance therapy. Ulcer relapse rates were significantly lower among patients on ranitidine as compared to those on cimetidine (8% vs 21% at four months, 14% vs 34% at eight months, and 23% vs 37% at 12 months, respectively)[18]. Ranitidine has also proved to be effective in the control of hypersecretory conditions and cimetidine-resistant ulcers[15,19].

Examination of the safety profile of ranitidine in 4532 patients indicated that the only convincingly drug-related adverse event was headache, which occurred in less than 2% of the patients and was generally mild, of short duration and well-tolerated[20]. Due to the known effect of cimetidine on the metabolism of other drugs, drug interactions with ranitidine have been closely scrutinized since clinical trials began in 1979[13]. Drug interactions with ranitidine are negligible, apparently for two reasons. The binding affinity of ranitidine for the cytochrome P-450 system is about 10% of that of cimetidine, and, due to its greater potency, the daily dose of ranitidine is only a quarter of that for cimetidine.

Ranitidine, like cimetidine, is also effective in inhibiting acid secretion in response to other known stimuli in addition to histamine. A study of the effects of H_2-antagonists on pentagastrin-stimulated acid secretion in healthy volunteers indicated that ranitidine is 13 times more potent than cimetidine on a molar basis[21]. Another study demonstrated that the plasma concentration of ranitidine required to inhibit food-stimulated gastric acid secretion by 50% was only one-fifth of the concentration of cimetidine necessary to produce similar effects[22].

The study comparing the effects of H_2-receptor antagonists on food-stimulated acid secretion revealed a longer duration of action of ranitidine as well as greater potency. A single oral dose of ranitidine 150 mg inhibited food-stimulated acid output by 86% at seven hours and by 44% at 12 hours after dosing, whereas an oral dose of cimetidine 300 mg inhibited food-stimulated acid secretion by 44% at seven hours and was ineffective after just ten hours[22]. The longer duration of action of ranitidine is possibly due to a slower dissociation from the parietal cell H_2-receptors[15] as the half-life of the two drugs after oral administration is similar (three hours for ranitidine and two hours for cimetidine[4]).

The combination of a greater specificity for the parietal H_2-receptor and a longer duration of action confers a considerable advantage to ranitidine over cimetidine in that equivalent treatment can be attained with lower doses and less frequent administration of medication. In fact, the current trend in the treatment of peptic ulcer disease is toward less frequent dosing.

In two foreign studies, the effects of twice-daily oral administration of ranitidine 150 mg and cimetidine 400 mg on 24-hour intragastric acidity were compared. The results indicated that in healthy volunteers[23] or in patients with active duodenal ulcer[24] ranitidine was significantly more effective in suppressing acid secretion, especially late in the afternoon and early in the morning.

In 1943 Dragstedt and Owens suggested that hypersecretion of gastric acid in the early morning hours was the primary factor in duodenal ulcer disease[25]. Recent reports offer support for the effectiveness of a single daily dose of H_2-antagonist administered at bedtime in the control of duodenal ulcer disease. In a study of twelve duodenal ulcer patients in remission, Gledhill and others found no difference in the reduction of intragastric acidity between twice daily or single daily doses of ranitidine (300 mg per day total) or cimetidine (800 mg per day total). In fact, the twice daily dose of cimetidine was significantly less effective than the other treatments[26].

In another study of 102 patients with active duodenal ulcer treated with ranitidine for four weeks, a single nocturnal dose of 300 mg was as effective as a twice

Table II

Possible Uses of H2-antagonists*

- Prevention of anaphylactoid drug reactions (when combined with H_1-antihistamines)
- Chronic urticaria (when combined with H_1-antihistamines)
- Prevention of acetaminophen overdose toxicity**
- Adjunct to pancreatic supplementation
- Prevention of aspiration pneumonitis
- Prevention of NSAID-induced gastric ulceration

* *Not approved by FDA*
** *Cimetidine only*

daily dose of 150 mg in healing the ulcers (96% and 84% healing rate, respectively)[27]. Very similar effects were seen in 48 patients treated with cimetidine 400 mg twice daily or 800 mg at bedtime[28].

Thus it appears that control of nocturnal acid secretion is the key to controlling peptic ulcer disease. Unopposed nocturnal acid secretion might be more damaging than acid secreted during the day which is buffered by the presence of food. Furthermore, the wisdom of inducing prolonged periods of hypochlorhydria has been questioned due to the possibility of gastric bacterial overgrowth and production of nitrosamines[12].

To date, H_2-receptor antagonists have FDA approval for short-term therapy of duodenal and gastric ulcers, for maintenance therapy in duodenal ulcer disease, and for treatment of hypersecretory disorders such as Zollinger-Ellison syndrome. The agents have been suggested for use in other disorders not yet included among the approved indications. Some of these suggested uses are listed in Table II. There is some documentation that H_2-antagonists may be useful in the treatment of reflux esophagitis or in preventing acute upper gastrointestinal bleeding in high-risk patients such as those with severe trauma, but they are not useful in controlling established upper gastrointestinal bleeding[5].

In summary, the availability of H_2-receptor antagonists since 1976 has dramatically improved the treatment of peptic ulcer disease. Both cimetidine and ranitidine have proved to be safe and effective for thousands of patients throughout the world. The extensive study of the effects of these agents has provided us with a better understanding of the pathological basis of peptic ulcer disease. Hopefully, this understanding will lead to further improvements and refinements in the control of acid-peptic disease.

REFERENCES

1. Kurata JH, Haile BM. Epidemiology of peptic ulcer disease. Clinics in Gastroenterology 13:289–307, 1984.
2. Brimblecombe RW, Duncan WA, Durant GJ, Emmett JC, Ganellin CR, Leslie GB, Parsons ME: Characterization and development of cimetidine as a histamine H_2-receptor antagonist. Gastroenterology 74:339–347, 1978.
3. Black JW, Duncan WA, Durant CJ, Ganellin CR, Parsons EM. Definition and antagonism of histamine H_2-receptors. Nature 236:385–390, 1972.
4. Brittain RT, Jack D. Histamine H_2-antagonists—past, present and future. J Clin Gastroenterol 5(Suppl.1):71–79, 1983. (27 ref.)
5. Freston JW. Cimetidine: I. Developments, pharmacology, and efficacy. Ann Internal Med 97:573–580, 1982.
6. Package insert. Tagamet. Smith Kline & French, Philadelphia, PA, March 1984.
7. Binder HJ, Cocco A, Crossley RJ, Finkelstein W, Font R, Friedman G, Groarke J, Hughes W, Johnson AF, McGuigan JE, Summers R, Vlahcevic R, Wilson EC, Winship DH. Cimetidine in the treatment of duodenal ulcer: A multicenter double blind study. Gastroenterology 74:380–388, 1978.
8. Akdamar K, Dyck W, Englert E, Belsito A, Sontag S, Vlahcevic Z, Strickland R, Achord J, Graham D, Kornfield R, Agrawal N. Cimetidine versus placebo in the treatment of benign gastric ulcer: A multicenter double blind study (Abstract). Gastroenterology 80:1098, 1981.
9. McCarthy DM, Collins SM, Korman LY, Jensen RT, Gardner JD. Long-term medical therapy in Zollinger-Ellison syndrome (Abstract). Gastroenterology 80:1227, 1981.
10. Spence RW, Celestin LR. Gynaecomastia associated with cimetidine. Gut 20:154–157, 1979.
11. Winters SJ, Banks JL, Loriaux DL. Cimetidine is an antiandrogen in the rat. Gastroenterology 76:504–508, 1979.
12. Freston JW. Cimetidine: II. Adverse reactions and patterns of use. Ann Intern Med 97:728–734, 1982.
13. Powell JR and Donn KH. The pharmacokinetic basis for H_2-antagonist drug interactions: concepts and implications. J Clin Gastroenterol 5(Suppl.1):95–113, 1983. (166 ref.)
14. Flind AC. Cimetidine and oral anticoagulants (Letter). Br Med J 2:1367, 1978.
15. Gaginella TS, Bauman JH. Ranitidine hydrochloride. Drug Intell Clin Pharm 17:873–885, 1983. (184 ref.)
16. Konturek SJ, Obtulowicz W, Kwiecien N, Sito E, Mikos E, Oleksy J. Comparison of ranitidine and cimetidine in the inhibition of histamine, sham-feeding and meal-induced gastric secretion in duodenal ulcer patients. Gut 21:181–186, 1980.
17. Zeldis JB, Friedman LS, Isselbacher KJ. Ranitidine: A new H_2-receptor antagonist. N Eng J Med 309:1368–1373, 1983.
18. Gough KR, Korman MG, Bardhan KD, Lee FI, Crowe JP, Reed PI, Smith RN. Ranitidine and cimetidine in prevention of duodenal ulcer relapse: A double-blind, randomised, multicentre, comparative trial. Lancet 2:659–662, 1984.
19. Collen MJ, Howard JM, McArthur KE, Raufman JP, Cornelius MJ, Ciarleglio CA, Gardner JD, Jensen RT. Comparison of ranitidine and cimetidine in the treatment of gastric hypersecretion. Ann Intern Med 100:52–58, 1984.
20. Simon B, Muller P, Dammann HG. Safety profile of ranitidine. In: Ranitidine, Proceedings of an international symposium held in the context of the Seventh World Congress of Gastroenterology. Riley AJ, Salmon PR (Eds.) Excerpta Medica, 181–189, 1982.
21. Sewing KF, Billian A, Malchow H. Comparative study with

ranitidine and cimetidine on gastric secretion in normal volunteers. Gut 21:750–752, 1980.

22. Brater DC, Peters MN, Eshelman FN, Richardson CT. Clinical comparison of cimetidine and ranitidine. Clin Pharmacol Ther 32:484–489, 1982.
23. Dammann HG, Friedl W, Muller P, Simon B. Effect of ranitidine and cimetidine twice daily on the 24 H intragastric acidity in man. Brit J Clin Pharmacol 16:461–462, 1983.
24. Corinaldesi R, Stanghellini V, Sacco T, Raiti C, Galassi A, Barbara L. Comparative effects of the twice-daily oral administration of ranitidine and cimetidine on 24-hour gastric hydrogen ion concentration and pH in duodenal ulcer patients. Curr Ther Res 34:92–97, 1983.
25. Dragstedt LR, Owens FM. Supradiaphragmatic section of the vagus nerves in treatment of duodenal ulcer. Proc Soc Exp Biol Med 53:152–154, 1943.
26. Gledhill T, Howard OM, Buck M, Paul A, Hunt RH. Single nocturnal dose of an H_2 receptor antagonist for the treatment of duodenal ulcer. Gut 24:904–908, 1983.
27. Ireland A, Colin-Jones DG, Gear P, Golding PL, Ramage JK, Williams JG, Leicester RJ, Smith CL, Ross G, Bamforth J, DeGara CJ, Gledhill T, Hunt RH. Ranitidine 150 mg twice daily vs 300 mg nightly in treatment of duodenal ulcers. Lancet 2:274–276, 1984.
28. Lacerte M, Rousseau B, Parent JP, Pare P, Levesque D, Falutz S. Single daily dose of cimetidine for the treatment of symptomatic duodenal ulcer: Results of a comparative two-centre clinical trial. Curr Ther Res 35:777–782, 1984. □

Chapter XVI

Newer Antihistamines and Histamine-Release Inhibitors

Philip N. Johnson, Ph.D.

ABSTRACT

Traditional H_1 receptor antagonists are a mainstay of drug therapy for the allergic state, but cause numerous discomforting side effects which often hinder compliance. Newer H_1 antagonists, including astemizole and terfenadine, appear remarkably free of central side effects and may provide a therapeutic breakthrough for clinicians. H_2 antagonists have revolutionized drug therapy for hypersecretory states. Ranitidine appears to have fewer side effects than cimetidine at this stage in its utilization history, but has not been used as extensively. Other antisecretory agents of promise include some tricyclic antidepressants, prostaglandin derivatives, and potassium-hydrogen ATPase inhibitors. Newer histamine-release inhibitors (ketotifen, oxatomide e.g.) are effective orally and offer better patient compliance.

INTRODUCTION

The profound physiological effects of a number of naturally-occurring substances with dissimilar structures, and widely varying pharmacological effects, have intrigued investigators and clinicians for decades. Histamine is the one autacoid, or hormone, which is the most familiar, and oldest-known of this diverse group of substances. Dale and Laidlaw studied histamine intensively over 70 years ago, noting its activity in stimulating numerous types of smooth muscle, and causing an impressive depressor action. The discovery of histamine's occurrence in the body, and that cellular injury, including antigen-antibody combination, could effect its release, only served to intensify interest in methods to blunt its profound effects. In following years, the discovery of two broad classes of histamine receptors further increased interest in the development of drugs to specifically antagonize the H_1 and H_2 receptor.

Blockade of many of the noxious actions of histamine was first achieved in 1937, when a diethylamine derivative was found to protect guinea pigs against lethal doses of histamine. This compound was too weak and yet too toxic for clinical use, but started an intense search for more suitable antagonists. The first drug found to have acceptable clinical use was Antergan, another diethylamine derivative. Shortly thereafter (1944), Neo-Antergan was introduced, and is still with us today, found in a plethora of OTC products as pyrilamine maleate. Diphenhydramine and tripelennamine were next (1946), and signalled the development of literally hundreds of compounds which were able to antagonize the H_1 receptor.

The H_1 blockers were developed in an early attempt to utilize structure-activity -relationships to antagonize the portion of the histamine molecule thought to be responsible for its actions: the ethylamine side chain. Over the past 30 years, five general structure groups have been synthesized which exhibit varying degrees of H_1 antagonism, as well as adverse effects. These structural classes include the ethanolamines, the ethylenediamines, the alkylamines, the piperazines, and the phenothiazines. All groups have been used to inhibit the effects of histamine

Associate Director, Department of Pharmacy, Rhode Island Hospital, 593 Eddy Street, Providence, Rhode Island 02906

on the H_1 receptor and blunt the effects of histamine on capillary permeability, on vascular, bronchial and other smooth musculature, and have been the mainstay of the clinician's armamentarium against the hypersensitive (allergic) state.

The adverse effects of the H_1 antagonists, while not seriously debilitating, have nonetheless caused consternation among clinicians and non-compliance among patients. The major side effects — seen within all drug classes in varying degrees — include sedation, the most common CNS side effect. Other central effects are dizziness, tinnitus, fatigue, incoordination, nervousness and tremors. The next most common adverse effects affect the gastrointestinal tract. Anticholinergic side effects are not uncommon among the H_1 blockers, and can be particularly noticeable in cases of "overcompliance," drug abuse, or frank overdose (especially likely with the OTC antihistamines.) Development of H_1 blockers devoid of these side effects, especially those of the CNS, has been an elusive goal for many years; two new drugs in particular, however, may have the potential to finally achieve efficacious H_1 antagonism without these adverse reactions: astemizole (Janssen Pharmaceutica) and terfenadine (Merrel-Dow).

Drowsiness is associated with all older H_1 blockers in varying degrees, and has been attributed to a number of mechanisms: inhibition of histamine-N-methyltransferase; blockade of central histaminergic receptors; preferential binding to central *vs* peripheral receptors; serotinergic antagonism, anticholinergic activity; and, perhaps, central alpha adrenergic blockade. Whatever the ultimate mechanism, or combinations thereof, it is necessary that the antihistamine cross the blood brain barrier. Most of the older H_1 antihistamines are highly lipophilic and cross the barrier with ease. Animal studies have shown that astemizole crosses the blood brain barrier with difficulty, and does not occupy central histamine receptors. Terfenadine, on the other hand, more readily enters the CNS, but has little if any anticholinergic activity, and apparently has a greater affinity for peripheral rather than central histamine receptors.

Clinical studies to date involving astemizole and terfenadine are relatively few, but are encouraging in that there appear to be remarkably few central side effects, and, that clinical H_1 antihistaminic efficacy (against seasonal hay fever, e.g.) is adequate. Final dosage strengths, indications, length of therapy, etc. are yet to be firmly established for either drug. Preliminary tolerance tests involving a battery of performance studies (visual-motor coordination, arithmetic ability, and digit symbol substitution) tested after astemizole (10 and 20 mg), terfenadine (60 mg), and triprolidine (10 mg sustained release) — each against placebo — have shown that the newer H_1 antagonists were essentially devoid of any effect on performance, while triprolidine caused a significant decrement in performance which lasted nearly four to five hours.

Another English clinical study compared terfenadine (60 mg twice daily) to 8 mg twice daily of chlorpheniramine (the most commonly used H_1 antagonist in the U.K. and generally considered not so prone to produce drowsiness), and to placebo in patients over twelve years old with active allergic rhinitis. One hundred thirty-two (132) patients in this one week test completed the trial and could be evaluated for side effects. Drowsiness and sleepiness, graded moderate to severe, occurred in only one patient on terfenadine (2%), in two patients on placebo (4%), but in 25% of the patients receiving chlorpheniramine.

Pharmacokinetically, the new H_1 antagonists offer equal if not superior characteristics for the patient and clinician. Terfenadine is rapidly absorbed, reaching a peak concentration in one to two hours. It is extensively metabolized in the liver, and has an elimination half-life of 16 to 23 hours, which permits convenient twice a day dosing. Of the newer H_1 antagonists, terfenadine is apparently the only one to have been studied in children under twelve, and an oral suspension is currently being investigated.

Astemizole is very interesting in a pharmacokinetic sense, exhibiting rapid absorption (time-to-peak, one hour), and is very slowly eliminated, with an elimination half-life of 104 hours, permitting the current dosing schedule of 10 mg once daily.

Finally, a new phenothiazine, mequitazine, has acceptable H_1 antagonism, minimal anticholinergic effects, and reasonable potency (5 mg dose). It crosses the blood brain barrier with difficulty, and preferentially occupies peripheral receptors, which apparently accounts for its low sedation.

NEWER H_2 ANTAGONISTS

The discovery in 1972 by Black and colleagues of agents which preferentially blocked gastric secretion, and other histaminergic responses refractory to traditional antihistamines, began a breakthrough in both clinical treatment, and pharmacological investigation of the H_2 receptor. The first examples of H_2 blockers, burimamide and metiamide, contained the imidazole structure characteristic of histamine, and a side chain incorporating a thiourea moiety; the imidazole moiety was believed to confer the H_2 specificity. Competitive inhibition of gastric acid secretion was demonstrated with these agents, including secretory effects induced by gastrin. Early on, fortunately, it was found that metiamide caused agranulocytosis and human testing was abandoned.

The important therapeutic breakthrough came with the introduction of cimetidine, which retained the imidazole moiety of histamine, but replaced the thiourea portion of the side chain with a cyanoguanidine. The successful use of cimetidine in peptic ulcer disease in the past six years requires little further comment, with the notable exception that its extensive worldwide use over these years has uncovered a number of infrequent, yet unpleasant side effects. These include antiandrogenic effects, CNS confusion (especially in the elderly), and inhibition of hepatic microsomal metabolism of a number of drugs, including benzodiazepines, theophylline, phenytoin, warfarin, lidocaine, and some beta-blockers.

Ranitidine, a very recent and efficacious entrant into the H_2 antagonist market, appears at this time to be devoid of many of the adverse effects associated with cimetidine. Apparently, the binding of ranitidine to androgen receptors, and to the P-450 hepatic microsomal enzyme sites is much less than with cimetidine, and to date, adverse effects have been few.

Ranitidine has a major structural difference from cimetidine, in that the substituted imidazole ring has been replaced with a furan. It thus appears that the imidazole moiety, common to both histamine and cimetidine, is not obligatory for H_2 specificity. Therapeutically, ranitidine has performed equally with cimetidine, but at lower doses and with less frequent dosing, and with many fewer adverse effects. On a molar basis, ranitidine is estimated to be four to nine times as potent as cimetidine. However, more extensive use of ranitidine in the future may uncover different, and perhaps more serious, adverse reactions.

An H_2 blocker chemically similar to cimetidine, still in investigational stages, is SKF 92994, or oxmetidine. It differs from cimetidine primarily in having an isocytosine ring instead of a cyanoguanidine group as a side chain. It appears to work as well as cimetidine in treating duodenal ulcer in the few studies so far published. There are major pharmacokinetic differences compared to cimetidine, however: total systemic clearance is less than cimetidine, and non-renal clearance is much greater (4% renal vs 60% for cimetidine). Oxmetidine is metabolized primarily by glucuronidation, whereas cimetidine is metabolized only to a small extent, and by sulfoxidation. Consequently, oxmetidine is almost completely metabolized and dependent on the intrinsic capacity of the liver. What, if any, therapeutic implications this may ultimately have remains to be seen.

OTHER ANTI-SECRETORY AGENTS

The parietal cell contains surface receptors for acetylcholine and gastrin, in addition to the H_2 histamine receptor. Anticholinergic therapy has long been a mainstay, albeit a relatively ineffective sole therapy for hypersecretory states. Some recent studies, primarily from the U.K. and Scandinavia, have stimulated interest in the use of an older class of drugs, which at first thought might seem an odd candidate for peptic ulcer disease. The tricyclic antidepressants, especially trimipramine and doxepin, have shown a remarkable *in vitro* ability to antagonize the histamine receptors, both H_1 and H_2. It is perhaps easily forgotten that imipramine and its congeners were originally classified as antihistamines; however, the discovery of the effectiveness of tricyclic structures as neuroleptics, and then as antidepressants, apparently overshadowed further pursuit of these compounds as antihistamines.

The tricyclic antidepressants are potent anticholinergics also, especially at the high doses occasionally required for antidepressant therapy, and this may be contributory to their apparent success in peptic ulcer disease. However, the potent H_1 and H_2 blocking activity demonstrated in *in vitro* animal brain models infers that antihistamine effects *per se* are more contributory. Trimipramine and doxepin have been shown to be more effective than placebo, and equipotent to cimetidine, in peptic ulcer disease in a number of European studies. Doses of the tricyclics used were considerably less than those used for depression: 100 or 50 mg h.s. A recent American study utilized doses of doxepin of 100 mg at h.s. in 12 patients with duodenal ulcer and one with an anastomotic ulcer. Eight of these patients had not responded to eight weeks of treatment with cimetidine and/or antacids. All 13 patients responded well to doxepin.

The precise mechanism of the apparent success of the tricyclics is uncertain; it is known however, that their inhibitory effect on acid secretion is small when compared to cimetidine. One major deterrent to unequivocal elucidation of the efficacy of the tricyclics is the difficulty in designing double-blind studies, due to their sedative and anticholinergic effects.

A new tricyclic antimuscarinic agent, pirenzepine, has been shown in foreign trials to be as effective as cimetidine in treatment of duodenal ulcers, at doses of 100 to 150 mg daily. Pirenzepine significantly suppresses basal, pentagastrin-stimulated, and insulin-stimulated acid secretion in a dose-related manner. In contrast to atropine and other anticholinergic drugs, pirenzepine is relatively selective for cholinergic receptors in the gastrointestinal tract, which avoids numerous adverse effects. None of the tricyclic drugs mentioned are approved for use in peptic ulcer disease in the United States.

Prostaglandins E_1 and A_1 are known to consistently reduce basal and stimulated acid secretion, but they are effective only when given intravenously. Methylated analogues (15, 15-dimethyl prostaglandin E_2, e.g.) however, are effective orally and cause an 80-90% inhibition of acid production. The mechanism of action of the prostaglandins is uncertain, but may involve stimulation of mucus production, or tightening of the gastric mucosal barrier.

Finally, drugs that inhibit the final common end point of stimulation of the parietal cell membrane receptors for histamine, acetylcholine, and gastrin — namely, secretion of the hydrogen ion — show great promise in treating hypersecretory states. The substituted benzimidazoles act as inhibitors of K^+ — H^+ ATPase. Animal studies have shown these drugs to be effective in inhibiting acid secretion stimulated by pentagastrin, histamine or vagal stimulation. Small clinical trials have begun with omeprazole, and have shown it to be an effective, potent, inhibitor of gastric acid secretion. A recent English study reported the results of a week long trial of 30 mg, once daily omeprazole in nine duodenal ulcer patients. Gastric acidity was virtually eliminated in all patients, with the median 24 hour intragastric pH rising from 1.4 to 5.3, while the mean hourly hydrogen ion activity fell from 38.5 to 1.95 mEq per liter. No unwanted side effects were observed in this brief trial. However, a recent Swedish investigation noted small transient rises in serum alanine aminotransferase (AAT) levels in some of their patients, and one patient was withdrawn from their trial because of a pronounced rise in AAT. Whether omeprazole was a causal factor will have to await further investigation.

INHIBITORS OF HISTAMINE RELEASE

The standard drug for suppression of mediator release from mast cells is cromolyn sodium (disodium cromoglycate). DSCG also is reported to block exercise-induced bronchospasm, as well as sulfur dioxide-induced bronchoconstriction, where mediator release may not be implicated. A major limitation to DSCG therapy has been that the only effective route of administration is insufflation, which many patients find uncomfortable. More recently developed drugs show therapeutic promise, and are effective by the oral route. Ketotifen is one such new oral antiasthmatic which has shown impressive antianaphylactic action, as well as antihistaminic action, in animal studies. Variable results as an asthma prophylactic reported in human studies may be a result of inadequate doses, or inadequate treatment time. The drug is very potent, however, one or two milligram doses being commonly used. Ketotifen has potent H_1 antagonism properties also, but appears to be devoid of anticholinergic activity. Consequently, its precise mode of action in the asthmatic remains uncertain. Clinical trials comparing ketotifen to DSCG, as well as to placebo, have produced equivocal results, but differing methodology makes comparison of the studies difficult. There is no question, however, that *in vitro* results have shown ketotifen to be a very potent antiasthmatic.

Oxatomide is another new oral antiasthmatic, effective in suppressing histamine release in hypersensitivity states. Preliminary studies indicate that it also antagonizes the effects of histamine, 5-HT and SRS-A. It might, therefore, prove to be of particular value in patients with both asthma and perennial rhinitis. A recent long term (52 weeks) clinical trial of oxatomide *vs* placebo in 60 patients with asthma, with or without perennial rhinitis, showed no statistical improvement over placebo, but there was a reduction in the use of bronchodilators, and in the symptoms of asthma and rhinitis for the oxatomide patients. Side effects most often seen were the (expected) drowsiness, and weight gain, perhaps a result of the anti-serotonin properties of oxatomide. Finally, a new benzothiazolinone derivative, tiaramide, has already been introduced in Japan. Tiaramide 200 mg tested against placebo in 12 adults successfully prevented a post-exercise (treadmill) fall in lung function associated with exercise-induced asthma; no side effects were reported in this brief trial.

The next few years may witness a plentitude of newer drugs being introduced to tame the multisystem effects seen when receptors for the ubiquitous hormone, histamine, are stimulated.

SELECTED REFERENCES

Historical Development of the Antihistamines

1. Douglas WW. Histamine and antihistamines; 5-hydroxytryptamine and antagonists. In Goodman LS, Gilman A (eds.) The pharmacological basis of therapeutics. 5th ed. New York: Macmillan 590, 1975.

Astemizole and Terenadine

2. Backhouse CI, Brewster BS, Lockhart JDF et al. Terfenadine in allergic rhinitis. A comparative trial of a new antihistamine versus chlorpheniramine and placebo. Practitioner 226:347-351, 1982.
3. Callier J, Engelen RF, Zanniello I et al. Astemizole [R43 512] in the treatment of hay fever, an international double-blind study comparing a weekly treatment (10 mg and 25 mg) with a placebo. Curr Ther Res 29:24-35, 1981.
4. Nicholson AN. Antihistamines and sedation. Lancet 2:211-212, 1983.
5. Nicholson AN, Stone BM. Performance studies with the H_1-histamine receptor antagonists, astemizole and terfenadine. Br J Clin Pharmacol 13:199-202, 1982.

H_2 Antagonists

6. Gugler R, Rohner HG, Somogyi AA. Gastric acid inhibition and oxmetidine kinetics in duodenal ulcer. Clin Pharmacol Ther 31:501-508, 1982.
7. Pando SJ. Treatment of gastric acid hypersecretion, pp 66-70. In: Jensen RT, moderator. Zollinger-Ellison syndrome: current concepts and management. Ann Intern Med 98:59-75, 1983.
8. Sorkin EM, Darvey DL. Review of cimetidine drug interactions. Drug Intell Clin Pharm 17:110-120, 1983.
9. Strum WB. Ranitidine. JAMA 250:1894-1896, 1983.
10. Zeldis JB, Friedman LS, Isselbacher KJ. Ranitidine: a new H_2-receptor antagonist. N Engl J Med; 309:1368-1373, 1983.

Other Anti-Secretory Agents

11. Berardi RR, Caplan NB. Agents with tricyclic structure for treating peptic ulcer disease. Clin Pharm 2:425-431, 1983 (47 Ref.).
12. Gustavsson S, Adami HO, Loof L et al. rapid healing of duodenal ulcers with omeprazole: double-blind dose-comparative trial. Lancet 2:124-125, 1983.
13. Lewis JH. Treatment of gastric ulcer. What is old and what is

new. Arch Intern Med 143:264-274, 1983 (132 Ref.).
14. Mangla JC, Pereira M. Tricyclic antidepressants in the treatment of peptic ulcer disease. Arch Intern Med 142:273-275, 1982.
15. Moshal MG, Spitael JM, Khan F et al. Pirenzepine, cimetidine and placebo in the long-term treatment of duodenal ulceration. A comparative study. S Afr Med J 62:12-14, 1982.
16. Richelson E. The use of tricyclic antidepressants in chronic gastrointestinal pain. J Clin Psychiatry 43(8 pt 2):50-55, 1982.
17. Richelson E. Tricyclic antidepressants and histamine H_1 receptors. Mayo Clin Proc 54:669-674, 1979.
18. Ruud TE, Hoff GS, Tonder M et al. Doxepin and cimetidine in the treatment of duodenal ulcer; an open clinical and endoscopic study. J Clin Psychiatry 43(8 pt 2):56-60, 1982. Adapted from Hoff GS et al. Scand J Gastroenterol 16:1041-1042, 1981.
19. Somerville KW, Langman MJS. Newer antisecretory agents for peptic ulcer. Drugs 25:315-330, 1983 (116 Ref.).
20. Walt RP, Gomes MFA, Wood EC et al. Effect of daily oral omeprazole on 24 hour intragastric acidity. Br Med J 287:12-14, 1983.

Inhibitors of Histamine Release
21. Flenley DC. New drugs in respiratory disorders: I. Br Med J 286:871-875, 1983 (76 Ref.).
22. Phillips MJ, Meyrick Thomas RH, Moodley I et al. A comparison of the *in vivo* effects of ketotifen, clemastine, chlorpheniramine and sodium cromoglycate on histamine and allergen induced weals in human skin. Br J Clin Pharmacol 15:277-286, 1983.
23. Sears MR. A double-blind comparison of ketotifen and disodium cromoglycate in atopic adult asthmatics. Clin Allergy 13:253-262, 1983.
24. Turner-Warwick M (for Brompton Hospital/Medical Research Council Collaborative Trial). A controlled trial of oxatomide in the treatment of asthma with or without perennial rhinitis. Clin Allergy 11:483-490, 1981. □

Chapter XVII

Treatment of Allergic Rhinitis with a New Selective H_1 Antihistamine: Terfenadine

C. Edward Buckley III, M.D.,° Stephen J. Klemawesch, M.D., Stephen K. Lucas, M.D.

ABSTRACT

The effectiveness of 60 mg b.i.d. of a novel antihistamine, terfenadine, was compared with an active control, 4 mg t.i.d. of chlorpheniramine, and placbo in 560 patients with seasonal allergic rhinitis. In contrast to the gradual decrease in seasonal symptoms observed over a 7 day period of study in placebo-treated patients, both antihistamines produced a prompt significant decrease in sneezing and rhinorrhea, and a gradual decrease in nasopharyngeal pruritis. Terfenadine-related sedation did not differ from that produced by the placebo and was less than the sedation produced by the active control.

INTRODUCTION

Seasonal pollen-induced allergic rhinitis is a significant source of morbidity among an estimated 19,000,000 persons each year.[1] Hay fever is especially distressing to patients who must rely on cognitive and communication skills, such as college students, who try to maintain normal scholastic activities despite the pollen seasons at the beginning and end of each school year. Pollen avoidance is impossible. The side effects of antihistamine therapy are often inconsistent with a reasonable quality of life. Antihistamine-induced drowsiness and airway dryness can be worse than the disease. The physician must frequently use pollen immunotherapy to control the patient's symptoms. Pharmacologic research has identified a potential solution for this problem.[2] Recent structural modifications of antihistamines and studies of the biologic properties of modified compounds suggest it is possible to reduce the soporific and anti-cholinergic side effects and retain pharmacologic effectiveness.

A novel antihistamine with these properties, terfenadine,[3] became available for renewed clinical trials in the United States in early 1982. Separate multi-centric studies of spring and fall allergic rhinitis were conducted. A population of perceptive college and graduate students with seasonal allergic rhinitis and an interest in the side effects of antihistamine therapy provided a unique opportunity to participate in this investigation. This report compares our local spring and fall experience with that of investigators at the other sites in each respective study and summarizes our collective experience with terfenadine in patients with seasonal allergic rhinitis.

METHODS

Patients. The study subjects were informed patients with a history of antihistamine responsive spring and/or fall allergic rhinitis and seasonal symptoms of two or

---

Departments of Medicine and Microbiology-Immunology, Duke University, Durham, North Carolina

---

°Corresponding author:
P.O. Box 3804, Duke Medical Center, Durham, NC 27710.
Presented at National Symposium on H_1 and H_2 Histamine Receptors, Brown University and Rhode Island Hospital, Providence, Rhode Island 02902, December 7, 1983.
Supported by a grant from: Merrell-Dow Pharmaceuticals, Inc. 2110 E. Galbraith Road, Cinn., Ohio 45215.

more years duration. Prior to entry into the study, each patient had positive skin tests to relevant spring or fall pollens and two or more symptoms and/or physical findings consistent with mild to severe allergic rhinitis and/or allergic conjunctivitis. Patients with respiratory infection and those with very severe allergic symptoms requiring progressive immunotherapy, systemic or inhaled corticosteroid therapy were excluded.

Design. The patients were entered into a randomized, parallel, double-blind comparison of three treatments: the experimental antihistamine; a positive antihistamine control; and, placebo. Each treatment was provided in the form of individually prepackaged doses mounted on a card. The packaged medications were designed to be taken three times daily for a period of seven days. The 60 mg unit dose of terfenadine was packaged for a b.i.d. delivery with placebo interposed between the active drug at noon. The 4 mg unit dose of chlorpheniramine, the active control medication, was packaged for a t.i.d. schedule. Identical placebo tablets were also packaged for a t.i.d. schedule. Treatment was initiated with the dose of medication due following the time of entry on the first day of therapy. Patients were requested to retain and not use overlooked doses of medication on their treatment cards. All unused medications were returned at the conclusion of the study.

Study Parameters. The observations summarized in this report were three symptoms of allergic rhinitis: rhinorrhea, sneezing, and nasopharyngeal pruritis. Each symptom was ranked as absent, mild, moderate or severe. Physician investigators evaluated each parameter prior to and after completion of treatment. Patients evaluated and scored each study parameter on a diary card at the end of each treatment day. Physician investigators also rated the overall outcome of treatment as worse, none, slight, moderate, marked or complete relief of symptoms at the end of the study. Patients rated their overall degree of symptomatic relief in terms of whether or not they would choose to use their particular treatment again for control of allergic rhinitis. The physician recorded all possible adverse effects that occurred during treatment at the final visit.

Analysis of Observations. All observations were collected and evaluated in order to assure completeness and adequacy for comparisons of drug efficacy. Separate summary tables were prepared of (a) all observations in order to assess drug safety and (b) observations considered adequate for comparisons of efficacy. For the purpose of this report, additional contingency tables were prepared in order to compare local observations with observations from the other study sites for each respective multicentric study. Local observations were verified from retained study records. All observations from the spring and fall collaborative studies were used in order to focus on the total experience with terfenadine in patients with seasonal allergic rhinitis.

Investigators at one site of a multicentric study have personal knowledge only of their own patients. This number of patients seen is usually too small to reliably corroborate or discard judgments about the outcome of the novel treatment. Our strategy in the evaluation of observations was focused on two concerns: (a) the effect of the experimental treatment; and (b) differences between the local site and the other study sites, e.g. the reproducibility of the findings. In making this assessment, we ignored prior assumptions about the respective study designs and separate analyses of the respective spring and fall studies. We independently evaluated all observations pertaining to allergic rhinitis in order to determine (a) whether or not detectable differences existed among the three treatments and (b) whether or not observations made at the local study site differed from those obtained by collaborating investigators. Tests of hypotheses were based on values of chi-squared and analyses of variance of contingency tables having two or more main effects.[4] The reliability of observed differences was accepted when the null hypothesis could be rejected with reasonable confidence ($p \leq 0.05$).

RESULTS

Review of the records of the 641 patients entered into the spring and fall collaborative multi-center studies of spring and fall allergic rhinitis revealed 81 (12.6%) patients whose records were not adequate for evaluation of efficacy. Failure to take the study medications and/or return within the specified time for evaluation was the cause of exclusion of 43 (6.6%) patients. The development of an intercurrent infection led to the exclusion of 26 (4.1%) of the patients. The inappropriate use of other antihistamines, decongestants or corticosteroids by 12 (1.9%) was the cause of exclusion of the remaining patients. This review process yielded 560 patients whose records were considered adequate for evaluation of the effect of antihistamine therapy. Safety evaluations were based on observations in all 637 patients; four patients were lost to follow-up after entry into the study.

Randomization and the exclusion of patients in whom interpretable observations were not available yielded 182 (32.5%) patients in the terfenadine treatment group, 190 (33.9%) patients in the chlorpheniramine treatment group, and 188 (33.5%) patients in the placebo treatment group. Table 1 summarizes the demographic characteristics of the study population. The ages of the 335 male and 225 female patients within the treatment groups were comparable and ranged from 12-80 years with a mean and standard deviation for all subjects of 30.8 ± 10.6 years. Differences among the subjects randomized into each treatment group with respect to race and sex were

Table I

Demographic Characteristics of Study Subjects

		Terfenadine	Chlorpheniramine	Placebo
Total Subjects		182	190	188
Age, years	Average	31.6	30.2	30.2
	S.D.	±11.6	±9.9	±10.1
Race	Cauc.	164	169	168
	Neg.	13	13	12
	Other	5	8	8
Sex	Female	74	69	82
	Male	108	121	106

Table II

Clinical Characteristics of Study Subjects

		Terfenadine	Chlorpheniramine	Placebo
Onset of First Episode of Allergic Rhinitis, years	Average	16.2	15.4	15.5
	S.D.	±6.9	±6.2	±6.7
Successive Years of Symptoms	Average	14.2	13.3	14.3
	S.D.	±6.6	±6.0	±6.8
Prior Immunotherapy	Percent	27.4	31.5	26.6
Duration of Present Episode, days	Average	5.7	6.0	7.4
	S.D.	±3.2	±3.5	±6.9
Current Drug Therapy	Percent	28.0	30.5	34.0

small and not significant. The mean age and standard error of the mean of the 58 locally studied patients was 28.00±0.54 years. This contrasted with a mean age and standard error of the mean of 31.08±0.45 years for the 502 patients studied at the other sites in each respective study. The small difference between the two mean ages was significant and suggests the average age of locally studied college and graduate student patients was less than patients studied elsewhere.

Table 2 summarizes the characteristics of the disease observed in the patients studied. The onset of symptoms of seasonal allergic rhinitis averaged 15.8 years prior to beginning the study; seasonal symptoms had persisted an average of 13.9 years during this interval. Allergen immunotherapy had been used previously by 28% of the patients and 31.9% had used other symptomatic medications for control of current symptoms during the 6.4 average number of days prior to entry into the study. Differences among the treatment groups in the number of patients having prior immunotherapy and need for current medications were small and not significant. The observations summarized in Table 1 & 2 suggest that the demographic characteristics and prior history of seasonal rhinitis were comparable among the three treatment groups.

Tables 3-5 summarize the evidence of the effectiveness of terfenadine and the positive control antihistamine in the treatment of seasonal allergic rhinitis. All 560 patients were categorized with respect to (a) the ranking indicated in each summary table, (b) their treatment group and (c) whether or not they were evaluated locally or at one of the other sites in the respective spring and fall studies. All contingency tables were analyzed in order to deduce whether the observations made at our local site differed significantly from those of other collaborating investigators and whether differences existed among the three forms of treatment. With the exception of comparisons based on the symptom scores provided by the patients on

Table III

Physicians Evaluation of Spring and Fall Hay Fever Symptoms

Symptom	Group	Percent of Patients with Moderate To Severe Symptoms	
		Pre-Treatment	Post-Treatment
Rhinorrhea	Terfenadine	67.0	22.5
	Chlorpheniramine	62.1	13.7
	Placebo	67.5	28.7
Sneezing	Terfenadine	45.6	10.4
	Chlorpheniramine	54.2	10.5
	Placebo	43.6	20.2
Pruritis	Terfenadine	45.6	15.9
	Chlorpheniramine	44.7	13.1
	Placebo	39.4	19.1

Table IV

Overall Evaluation of Efficacy of Terfenadine

Treatment	Percent of Patients With Slight To Complete Relief	Percent of Patients Who Would Use The Medication Again
Terfenadine	82.5	62.6
Chlorpheniramine	85.3	65.3
Placebo	60.1	39.9

all seven days of treatment (Table 5), differences related to the site at which the patients were studied were not significant and are not presented in the summary tables.

Separate contingency tables were prepared from the physicians' estimates of severity of illness before and after treatment. The patients were categorized as having either absent to mild, or moderate to severe sneezing, rhinorrhea, and nasopharyngeal pruritis. Each contingency table was evaluated and used to prepare the summary presented in Table 3, where the trends and differences in the severity among the three symptoms are presented as the proportion of patients with moderate to severe symptoms. Prior to treatment, the physicians detected highly significant variation between the different symptoms used to estimate the severity of the disease ($p \leq 0.0001$). The physicians identified rhinorrhea as more severe than sneezing and nasopharyngeal pruritis. Pre-treatment estimates of differences in symptoms related to the assignment to treatment groups ($p \leq 0.3211$) were small and not significant. This suggests the physicians' overall pre-treatment estimates of the severity of symptoms were comparable in all three treatment groups.

Despite the reduction in symptoms on treatment, the physicians were able to detect significant post-treatment differences in the relative severity of the three symptoms ($p \leq 0.0001$). Rhinorrhea remained the most severe symptom. Following antihistamine therapy, the physicians' observed a 44.5-48.4% reduction in the prevalence of moderate to severe rhinorrhea, a 35.2-43.7% reduction in sneezing, and a 29.7-31.6% reduction in nasopharyngeal pruritis. Following placebo therapy, the physicians detected a 38.8% reduction in moderate to severe rhinorrhea, a 23.4% reduction in sneezing, and a 20.3% reduction in nasopharyngeal pruritis. The post-treatment differences in the severity of symptoms related to assignment to the three treatment groups were highly significant ($p \leq 0.0001$). This suggests that the physicians were able to identify a clinically significant change in the patient's symptoms on antihistamine therapy.

Additional contingency tables were prepared respec-

Table V

Summary of Patients Daily Evaluation of 3 Symptoms*

— Main Effects —		Moderate to Severe Symptoms, Percent of All Observations	p≤
Site of Study	Local	22.8	0.0002
	Others	29.4	
Symptoms	Sneezing	25.4	0.0001
	Pruritis	26.7	
	Rhinorrhea	33.9	
Day of Treatment	Day 1	41.9	0.0001
	Day 2	81.0	
	Day 3	27.6	
	Day 4	24.5	
	Day 5	25.9	
	Day 6	24.7	
	Day 7	24.1	
Treatment	Terfenadine	25.5	0.0001
	Chlorpheniramine	24.4	
	Placebo	36.1	

* *An analysis of variance was done on a contingency table categorizing patients with respect to either absent to mild symptoms or with respect to moderate to severe symptoms. The percentages represent the portion of observations of symptoms ranked as moderate to severe during the 7 day treatment period (see text).*

tively from the results of the physician's overall evaluation of the effectiveness of treatment and from the patient's stated desire to use the medication again. The results of evaluation of both contingency tables are summarized in Table 4. In the physician's assessment, the patients were categorized either as exhibiting no improvement, or slight to complete relief. Physicians estimated that 82.5-85.3% of the patients obtained slight to complete relief on antihistamine therapy. In contrast, this estimate was made in only 60.1% of the patients on placebo therapy. Overall, the physicians detected highly significant differences between the three forms of treatment ($p \leq 0.0001$). In the evaluation of the patient's assessment, each subject was categorized with respect to their desire to use their particular medication again. Among the patients, 62.6-65.3% of those receiving the antihistamines desired to use the medication again, while only 39.9% wanted to use the placebo again. The difference among the three treatments was also highly significant ($p \leq 0.0001$). Table 4 suggests that differences between the placebo and the two antihistamines accounted for these findings. The observations summarized in Table 4 reveal that the physicians and the patients agreed in their overall assessment of the effectiveness of terfenadine and the active control medication.

The patient's daily evaluation of the symptoms of allergic rhinitis yielded a much more complex contingency table. Each patient recorded symptom scores for rhinorrhea, sneezing and nasopharyngeal pruritis for a minimum of seven days of treatment. The scores for each symptom were categorized in one of two categories, either absent to mild, or moderate to severe. Inspection of this table identified possible differences in the relative severity of symptoms based on four independent sources of variation: (a) the study site, (b) the particular symptom, (c) the day of the observation, and (d) the experimental treatment group. Table 5 summarizes the evaluation of these four sources of variation. Differences related to the site of study were evaluated as the number of times each symptom was ranked in one of the two categories of severity, by summing over all symptoms, days and treatments. Differences among the three symptoms were evaluated as the number of times each symptom was ranked in the two categories of severity, by summing over all days, sites and treatment groups. Differences in the daily variation of the symptoms were evaluated by summing the two categories of severity on each day over all symptoms, sites and treatment groups.

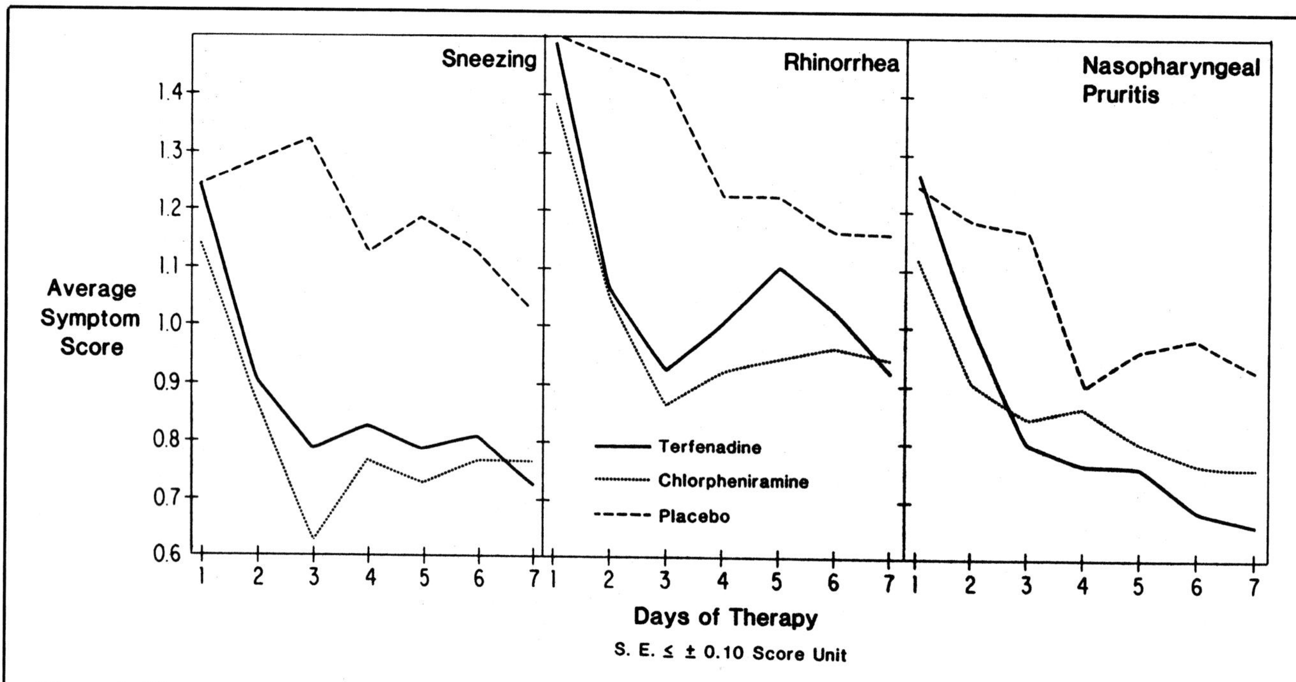

Figure 1. The average symptom scores for sneezing, rhinorrhea and nasopharyngeal pruritis in 560 patients with seasonal allergic rhinitis changed during seven days of observation. The patients' symptoms were assigned a numerical value of 0 if absent, one if mild, two if moderate and three if severe. Scores for each treatment group (terfenadine, chlorpheniramine, placebo) were averaged by day of the study. Patients treated with placebo exhibited a gradual decrease in their symptoms, changes consistent with the seasonal nature of the illness. Patients treated with terfenadine and the active control antihistamine, chlorpheniramine, noted a prompt and persisting decrease in sneezing and rhinorrhea by the second and third days of treatment and a gradual decline in nasopharyngeal pruritis during the seven day course of therapy. The differences between terfenadine and the positive control antihistamine were small and not significant.

Differences among patients treated with terfenadine, the active control antihistamine and placebo, were evaluated by summing categories of severity over all symptoms, days and sites of study. Table 5 presents the comparisons of these four main sources of variation as the percentage of reports of moderate to severe symptoms. The estimates of the significance of the differences compared in Table 5 are based on values of chi-squared obtained from the contingency table and an analysis of variance.

Although the 6.6% difference between the 22.8% occurrence of moderate to severe symptoms in the local college and graduate student population and the 29.4% occurrence in patients studied at other sites was small, the site-related effect was significant ($p \leq 0.0002$). Overall our local patient population ranked their symptoms as less severe than patients at the other study sites. This suggests the method used to evaluate symptoms and the analysis of observations was sensitive to differences between the local site and all other study sites. The patients also reported significant differences in severity among the three symptoms ($p \leq 0.0001$). Rhinorrhea was ranked as moderate to severe 33.9% of the time. This compared with the 25.4% occurrence of moderate to severe sneezing and 26.7% occurrence of moderate to severe nasopharyngeal pruritis. Significant daily variation ($p \leq 0.0001$) in the severity of symptoms occurred over the treatment period. The overall occurrence of moderate to severe symptoms decreased from 41.9% on the first day to 24.1% on the seventh day of treatment. The site-related variation, the differences in severity among the three symptoms and the daily variation in the symptoms were not unexpected. The effect of these three extraneous sources of independent variation was identified and distinguished from the effects of antihistamine and placebo treatment. Highly significant treatment-group-related differences were detected in the occurrence of moderate to severe symptoms of allergic rhinitis ($p \leq 0.0001$). The 25.5% occurrence of moderate to severe symptoms in the terfenadine-treated group was approximately equivalent to the 24.4% occurrence of similar symptoms in the patients treated with chlorpheniramine. The 36.1% occurrence of moderate to severe symptoms in the

Table VI

Antihistamine Sedation and Dryness

Treatment Group	Sample Size	Sedation No.	Sedation %	Dryness No.	Dryness %
Terfenadine	213	12	5.6	7	3.3
Chlorpheniramine	217	32	14.7	7	3.2
Placebo	211	5	2.4	4	1.9

placebo-treated group was greater than the frequency of similar symptoms in both antihistamine-treated groups.

Although the observations summarized in Table 5 reveal that highly significant differences could be detected in the severity of symptoms related to antihistamine therapy, the summary percentages presented do not provide a clear understanding of how the symptoms in the three treatment groups varied over the course of treatment. This information is shown in Figure 1, which summarizes and describes the average effect of each treatment on the symptoms of all 560 patients with spring and fall allergic rhinitis. The averaged scores in Figure 1 were obtained directly from the primary data tabulated by each patient on the daily diary card. Even though the daily symptoms scores were not normally distributed, the standard error of each averaged daily score was less than ±0.1 symptom score unit. This observation and the comparisons presented in Table 5 suggest confidence can be placed in the differences described in Figure 1.

Using this conservative criteria to evaluate the averaged symptom scores, Figure 1 reveals several interesting highly significant trends. First, highly significant variation in the primary symptoms of allergic rhinitis occurred over the seven days of observation. This included a gradual decrease in the symptoms of patients treated with the placebo. This observation is consistent with the transient seasonal nature of the natural history of spring and fall allergic rhinitis. The observations in the placebo group suggest the experimental treatment was initiated close to the onset of the symptoms. A second interesting finding can be deduced from a comparison of the symptom scores of terfenadine and chlorpheniramine-treated patients with one another and with the placebo-treated patients. In comparison to the placebo, treatment with both antihistamines had a significant effect on sneezing, rhinorrhea and nasopharyngeal pruritis. By inspection, this effect of treatment was detectable by the second day of treatment, became maximum by the third day and remained essentially unchanged thereafter. Averaged symptom scores in the antihistamine-treated patients remained less than in the placebo-treated controls throughout the study. The maximum immediate effect of antihistamine therapy noted by the patients was a decrease in the severity of sneezing. The modest decrease in nasopharyngeal pruritis appeared to take longer. Finally, Figure 1 reveals no remarkable differences between the averaged scores of patients treated with the two antihistamines. This suggests the effect of terfenadine therapy on the symptoms of seasonal allergic rhinitis was comparable to the therapeutic effect of the positive control.

Table 6 summarizes the reports of the relative incidence of side effects of antihistamine therapy in 637 of the 641 patients. Reports of sedation occurred in 14.7% of the patients receiving the active control medication, in 5.7% of the patients taking terfenadine, and in 2.4% of the patients on the placebo. The relative incidence of sedation on chlorpheniramine, the active control medication, was significantly greater than with the placebo (chi-squared = 20.751, $p \leq 0.0001$) and terfenadine (chi-squared = 9.718, $p \leq 0.0022$). Differences in the relative incidence of sedation between terfenadine and the placebo were small and not significant (chi-squared = 2.934, $p \leq 0.0828$). Dryness was reported in 1.9% of patients on the placebo and on 3.2-3.3% of the patients receiving the antihistamines; these differences were small and not significant.

DISCUSSION

The three symptoms of seasonal allergic rhinitis selected for evaluation in this report clearly provide reliable clinical evidence of the activity of histamine in the nasopharynx of patients. This observation is consistent with prior observations.[2] The summarized observations indicate that terfenadine therapy provides effective control of these symptoms. The data presented in Tables 3-5 and Figure 1 reveal that the efficacy of terfenadine therapy did not differ from the positive control antihistamine, chlorpheniramine. In contrast to the positive control, terfenadine produced significantly less sedation.

The clinical utility of terfenadine stems from the needs of patients who become impaired on conventional antihistamine therapy. Side effects, such as drowsiness, are a source of morbidity. Psychophysiologic studies suggest terfenadine causes no significant impairment of central nervous system function.[5]

Terfenadine is a novel piperidine-type antihistamine.[3] The structural basis for terfenadine's lack of side effects may reside in the tertiary butyl group and hydroxyl group proximate to the phenyl ring.[6] The tertiary butyl group may retard the ability of terfenadine to pass the blood brain barrier. Perhaps the most compelling demonstration of the compound's inability to reach central nervous system tissues can been seen in studies of the distribution of radiolabeled drug in experimental animals. Autoradiographs of sagittal sections of frozen rats reveal no appreciable evidence of the compound in the brain and other neural tissues.[7] The relative absence of drowsiness detected in these studies of seasonal allergic rhinitis suggests terfenadine will be useful in those patients who are impaired by the side effects of available antihistamines.

The persistence of terfenadine in blood and other body tissues permits the twice daily dose schedule used in these studies.[8] Studies of the plasma concentration of terfenadine reveal the half-lfe of the rapid alpha phase of drug distribution is 3.6 hours; the more prolonged beta phase varies between 16.1-22.7 hours[9]. The studies of seasonal allergic rhinitis presented in this report suggest the antihistaminic activity of terfenadine taken twice daily was not different from chlorpheniramine taken three times each day. The ability to use terfenadine on a morning and evening schedule should facilitate compliance and improve the outcome of antihistamine therapy. Despite this advantage, terfenadine-induced inhibition of histamine-provoked skin wheals appears to decrease by 24 hours and subside by 48 hours.[10] If this desirable property can be documented for flare and wheal of the allergen-induced skin test, terfenadine could be extremely useful to the physician who wishes to skin test the patient with severe allergic rhinitis shortly after pharmacologic therapy of the acute symptoms.

The primary goal of a multi-centric study of a novel therapy is the rapid acquisition of more observations than could be obtained at a single study site. Secondary goals, such as the extent to which the outcome varies over time, the age and sex of the patients studied, and the study site are often ignored. From the perspective of the patient and the physician, this additional information could be very important. For example, evaluation of the small overall site-related decrease in the ranking of the severity of symptoms by our local population of predominantly college and graduate students revealed several interesting findings. First, the average ranking of all symptoms was slightly more severe during the spring season than at all other sites. In contrast, the average ranking of all symptoms was much less severe during the fall season than at all other sites. These trends were consistent with increased rainfall and an abortive ragweed season in the piedmont region of North Carolina during the fall study. Seasonal site-related differences of this type are not unexpected in multicentric studies of antihistamines. Second, the average ranking of sneezing among our college and graduate student population was proportionately greater than among the patients at all other study sites. Climatic and exposure-related site differences would be expected to have a proportionate effect on other symptoms as well. This suggests that the predominant symptoms of allergic rhinitis and clinical outcome of therapy might differ in young as opposed to older adults. This possibility is especially important in view of the increasing portion of older adults in the population who may rely on terfenadine to control their symptoms. If these provocative symptomatic trends are reproducible, physicians would want to be aware that the outcome of antihistamine therapy may differ in young and older adults. Finally, the site-related difference was detected with the patient's symptom scores, but not with the estimates of severity made by the physicians. This suggests that the symptom scores provided directly by patients may provide a more reliable measurement of the illness and the efficacy of the drug. An awareness of the utility of patient's symptom scores could be extremely useful in the design of other multicentric studies.

REFERENCES

1. Buckley CE. Allergy and Atopy, chapter 21 in "Zinsser Microbiology", 18th Edition, ed. by Joklin WK, Willet HP, Amos DB. Appleton-Century Crofts. New York pp. 403-21, 1984.
2. Trzeciakowski JP, Levi R. Antihistamines, in "Allergy Principles and Practice", 2nd edition, edited by Middleton E Jr., Reed CE, Ellis EF, Mosby CV. Saint Louis p575-592, 1983.
3. Cheng HC, Woodward JK. Antihistamine effect of terfenadine. Drug Dev Res 2:181-196, 1982.
4. Mather K. Statistical analysis in biology. Interscience NY, 1948.
5. Nicholson N, Stone BM. Performance studies with the H_1-histamine receptor antagonists, astemizole and terfenadine. Br J Clin Pharmacol 13(2):199-202, 1982.
6. Carr AA, Meyer DR. Synthesis of terfenadine. Arzneimittel Forsch 32 9a p1157-1159, 1982.
7. Leeson GA, Chan KY, Knapp WC, Biedenbach SA, Wright GJ, Okerholm RA. Metabolic disposition of terfenadine in laboratory animals. Arzneimittel Forsch 32 p1173-1178, 1982.
8. Okerholm RA, Weiner DL, Hook RH, Walker BJ, Leeson GA, Biedenbach SA, Cawein MJ, Dusebout TD, Wright GJ, Myers M, Schindler V, Cook CE. Bioavailability of terfenadine in man. Biopharm DRug Dispos 2:185-190, 1981.
9. Garteiz DA, Hook RH, Walker BJ, Okerholm RA. Pharmacokinetics and biotransformation studies of terfenadine in man. Arneimittel Forsch 9a p1185-1190, 1982.
10. Huther KJ, Renftle G, Barraud N, Burke JT, Koch-Weser J. Inhibitory activity of terfenadine on histamine-induced skin wheals in man. Eur J Clin Pharmacol 12:195-199, 1977. □

Chapter XVIII

Treatment of Upper and Lower Airway Disease with Azelastine

James L. Perhach, Ph.D., John T. Connell, M.D., James P. Kemp, M.D.

ABSTRACT

Azelastine is capable of interfering with a wide variety of mediators of airway hyperreactivity and provides significant protection and bronchodilation in allergic hay fever and allergic asthma, respectively. Clinical studies have shown that azelastine produces clinically significant bronchodilation of long duration in moderate to severe reversible lower airway disease. In addition, azelastine has been shown to have an effect on the upper airways by effective symptom relief in patients with seasonal allergic rhinitis; furthermore, azelastine affords protection against exercise and allergen provocation.

I. PHARMACOLOGIC PROFILE

Azelastine, a phthalazinone derivative (Figure 1), is a chemically novel, orally effective and long-acting drug with histamine (H_1)-receptor blocking properties[1]. Azelastine also exerts receptor blocking activities towards SRS-A (leukotrienes), serotonin (5-HT), acetycholine and bradykinin, but at concentrations greater than that required to block H_1-receptors.[2–4] Dissociation of azelastine's antiallergic activity from its H_1 and 5-HT blocking activities has been shown.[5] In several *in vivo* and *in vitro* model systems azelastine is a potent inhibitor of the allergic and nonallergic chemical mediator release.[6–8] Azelastine is exceptionally effective in providing protection against histamine and antigen (aerosol)-induced bronchospasm as well as SRS-A (leukotriene) mediated allergic bronchospasm in guinea pigs.[9]

Since azelastine is capable of inhibiting the synthesis and release of chemical mediators coupled with long-lasting receptor blockade of many of the mediators of immediate hypersensitivity, clinical investigators were undertaken to determine if azelastine could provide effective therapy and prophylaxis for acute, subacute or chronic forms of allergic airway disease.

II. CLINICAL ACTIVITY

A. Upper Airways

Connell et al.[10] studied the efficacy and safety of azelastine over an eight-fold dose range in a randomized, double-blind, placebo- and positive-controlled study conducted at five study centers during the ragweed season. Two hundred two patients were treated with either azelastine (0.5, 1, 2 or 4 mg b.i.d.), chlorpheniramine (4 mg q.i.d.) or placebo for two days. There were 31 to 35 patients in each treatment group. Uniform environmental exposure was maintained by having patients remain in the same outdoor area from 9:00 a.m. to 5:00 p.m. for two consecutive days during treatment.

Nose blows, sneezes, nasal-eye-throat pruritus, runny nose and eyes and sniffles (the major hay fever symptom complex) were reported hourly on IBM mark sense cards. Patients who received azelastine at any dose and

Wallace Laboratories, Cranbury, NJ, Nasal Disease Study Center, Engelwood, NJ and University of California, San Diego, CA

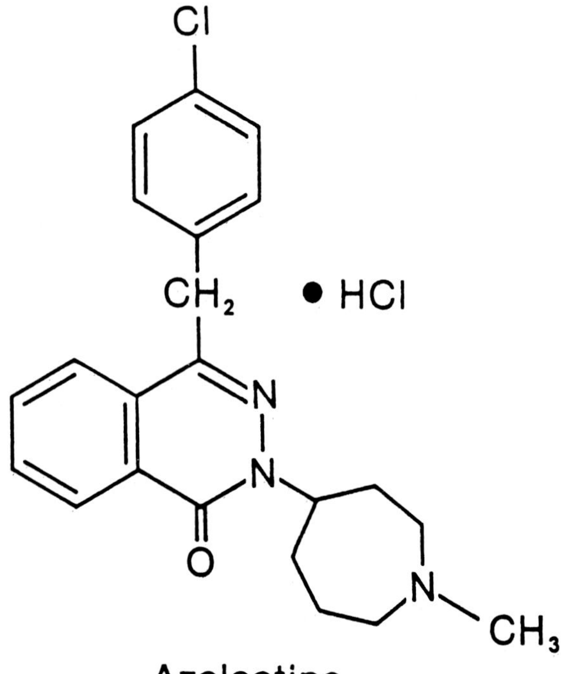

Azelastine

Figure 1. *Azelastine*

those who received chlorpheniramine achieved improvement in allergy symptoms which was significantly better than placebo. No dose response was identified among the azelastine treatment groups. Onset of improvement (30% of patients) was apparent during the first four hours following azelastine administration and by the evening of the first day all treatment groups were significantly better (50%) than placebo. Improvement continued throughout the second day (60–70%) in the azelastine treatment groups, but the placebo-treated patients were worse than at their pretreatment levels.

In another study 214 patients were enrolled during the grass pollinating season in a multicenter, randomized, double-blind, placebo- and positive-controlled study to determine the efficacy of azelastine on seasonal allergic rhinitis symptoms[11]. Patients received either azelastine (1, 2 or 4 mg b.i.d.), chlorpheniramine (4 mg q.i.d.) or placebo for two days. In order to maintain uniform environmental exposure to grass pollen, the patients stayed at a central outdoor location at each study center during the two-day treatment period. Nose blows, sneezes, itchy nose, rhinorrhea, sniffles, itchy eyes and lacrimation (the major hay fever complex) were reported hourly on IBM mark sense cards.

All treatment groups were statistically superior ($p < 0.05$) to placebo for the major hay fever complex. Azelastine 2 mg was superior to placebo at every hourly reporting period from the second hour post-treatment through the final hour of the study. Azelastine (1 and 4 mg) and chlorpheniramine were superior to placebo at many of the hourly reporting periods. The rank order of efficacy was azelastine 2 mg > 1 mg > 4 mg > chlorpheniramine 4 mg > placebo.

Patients reported adverse experiences, if any, at each hourly interval. There were no statistically significant differences among treatment groups relative to the frequency of adverse experiences at any hourly assessment.

The effects of azelastine over an entire pollinating season were studied by Weiler et al.,[12] who examined azelastine for its ability to treat allergic rhinitis and for safety in a four-week study in 99 patients during spring(grass) or fall(ragweed) pollen season. Azelastine (0.5, 1 or 2 mg b.i.d.), chlorpheniramine (4 mg q.i.d.) or placebo was administered in a double-blind, placebo- and positive-controlled trial in prescreened subjects. Symptoms were reported twice daily using a pencil scored computer card that was analyzed using an Apple IIe computer. Symptoms examined were stuffiness, nose blows, sneezes, itchy eyes, itchy throat and cough.

During the pretreatment period there were no differences in symptoms among the five treatment groups. At weeks one and two the active treatment groups all had significantly fewer symptoms than did the placebo treated group, although there were no differences among the groups given active treatment. Adverse experiences reported were drowsiness, headache, dizziness, jitteriness and nausea. Except for a slightly higher incidence of drowsiness in the chlorpheniramine group and in the higher dose of azelastine, there were no significant differences in adverse experiences among the treatment groups.

Azelastine was found to be an effective and safe medication for patients with allergic rhinitis treated during an entire pollen season.[12]

B. Lower Airways

Kemp et al.,[13] investigated the bronchodilator effect of azelastine in a randomized, double-blind, placebo-controlled, multicenter study; in 150 patients aged 12–60 years with moderate to severe asthma. Patients received a single oral dose of 2, 4, 8, 12 or 16 mg of azelastine or placebo. Theophylline was discontinued 24 hours before and other bronchodilators eight hours before a study day. Patients were evaluated for eight hours postdose by spirometry and were monitored for adverse effects. The mean maximal increases in the following variables were determined: FEV_1, FEF_{25-75}, PEFR, as well as the duration of bronchodilation. All doses of azelastine produced clinically significant bronchodilation with 4 mg > 2 mg > P; higher doses did not increase magnitude or duration of effect. There were no significant adverse experiences. The optimal dose appears to be 4 mg for adolescent and adult patients with asthma.

As a component of the study reported by Kemp, Spector et al.,[14] obtained blood samples at each pulmonary function measurement time for determination of azelastine and N-desmethylazelastine, an identified metabolite in man. Assay was accomplished by high power liquid chromatography with fluorescence detection and was sensitive to a 0.1 μg/mL for each. Azelastine and N-desmethylazelastine displayed linear pharmacokinetics for AUC_{0-8} hours and C_{max}; the C_{max} occurring approximately four hours after dosing. This corresponded to the time of maximum increase in FEV_1. An earlier onset of action was observed with the higher doses (12–16 mg). The dimination half-life for azelastine is estimated to be 20 hours.

In a study which looked at longer term treatment of asthmatics, Storms, et al.,[15] examined a total of 70 adult patients with a predictive FEV_1, 50–80% and at least a 15% improvement in response to an aerosolized bronchodilator. After a baseline (placebo treatment) week, patients received oral medication of either azelastine (4 mg, b.i.d.), albuterol (4 mg, t.i.d.) or placebo. Medications continued for two weeks and pulmonary function was tested hourly for six hours after initial dosing and then weekly.

Azelastine and albuterol both produced a statistically and clinically significant increase in FEV_1 after a single dose. The FEV_1 response for azelastine was sustained after two weeks. Significant reductions in the mean number of daily asthma attacks occurred in the azelastine patients. Backup medications (theophylline and/or aerosol beta agonist) were also reduced in azelastine patients. Other symptoms associated with asthma (wheezing, dyspnea, cough) showed reductions in severity and occurrence with azelastine. Blood pressure and EKG evaluations revealed azelastine to have no influence. Adverse experiences related to excitation were most common with albuterol, while a bitter taste with azelastine was the most frequent.

III. AIRWAY CHALLENGES

Gould et al.,[16] investigated the effect of azelastine on allergen induced asthma in a double-blind, random order, crossover, placebo-controlled study. Twenty extrinsic asthmatic patients were randomly allocated to receive either 2 or 4 mg of azelastine. Patients received randomized test drug or placebo twice daily for 21 days, then placebo for 21 days, followed by test drug or placebo for a further 21 days. Allergen provocation was carried out using *D. pteronyssinus* prior to treatment and after single- and multiple-dose therapy with azelastine or placebo. Response to challenge was measured by changes in specific airways conductance. Azelastine 4 mg, but not 2 mg, administered twice daily for 21 days significantly increased the amount of inhaled allergen required to produce a 35% fall in specific airway conductance on allergen provocation when compared with placebo.

Motojima, et al.,[17] studied the effects of azelastine on allergen- and exercise-induced asthma. In six allergen inhalation tests in five asymptomatic asthma patients treated with placebo, the maximum percentage fall in FEV_1 immediately after inhalation of allergen extract was 37.2%. The maximum percentage fall in FEV_1 with azelastine after inhalation of allergen extract in the same manner as with the placebo was 17.3%. The difference was statistically significant ($p < 0.05$). The percentage fall in FEV_1 with placebo and azelastine in late asthmatic response was 36.0% and 10.0%, respectively. This difference was also statistically significant ($p < 0.01$). An exercise test was carried out on seven asymptomatic asthmatic patients using an inclined treadmill. The maximum percentage fall in FEV_1 without drugs, with diphenhydramine and with azelastine was 38.9%, 20.1% and 11.3%, respectively. Statistically significant differences were found among each group ($p < 0.05$). These results suggest that chemical mediator release may be involved not only in allergen-induced asthma but also in exercise-induced asthma.

Mandi, et al.,[18] in a double-blind study compared azelastine to ketotifen. The parameters used were airway resistance, intrathoracic gas volume, as well as blood pressure, heart rate, subjective and associated side effects. Azelastine protected against histamine bronchospasm to a greater degree than that exerted by ketotifen. After administration of azelastine and ketotifen, a slight but significant bronchodilatory effect appeared.

IV. SUMMARY

The clinical response reported with azelastine may be related to apparent dual mode of action which includes inhibition of synthesis and release as well as antagonism of chemical mediators implicated in airway hyperreactivity. Azelastine is a non-steroid drug which provides clinically meaningful bronchodilation in asthmatic patients and relief of symptoms in those with allergic rhinitis.

REFERENCES

1. Zechel HJ, Brock N, Lenke D, Achterrath-Tuckermann U. Pharmacological and toxicological properties of azelastine, a novel antiallergic agent. Arzneimittelforsch 31ptII:8, 1184–1193, 1981.
2. Chand N, Harrison JE, Rooney SM, Sofia RD, Diamantis W. Inhibition of passive cutaneous anaphylaxis (PCA) by azelastine: dissociation of its antiallergic activities from antihistaminic

and antiserotonin properties. Int J Immunopharmacol 7:6, 833–838, 1985.

3. Kataymа S, Akimoto N, Shionoya H, Morimoto T, Katoh Y. Anti-allergic effect of azelastine hydrochloride on immediate type hypersensitivity reactions *in vivo* and *in vitro*. Arzneimittelforsch 31ptII:8, 1196–1203, 1981.
4. Chand N, Diamantis W, Sofia RD. Antagonism of leukotrienes, calcium and histamine by azelastine. Pharmacologist 26:3, 152, 1984.
5. Diamantis W, Chand N, Harrison JE, Rooney SM, Sofia RD. Dissociation of antiallergic (Anti-PCA) activity from the antihistaminic and antiserotonin activities of azelastine. Pharmacologist 26:151, 1984.
6. Fields DAS, Pillar J, Diamantis W, Perhach JL, Sofia RD, Chan N. Inhibition by azelastine of nonallergic histamine release from rat peritoneal mast cells. J Allergy Clin Immunol 73:3, 400–403, 1984.
7. Chand N, Pillar J, Diamantis W, Perhach JL, Sofia RD. Inhibition of calcium ionophore (A23187)-induced histamine release by a novel anti-allergic agent, 4-(p-chlorobenzyl)-2-(hexahydro-1-methyl-1H-azepine-4yl)-(2H)-phthalazinone hydrochloride (azelastine; A5610). Int J Immunopharmacol 4:4, 342, 1982.
8. Chand N, Pillar J, Diamantis W, Sofia RD. Inhibition of IgE-mediated allergic histamine release from rat peritoneal mast cells by azelastine and selected antiallergic drugs. Agents Actions 16:5, 318–322, 1985.
9. Chand N, Nolan K, Diamantis W, Sofia RD. Inhibition of acute bronchial anaphylaxis by azelastine in aerosol-sensitized guinea pig (GP) asthma model. Ann Allergy 55:393, 1985.
10. Connell JT, Perhach JL, Weiler JM, Rosenthal R, Hamilton L, Diamond L, Newton JJ. Azelastine (AZ) a new antiallergy agent: efficacy in ragweed hay fever. Ann Allergy 55:2, 392 1985.
11. Perhach J, Connell J, Hamilton L, Diamond L, Weiler J, Melvin J. Multicenter trial of azelastine in allergic rhinitis. J Allergy Clin Immunol 73:144, 1984.
12. Weiler JM, Rhodes BJ, Iwamoto PKL, Donnelly AL, Perhach JL. Effectiveness and safety of azelastine in a chronic study in patients with allergic rhinitis. J Allergy Clin Immunol 77:180, 1986 (abstract).
13. Kemp JP, Meltzer EO, Orgel HA, Welch MJ, Lockey RF, Middleton E Jr, Spector SL, Perhach JL, Newton JJ. A dose-response study of the bronchodilator action of azelastine (AZEL) in asthma. J Allergy Clin Immunol 77:249, 1986 (abstract).
14. Spector S, Rohr A, Rachelefsky G, Katz R, Siegel S, Perhach JL, Newton JJ. Pharmacodynamic evaluation of azelastine in asthmatics. J Allergy Clin Immunol 77:249, 1986 (abstract).
15. Storms W, Middleton E, Dvorin D, Kemp J, Spector S, Newton JJ, Perhach JL. Azelastine (AZEL) in the treatment of asthma. J Allergy Clin Immunol 75:167, 1985.
16. Gould CAL, Ollier S, Davies RJ. The effect of single and multiple dose therapy with azelastine on the immediate asthmatic response to allergen provocation testing. Ann Allergy 55:232, 1985.
17. Motojima S, Ohashi Y, Otsuka T, Fukuda T, Makino S. Effects of azelastine on allergen- and exercise-induced asthma. Asian Pacific J Allerg Immun 3:174–178, 1985.
18. Mandi A, Galgóczy G, Galambos E, Aurich R. Histamine protection and bronchodilation with azelastine, a new antiallergic compound. Bull Eur Physiopathol Respir 17:5, 1981. □

Chapter XIX

The Development of a New Antihistamine: Astemizole

James A. Ray, D.V.M., Ph.D.

ABSTRACT

As compared with reference antihistamines, the action of astemizole is characterized by several unusual properties: highly pronounced and very specific histamine H_1 antagonism, long duration of action and absence of central and sedative effects.

The classic antihistamines not only show a great physicochemical and structural similarity to each other, but they also have similar pharmacological characteristics. On further consideration, however, there appear to be large differences between the various antihistamines.

There are quantitative differences. Antihistamines have different affinities for H_1 receptors. Additionally, they do not match the cellular histamine receptors equally well, so that marked potency differences appear among them. Furthermore, the binding to the receptors may be relatively firm or loose, a property which affects their duration of action.

There are also qualitative differences among antihistamines. Most antihistamines not only have an affinity for histamine receptors but also for other cell receptors, so that there are differences in specificity.

Finally, all antihistamines exert a number of effects, of which not all are immediately related to histamine or other receptors. Upon clinical application these manifest themselves as side-effects.

Astemizole's chemical structure (Figure 1) is unrelated to that of histamine and the classic antihistamines. It also presents pronounced pharmacological differences. Astemizole is by far the most potent and specific H_1 antagonist known at this moment. It has an extraordinarily long duration of action and is devoid of central (sedative) effects[1,2].

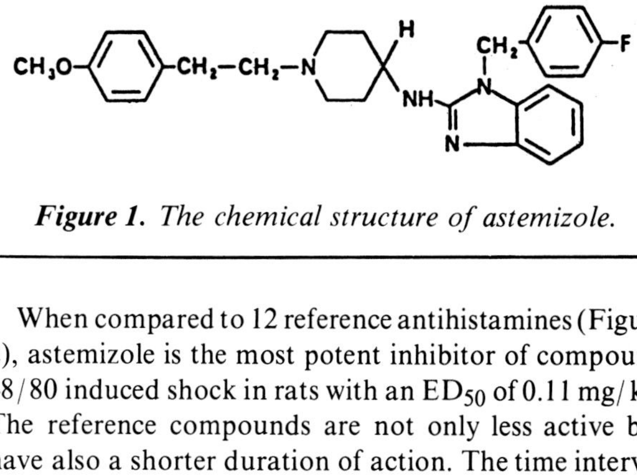

Figure 1. The chemical structure of astemizole.

When compared to 12 reference antihistamines (Figure 2), astemizole is the most potent inhibitor of compound 48/80 induced shock in rats with an ED_{50} of 0.11 mg/kg. The reference compounds are not only less active but have also a shorter duration of action. The time interval of effective protection covered by a dosage equal to three times the lowest effective dose ranges only from three to eight hours for the reference compounds, but is 24 hours for astemizole.

Astemizole's high potency and long duration of action were confirmed by several clinical pharmacological studies in man using skin, nose, and bronchial challenges with histamine and allergens. Astemizole produced a dose-related and long-lasting inhibition of the wheal and flare response to intradermal histamine (Figure 3). The degree of inhibition is dose-related with a single oral dose of 10 mg of astemizole causing a maximal inhibition of 68%[3,4].

The duration of inhibition is also dose-dependent and increases with repeated administration. During a 20-day treatment at a daily dose of 10 mg, inhibition of the flare response reaches 89% after six days and is maintained

Presented by: J.A. Ray, D.V.M., Ph.D., Janssen Pharmaceutica, Inc., 40 Kingsbridge Road, Piscataway, NJ, 08854

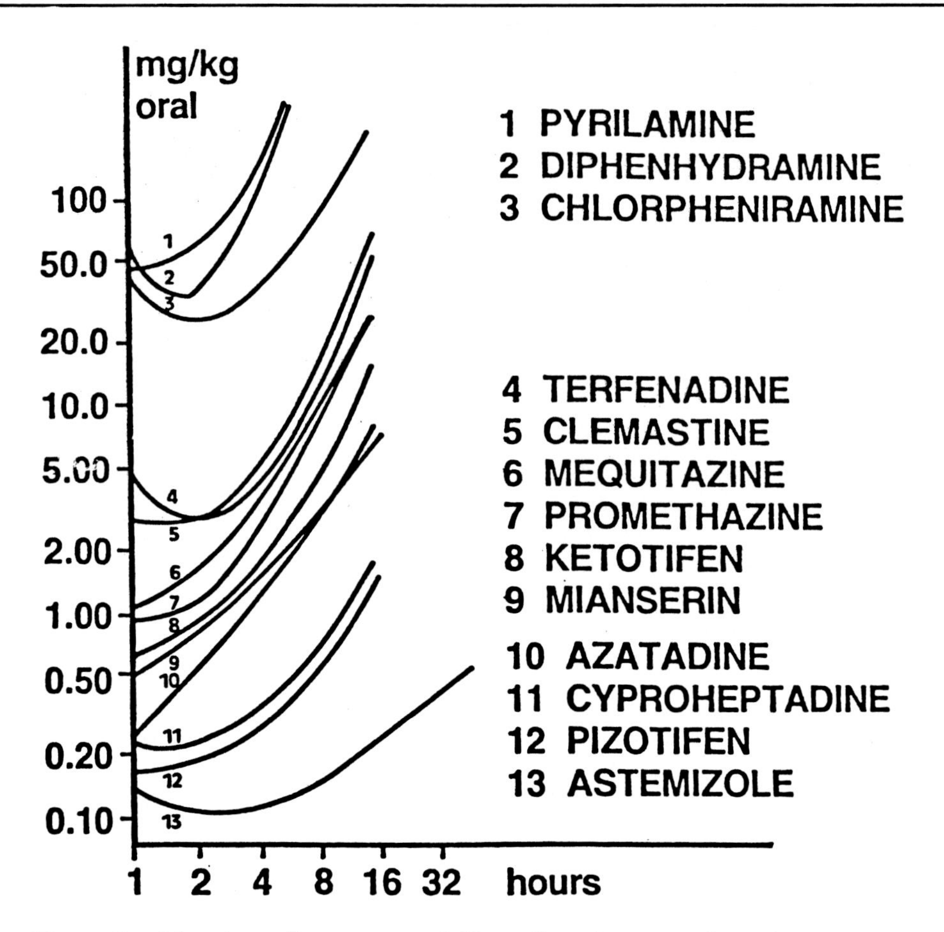

Figure 2. *The time-effect curves of 13 orally administered antihistamines in inhibiting compound 48/80 induced shock in rats.*

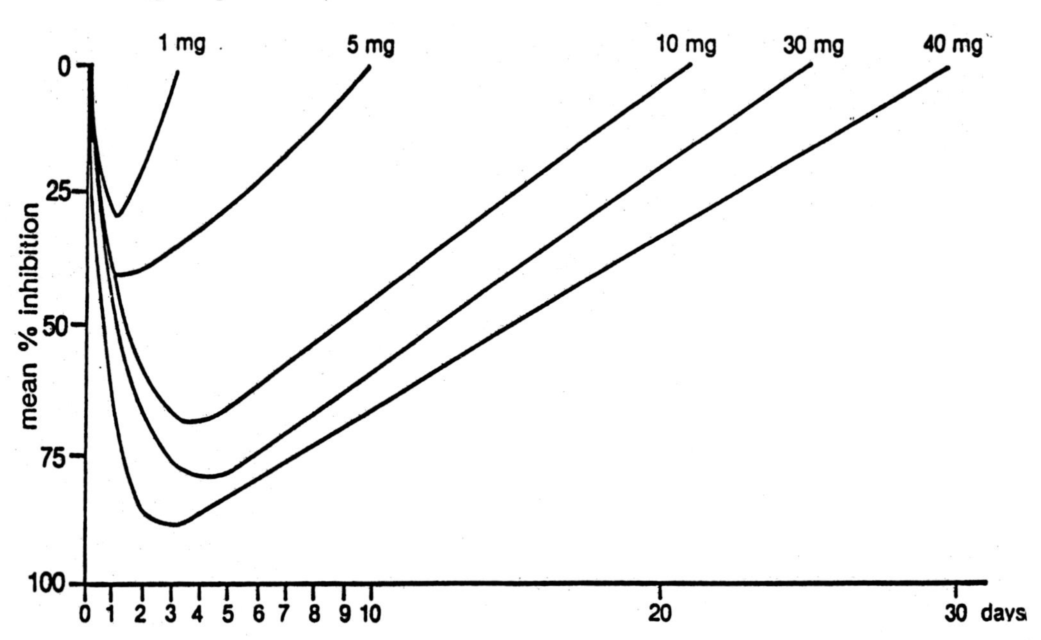

Figure 3. *The mean percent inhibition of the flare reaction induced by intradermally injected histamine (5ug) following single doses of astemizole administered orally to man.*

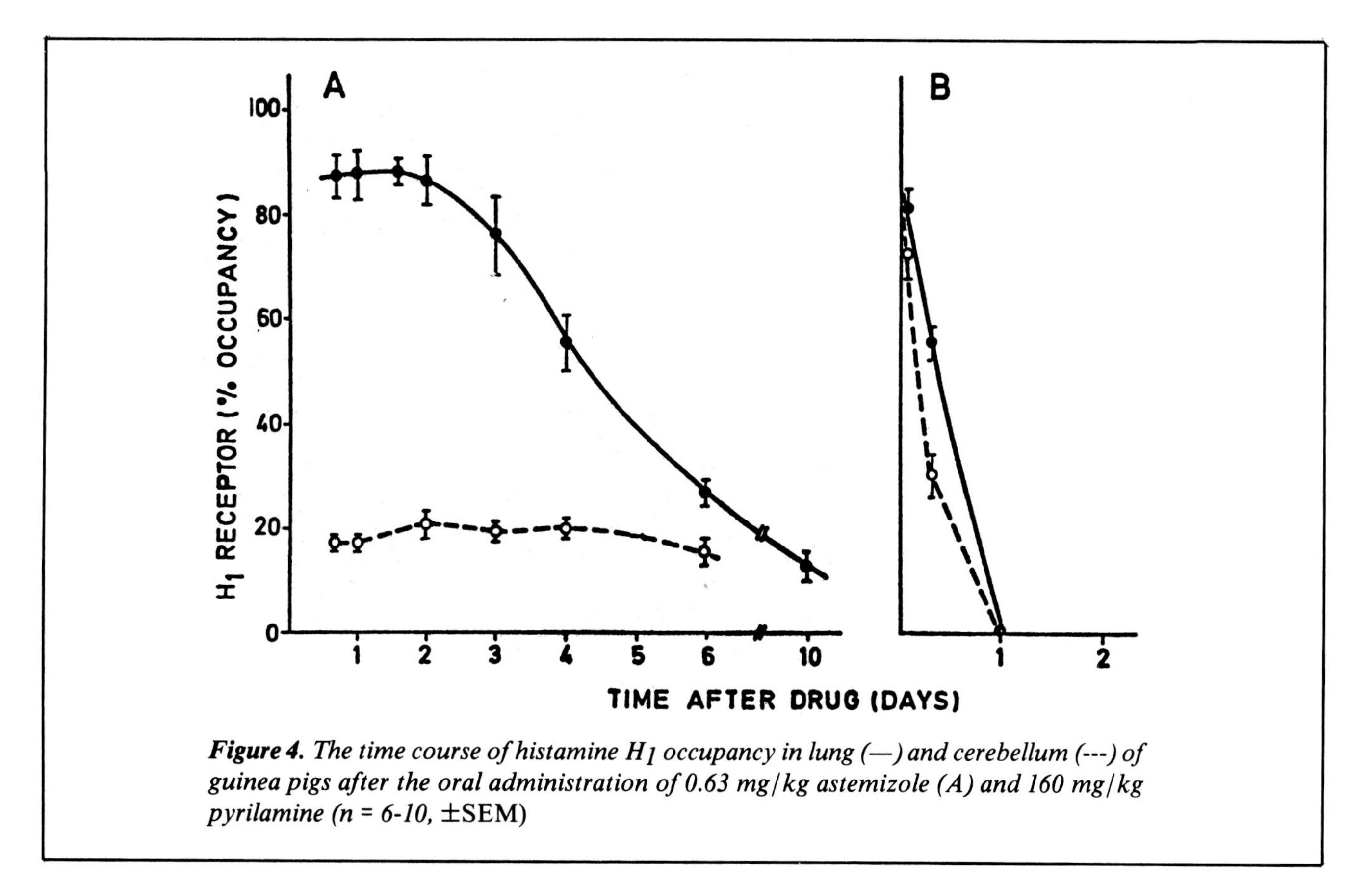

Figure 4. The time course of histamine H_1 occupancy in lung (—) and cerebellum (---) of guinea pigs after the oral administration of 0.63 mg/kg astemizole (A) and 160 mg/kg pyrilamine (n = 6-10, ±SEM)

during the remaining 14 days of treatment.

There are a number of molecular events that may play a role in astemizole's potency and in particular in the large differences in the time course of action of astemizole when compared with other antihistamines.

Astemizole has a strong affinity for histamine H_1 receptors[5]. After oral administration to guinea-pigs in a dosage of 0.63 mg/kg, over 80% of the H_1 receptors in the lungs of the animals were found to be occupied (Figure 4). To obtain a similar occupancy with pyrilamine, a dosage as high as 160 mg/kg is needed. The blockage of the H_1 receptors was furthermore shown to remain maximal for 3 days with astemizole but disappeared completely within a few hours with pyrilamine.

Astemizole forms extremely stable receptor-drug complexes. The mechanism of this stability, presumably thermodynamic, is difficult to explore directly because astemizole also binds non-specifically to tissues. This phenomenon has important consequences. Maximal occupancy of H_1 receptors is slower than expected from the drug's affinity for these specific receptors and is very persistent as tissue-bond drug remains available for occupancy of free receptors. It is very likely that a tissue reservoir of astemizole also plays this double role *in vivo*. In addition, the *in vivo* breakdown of astemizole yields two active compounds i.e. desmethyl-astemizole and nor-astemizole. These compounds have pharmacologic properties closely approximating those of astemizole.

Astemizole also has a highly specific histamine-antagonism. In Table 1 are presented the ED_{50} values of various antihistamines in the rat histamine skin reaction test, the serotonin skin reaction test (antiserotonin activity), and the induction of mydriasis, (anticholinergic activity). As indicated, astemizole is approximately 100 times more potent as an antihistamine than as an antiserotonin agent. Moreover, it completely lacks any anticholinergic activity. This is in contrast to properties of other antihistamines tested[1].

Astemizole's lack of anticholinergic activity was confirmed in man. A single oral 40 mg dose of astemizole did not induce significant changes in salivary flow in volunteers as compared with placebo, whereas, 16 mg of chlorpheniramine significantly reduced salivary flow between four and eight hours after intake[4].

Pharmacological studies had indicated that astemizole was devoid of direct central effects in rats and that it also does not interact with other agents that affect the CNS activity such as hypnotics, neuroleptics and analgesics[1]. Astemizole's central and sedative effects were also studied in dogs and man.

Wauquier et al[6] used EEG recordings to measure the effect of astemizole and two reference antihistamines (terfenadine and ketotifen) on the sleep-wakefulness patterns of dogs[6]. Astemizole did not change any of the

Table I

ED_{50} Values Determined 2 Hours Following Oral Administration of the Compound to Rats

Compounds	Histamine skin reaction (50 ug intradermal)	Serotonin skin reaction (0.1 ug intradermal)	Mydratic activity
astemizole	0.13	14.2	160
azatadine	0.77	18.8	5.39
chlorpheniramine	>40	>40	8.15
cyproheptadine	0.89	2.35	9.36
diphenhydramine	>40	>40	24.7
ketotifen	1.17	28.4	40
pyrilamine	>40	>40	56.5

sleep stages (Figure 5). Ketotifen significantly increased slow wave sleep and significantly decreased REM sleep. Terfenadine, at a dose producing a much weaker peripheral antihistamine activity in the Ascaris allergy test than the same dose of ketotifen and astemizole, significantly descreased wakefulness and significantly increased both slow wave sleep and REM sleep. With both ketotifen and terfenadine, REM-latency was prolonged.

These studies indicate both directly and indirectly that astemizole up to very high dose levels is devoid of effects which are not related to reactions mediated by exogenous or endogenous histamine.

Moreover, astemizole seems to cross the blood-brain barrier only with great difficulty. The occupancy of histamine H_1 receptors in the lung and cerebellum of guinea-pigs two days after oral treatment with astemizole is depicted in Figure 6. At the low dose of 0.02 mg/kg the H_1 receptors in the lung were occupied and the occupancy is dose-dependent. At 0.31 mg/kg nearly maximal occupancy of the lung H_1 receptors was reached, whereas, cerebellar receptor occupancy was minimal[5].

On the basis of these pharmacological studies, it was predicted that astemizole would be devoid of sedative effects in man. Several especially designed clinical-pharmacological studies using both subjective and objective methods confirmed that single and repeated doses of astemizole do not affect the psychophysiological performance of healthy volunteers[7]. Nicholson and Stone[8] from the RAF Institute of Aviation Medicine in Farnborough (U.K.) evaluated the effects of terfenadine (60 mg) and astemizole (10 and 20 mg) on performance in healthy volunteers in a double-blind placebo-controlled study. The sedating drug triprolidine was used as a positivie reference drug. Performance was significantly impaired from 0.5-3.5 hours after ingestion of 10 mg triprolidine. There were no changes in performance after terfenadine 60 mg and after astemizole 10 and 20 mg.

Bateman and Rawlins[4] studied the possible sedative effects of 40 mg of astemizole and 16 mg of chlorpheniramine in volunteers in a randomized, single-blind, placebo-controlled cross-over study. Visual discrimina-

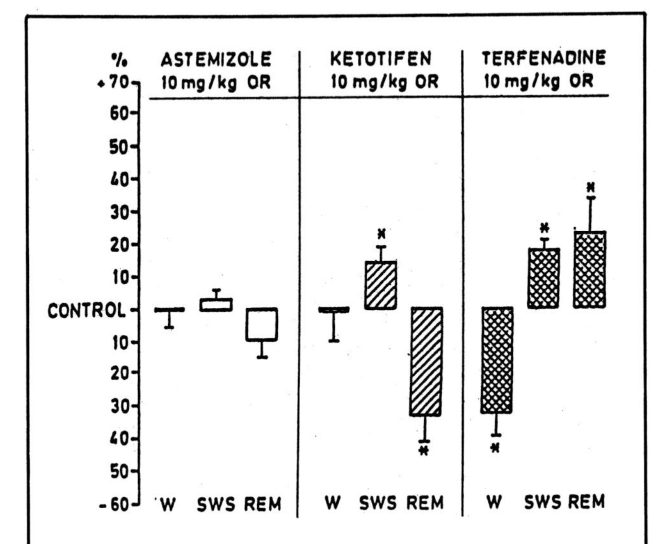

*Figure 5. The mean percent(± SEM) change from pretreatment values following the oral administration of 10 mg/kg astemizole, ketotifen or terfenadine to beagles: EEG determined duration of wakefulness(W), 'slow wave sleep (SWS) and rapid eye movement sleep (REM) during 16 hour periods. (n=6) *p<.05, Wilcoxon matched-pairs signed ranks test, two tailed probability.*

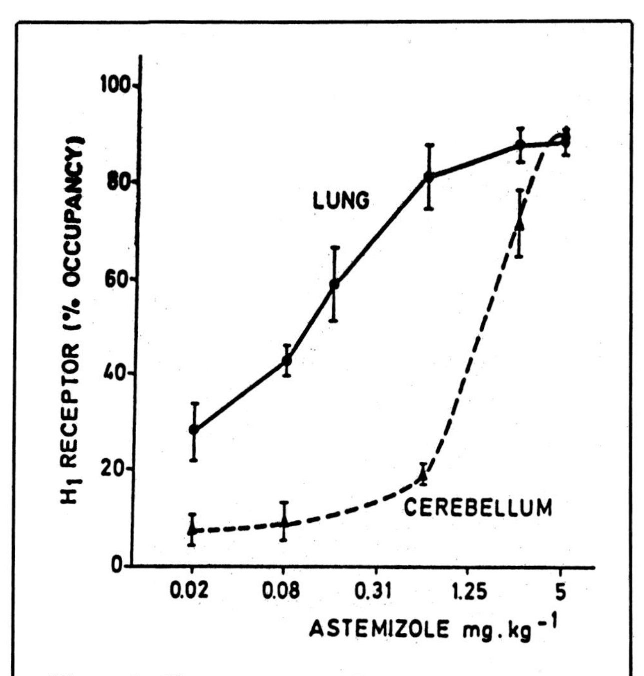

Figure 6. The occupancy of histamine H_1 receptors in the lung and cerebellum of guinea pigs two days after the oral administration of astemizole at various dose levels. (means [±SEM], n=6-10).

tion and alertness measured by a letter crossing-out test was significantly reduced at two hours and four hours after chlorpheniramine. Astemizole did not significantly change alertness. Visual analogue scale rating of sedation showed that individuals were significantly more sedated on chlorpheniramine than on placebo. Astemizole did not produce any significant sedation and individuals on astemizole were significantly more awake between two and eight hours after ingestion than when on chlorpheniramine.

N. Rombaut conducted a double-blind randomized cross-over study in which 12 volunteers were given daily doses of either 60 mg astemizole, 3 mg of ketotifen or placebo for 3 consecutive days. Between each treatment period an interval of one week was provided. Daytime sedation as assessed by a visual analogue scale could not be shown three and six hours after astemizole, and no difference could be seen between astemizole and placebo. At three and six hours after ketotifen, however, significant daytime sedation was demonstrated (Figure 7). Evening somnolence evaluated at least eight hours after dosing was reported by eight ketotifen, four astemizole and three palcebo-treated volunteers.

Smith[9] evaluated EEG and mood changes in 40 healthy volunteers receiving placebo, diphenhydramine (50 mg)

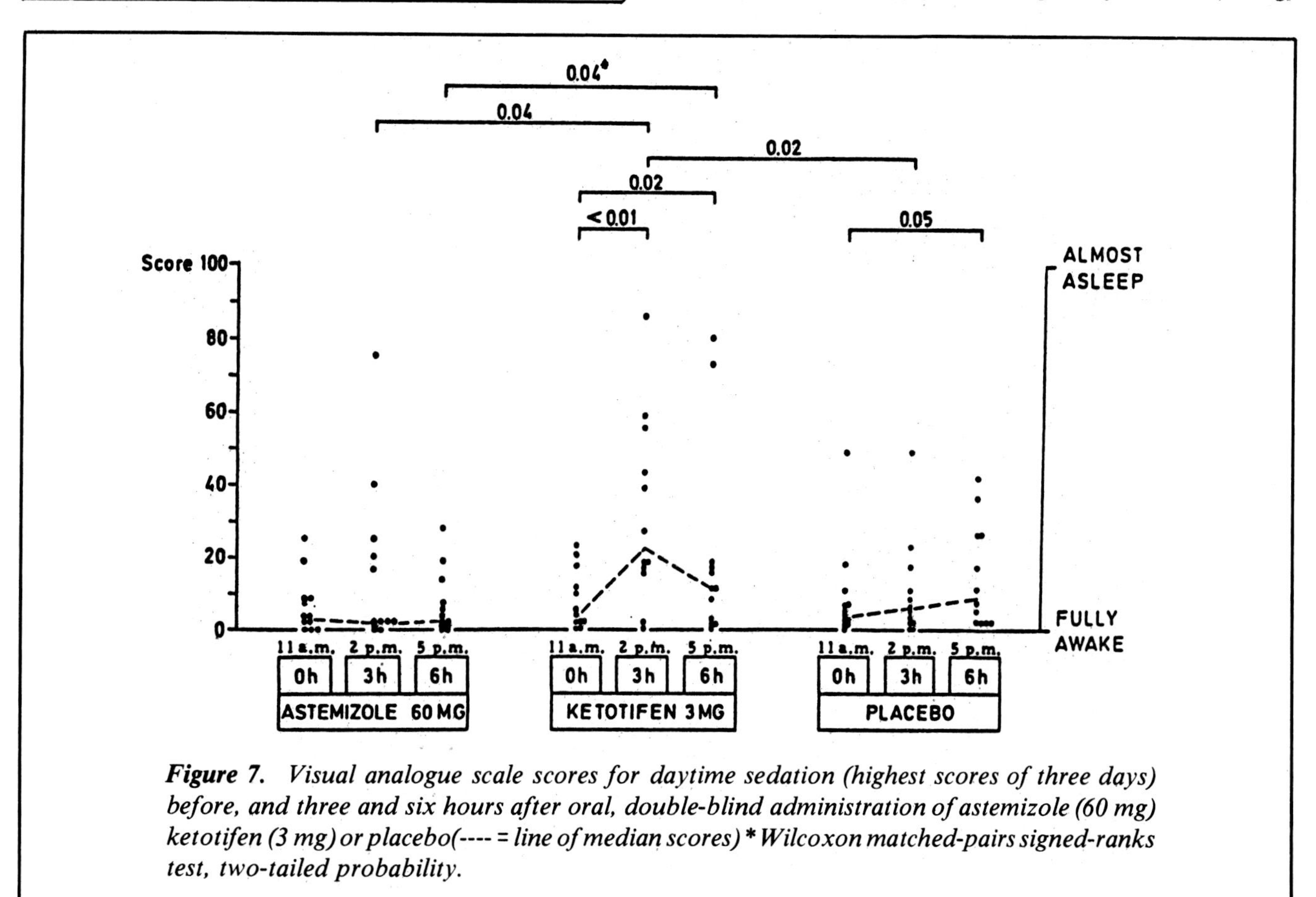

*Figure 7. Visual analogue scale scores for daytime sedation (highest scores of three days) before, and three and six hours after oral, double-blind administration of astemizole (60 mg) ketotifen (3 mg) or placebo(---- = line of median scores) * Wilcoxon matched-pairs signed-ranks test, two-tailed probability.*

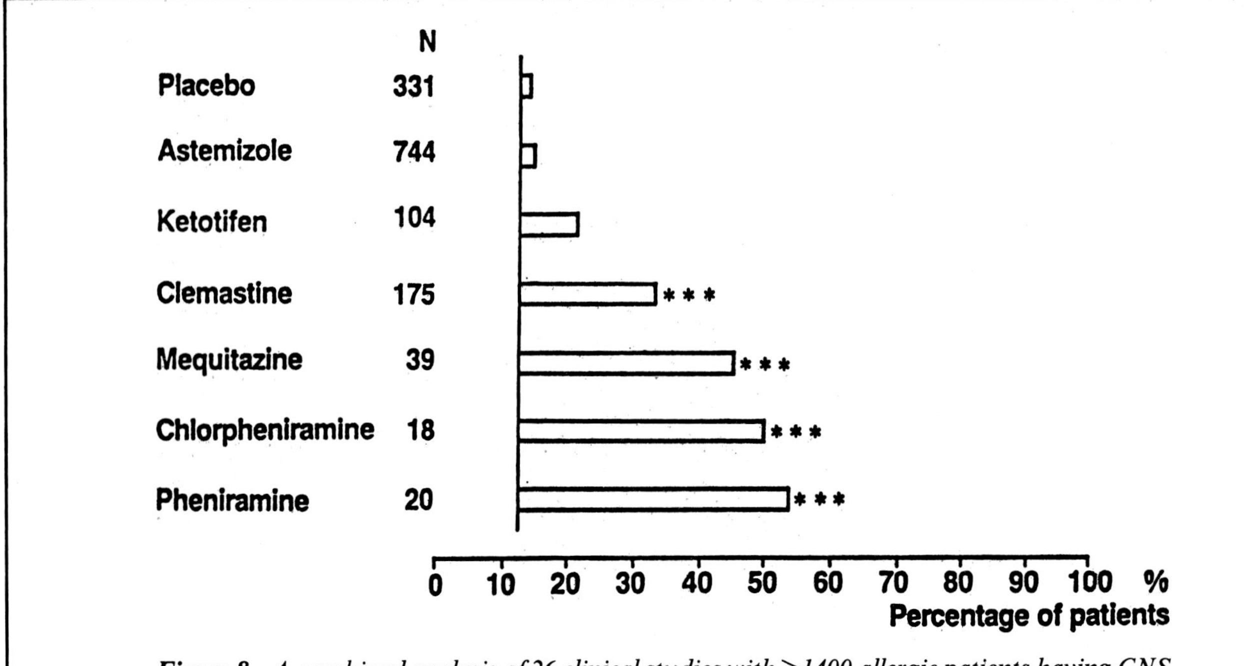

Figure 8. A combined analysis of 26 clinical studies with >1400 allergic patients having CNS depression during treatment with placebo or clinical dosages of astemizole, ketotifen, clemastine, mequitazine, chlorpheniramine or pheniramine.
n = number of patients
****p <.001 vs. astemizole (chi-square test).*

or astemizole in a double-blind randomized cross-over order. A total dose of 250 mg of astemizole (60 mg/day for 3 days + 30 mg for 1 day + 10 mg/day for 4 days) was administered to reach steady-state plasma levels. The evaluations used an aperiodic analysis of the EEG, each wave being identified and mapped according to its frequency, amplitude, and time of occurrence; and a profile-of-mood-state (POMS) test evaluating via a questionnaire several characteristics of mood, vigor, fatigue, confusion elation and friendliness. Using the detailed EEG analysis, no changes produced by astemizole could be detected either on the short terms (1 or 2 hours) or the long terms (1 week). On the other hand, several changes produced by diphenhydramine, particularly after two hours, were significantly different from placebo and from astemizole. The POMS evaluation essentially confirmed the EEG analysis. Most of the changes observed were related to diphenhydramine vs. placebo or diphenhydramine vs. astemizole. The principle variables affected were fatigue (increased) and vigor (decreased).

The absence of sedative effects was confirmed in atopic patients treated with astemizole. A combined analysis of 26 clinical studies in over 1400 patients with various allergic diseases showed that the percentage of patients with CNS depression was the same in the placebo (13.3%) and astemizole groups (14.7%). These were significantly lower than the incidences observed with the other active agents[10]. Differences with clemastine, mequitazine, chlorpheniramine and pheniramine were statistically highly significant (Figure 8). Also the incidence of dry mouth was comparable in astemizole and placebo-treated patients and the same applies to the remaining adverse experiences (Table 2).

In a combined analysis of clinical efficacy, investigator's global evaluations of astemizole treatment in 362 hay fever sufferers were good or excellent in 67% of the patients. These results were significantly superior to those of placebo (30%), clemastine (46%) and ketotifen (56%). Nasal symptoms responded in 60% to 70% of the cases and ocular symptoms appear to respond even better with 70% to 90%.

The same high activity for astemizole was observed in the treatment of perennial rhinitis i.e., good or excellent overall results in 81% of the patients vs. 28% in the placebo group, 59% of the clemastine and 55% of the chlorpheniramine treated patients[23].

Patients with allergic conjunctivitis responded favorably to astemizole in 70% of the cases against only 25.9% to placebo. The overall results of astemizole in the treatment of chronic urticaria were rated good to excellent in 76% of the patients, being significantly superior to the results of 25% in the placebo control group.

Table II

Adverse Experiences Found In 26 Clinical Studies Astemizole vs. Placebo (in %)

	Astemizole	Placebo
Number of patients	744	331
CNS depression	14.7	13.3
CNS stimulation	0.7	1.2
Headache	4.8	6.0
Dry mouth	5.0	4.5
Nausea	2.2	2.4
Abdominal pain	0.5	1.5
Flatulence	0.5	0
Diarrhea	0.9	2.1
Rash	1.2	0.3
Eczema	0.4	1.2
Increased appetite	0.5	0.6
Increased weight	0.4	0.3

CONCLUSION

As compared with reference antihistamines, the action of astemizole is characterized by several unusual properties: highly pronounced and very specific histamine H_1 antagonism, long duration of action and absence of central and sedative effects.

Astemizole's efficacy in preventing and relieving typical symptoms of hay fever, allergic perennial rhinitis, conjunctivitis, and urticaria was shown in carefully controlled clinical trials. The expected absence of sedation was clearly confirmed.

Thus, astemizole does not appear to be limited in its clinical action by CNS depressant effects. This is a major step forward in the development of new antihistamine and anti-allergic drugs.

REFERENCES

1. Awouters FHL, Niemegeers CJE, Janssen PAJ. Pharmacology of the specific histamine H_1-antagonist astemizole. Arznein Forschung/Drug Research 33(3): 381-388, 1983.
2. Van Wauwe J, Awouters F, Niemegeers CJE, Janssens F, Van Nueten JR, Janssen PAJ. *In vivo* pharmacology of astemizole, a new type of H_1-antishistamine compound. Arch. Int. Pharmacodyn. Ther. 251:(1) 39-51, 1981
3. Brugmans J, Vanden Bussche G, Scheijgrond H. Inhibitory activity of astemizole on histamine-induced skin reactions in humans.In: "Current Chemotherapy and Immunotherapy" (International Congress of Chemotherapy, 12th, Florence Italy) P. Periti and G.G. Grassi, eds. American Society for Microbiology) Vol II, pp 1102-1168, 1982.
4. Bateman DN, Rawlins RD. Clinical pharmacology of astemizole in: Astemizole: A New, Non-sedative, long-acting H_1-antagonist, (Medicine Publishing Foundation Symposium Series II). Oxford: Medical Education Services 1984: pp 43-53.
5. Laduron PM, Janssen PFR, Gommeren Leysen JE. *In vitro* and *in vivo* binding characteristics of a new long-acting histamine H_1 antagonist, astemizole Mol. Pharmacol. 21 (2):294-300, 1982.
6. Wauquier A. Sleep-wakefulness profiles of astemizole and other antihistamines. In: Astemizole, a New, Non-sedative, Long-acting H_1-antagonist. (Medicine Publishing Foundation Symposium Series II) Oxford: Medical Education Services pp35-41, 1984.
7. Vanden Bussche G, Rombaut N, Roens R, Schuermans V. Astemizole and psychophysical performance: lack of control and sedative effects. Pharmatherapeutica 3, Suppl 2: 3-9, 1984.
8. Nicholson AN, Stone BR. Performance studies with the H_1-histamine receptor antagonists, astemizole and terfenadine. Brit. J. Clin. Pharmacol. 13: 199-202, 1982.
9. Smith TN, Janowsky D, Quinn R, Silber RN. A comparison of the effects of astemizole, diphenhydramine and placebo on the EEGs of healthy volunteers. Presented at the Symposium: Antihistamine therapy, current clinical concepts. Chicago, March 7, 1984.
10. Vanden Bussche G, Rombaut N, Schuermans V, Gypen L, Dom J, Roens M. Clinical activity of astemizole. A review of worldwide data. In: Astemizole, a New, Non-sedative, Long-acting H_1-antagonist, (Medicine Publishing Foundation Symposium Series 11). Oxford: Medical Education Services: pp 101-111, 1984.

□

Chapter XX
A Multicenter Study with Ketotifen (Zaditen®)

Robert B. P. Burns, M.D.

ABSTRACT

Seven hundred and thirty-three atopic asthmatic patients were entered into two multicenter double-blind double-placebo controlled studies comparing the prophylactic effects of ketotifen (445 patients), placebo (143 patients), disodium cromoglycate (72 patients) and theophylline (73 patients). The primary measure of therapeutic effects was a decrease in concomitant medication without a significant increase in symptomatology or a decrement in pulmonary function: in both studies ketotifen was shown to be an effective and safe therapeutic agent at an oral dose of 1 mg bid. The positive control, DSCG, was also shown to be effective when used properly, while theophylline did not show a significant prophylactic effect.

Before presenting the data on our multicenter clinical trials, I would like to review the background on ketotifen, and define where these two studies fit in the overall research program. Ketotifen, or Zaditen,® as the trade name will be, is a benzocycloheptathiophene derivative which is orally active. Structurally the compound resembles cyproheptadine and azadatine. The three compounds are all tricyclic with the similar side chain; however, in ketotifen the typical benzene ring has been replaced by a 5-membered sulphur-containing thiophene ring. The compound with this modification retains its antihistaminic effect, but acquires: the ability to stabilize mast cells and inhibit the release of histamine and SRS-A; the ability to effect beta-receptor mediator responses in a manner similar to corticosteroids; the ability to prevent anaphylactic reactions in animals rendered tachyphylactic to DSCG or isoprenoline; and the ability to inhibit calcium transport across most cell and smooth muscle membranes. The activity of ketotifen in the prophylaxis of asthma is probably due to a combination of these effects. For example, the restoration of the response to isoprenoline may be relevant in asthma when improving the sensitivity or actually restoring the normal sensitivity of bronchial beta-receptors would prove therapeutically beneficial. This is seen with the use of the corticosteroids in this situation. We are now investigating a similar situation, the effect of ketotifen in reversing the reduced sensitivity seen with repeated doses of terbutaline in humans.

Ketotifen has been the subject of extensive clinical trials in Europe, South America, and Asia, and based upon the results of these trials, it is now currently on the market in approximately 35 countries throughout the world. The overall impression of the efficiency of ketotifen based upon the European trials has been a reduction in both the frequency and intensity of asthmatic attacks. In addition, concomitant bronchodilator and/or steroid therapy could be gradually reduced and even discontinued while the lung function remained the same or even improved. While the drug was used in both intrinsic and extrinsic asthma, it was both more effective and began its

---

Director of Clinical Research, Sandoz, Inc., East Hanover, New Jersey, 07936. *Presented at the National Symposium on H_1 and H_2 Histamine Receptors, Rhode Island Hospital, December 7, 1983*

therapeutic action more rapidly in extrinsic asthma. In the usual clinical trial, the true full therapeutic effect of Zaditen was not seen for anywhere from 4-12 weeks. A recent review article covers the data on Zaditen quite succinctly and provides reference for its various activities.[1]

With the extensive experience with Zaditen in Europe in clinical research, and with the post-marketing surveillance program in Great Britain clearly demonstrating both the safety and efficacy of the compound, the objective of the U.S. trial program was to confirm and expand these data in U.S. patients.

The program encompassed seven studies in addition to that of the multicenters. A preliminary dose range or dose toleration study insured that the formulation used in our studies had the same safety profile as that used overseas. Four bioavailability and metabolism studies were performed to compare the tablet, capsule and syrup forms to a standard solution to document equal bioavailability. Two special studies were an antigen-challenge study which showed an ordered dose response from placebo to 1mg-2mg of ketotifen and an exercise-induced asthma study in which ketotifen was shown to be superior to DSCG.

A total of 873 subjects were involved in these U.S. studies, of whom 733 were in the main portion of the program — the two year-long multicenter clinical trials designed to show the prophylactic effect of oral Zaditen lmg bid over a 12-month period. For each patient, the trial would encompass all the various allergen-irritant challenges normally encountered in their personal environments — pollen, cold, dust, infections, etc. They would also document the safety of prolonged administration of the compound.

These were multicenter, double-blind, double-placebo controlled clinical trials of similar design comparing Zaditen 1mg bid, an active control, and placebo. The basic difference was the active control medication used. In one study disodium cromoglycate (DSCG) was the control, involving 14 investigators, primarily mid-west and west coast; and in the other theophylline sodium glycinate, involving 13 investigators, primarily on the east coast.

At the initial visit a complete history, physical examination, clinical laboratory evaluation, and pulmonary function tests were performed. All patients were to have a history of extrinsic or atopic asthma which was being reasonably controlled on their present regimen. Either at the initial visit or sometime in the last year the patient must have had an FEV_1 which was 85% or less than the predicted normal for that patient, and this must have been reversed by at least 15% with a standard dose of isoproterenol or equivalent. Signed informed consent was obtained from all patients and from guardians of those patients who were minors.

Table I

A Multicenter Study with Ketotifen

DESIGN	A) Parallel Group B) Double-blind C) Double Placebo
DURATION	1 Year
BASELINE	2 Weeks
VISITS	Monthly
EFFICACY PARAMETERS	1. Concomitant Medication 2. Symptomatology 3. Pulmonary Function 4. Physician's Global
SAFETY PARAMETERS	1. Physical Examination 2. Laboratory Evaluation 3. Adverse Reaction Questionnaire
POSITIVE CONTROL	DSCG - Theophylline

Table 1 shows the efficacy and safety parameters which were evaluated. An initial two week baseline period was designed during which the patients maintained their current medication, and added the new agent, Zaditen, DSCG, theophylline or placebo. Of the 733 patients entered, 445 received Zaditen, 143 placebo, 72 DSCG and 73 theophylline as the study drug. The Zaditen group was deliberately three times the size of the other groups to generate sufficient long-term data for the NDA submission. During this baseline period and all subsequent periods the patient maintained a daily diary of his/her symptoms and all concomitant antiasthmatic medications. The specific details of both these studies will be presented as two separate publications, both of which are now in the final manuscript phase; the following is a summary of the principal overall results of the two studies. Initially I would like to start with some of the rationale for the specific data that we collected.

At the multicenter meetings before the study, we attempted to arrive at a workable definition of an asthmatic attack, since this was the principal efficacy parameter used in the European trials, but we had as many definitions as we had investigators. We elected to have the patients record their actual symptoms. The combination of the symptoms of cough, shortness of breath and wheeze combined as the "sum of three symptoms" was felt to give an indication of not only the relative frequency, but also the severity of the patient's asthma. Information was also gathered on the sleep patterns of the patients, whether they slept better or worse, their energy levels and their overall feelings about their asthma. Using the same diary, they also documented the medications they were taking on a daily basis. From just this one piece of paper - the patient diary - we generated a grand total of over one million, 500 thousand data points.

The other problem we encountered was that there was no meaningful yardstick to equate decreases in concomitant medications, either within a single patient over time, or between patients, when they are taking a variety of different medications. Combining the two studies, during baseline we had 43 patients taking beta agonists only, 75 xanthines only, 11 steroids only, 23 steroids plus beta agonists, 29 xanthines plus steroids, 202 xanthines plus beta agonists, and 211 xanthines/plus both steroids and beta agonists. The problem was how to compare the changes in two patients, for example, one on xanthines who decreases the beta agonist and another on xanthines who decreases the steroid; how do you weight the differences between the two? The average mg/day consumption of concomitant medications for these patients showed variations from visit to visit, and highlighted the problem of correlating the changes in types of medication. Our approach to this problem has been published in the Journal of Asthma.[2] We defined a unit dose of the various compounds, that is, within the various classes of beta agonists, steroids, xanthines. We determine the actual mg weight of equivalent doses of the various members of the class, and then developed a conversion factor for the between-drug comparison. The beta agonist unit was arbitrarily assigned a value of one, and we felt that a xanthine unit was 1½ times as potent as a beta agonist unit and gave it a factor of 1.5 and a steroid unit was given a factor of 5. Each medication a patient received was then listed and factored into a single number and the different medications were summed to give the Asthma Medication Index (AMI). This figure allows comparison of the changes in concomitant medication in a single patient during the study and also between patients at any time point. The other major efficacy parameters were straight-forward measurements, FEV_1 and physician's global evaluation.

For each study, four figures summarize the major parameters evaluated. Figures 1-4 present the data for the four efficacy parameters measured during the study with theophylline at various time points months 1, 2, 3 and then at 6, 9 and 12 months. We have the actual data for the intervening months, but these points show the initial onset of activity and the maintenance of the effect over time.

The overall efficacy of the compounds in these studies can be determined only by correlating the interdependent variables measured. That is, pulmonary function and symptomatology should improve with an increase in concomitant medication and the attending physician should interpret this as a positive effect of the concomitant medication. If an added variable, in this case the experimental drug, is able to alter this relationship, and cause an improvement in pulmonary function, symptomatology, and physician's evaluation at a time when the concomitant medication is being decreased, it must then be exerting a therapeutic effect equal to the sum of the amount of the decreased medication, plus that amount of additional medication which would have been necessary to cause the observed improvement.

This inter-relationship is clearly shown in the graphs. Figure 1 shows that for all test groups the FEV_1's were fairly stable; in fact, they all increased slightly, but not significantly. The second figure shows the Asthma Medication Index for the three groups. From month two onward, the ketotifen patients used less concomitant medication than during baseline, while the other two groups used more. At the same timepoint in Figure 3, the ketotifen patients showed a consistent decrease in symptoms and this interpreted as improvement in the physician's global evaluation (The value listed as Month 13 is really the end of the study of overall global evaulation.)

The time course seen here, (about 2-3 months for the effects to become apparent), confirms the previous observations that were made with ketotifen that there is a delay of anywhere from 4 to 12 weeks in the onset of observable clinical therapeutic effects when measured using a symptomatology rating scale. The specific reason for this delay has not yet been elucidated, but is under investigation. In the original clinical trials in Europe, this fact was not appreciated and negative data was generated because the pre-treatment time was insufficient to allow the drug to exert its full effect.

In this study, the theophylline patients experienced greater symptomatology at the time they were taking the double-blind medication and the physician, therefore, rated the medication as being less effective than ketotifen. The placebo group naturally had the greatest increase in concomitant medication, and as would be expected, had a decrease in symptoms secondarily to this except at month 12, but this was properly interpreted by the investigator as a lack of efficacy, especially in the overall rating. It is, therefore, quite evident that patients receiving ketotifen were able to decrease their concomitant medication and at the same time experience an improvement in their pulmonary function and symptomatology. This was not true in the case of the placebo group.

Figures 5-8 show the data from the study with DSCG. Comparing these figures with those of the previous study, there are obviously greater differences between the two active agents and placebo in the AMI. This was one of those strange phenomenon which make clinical research so interesting. Here we have two groups of patients with similar instructions from their physicians to try to decrease their concomitant medication until their symp-

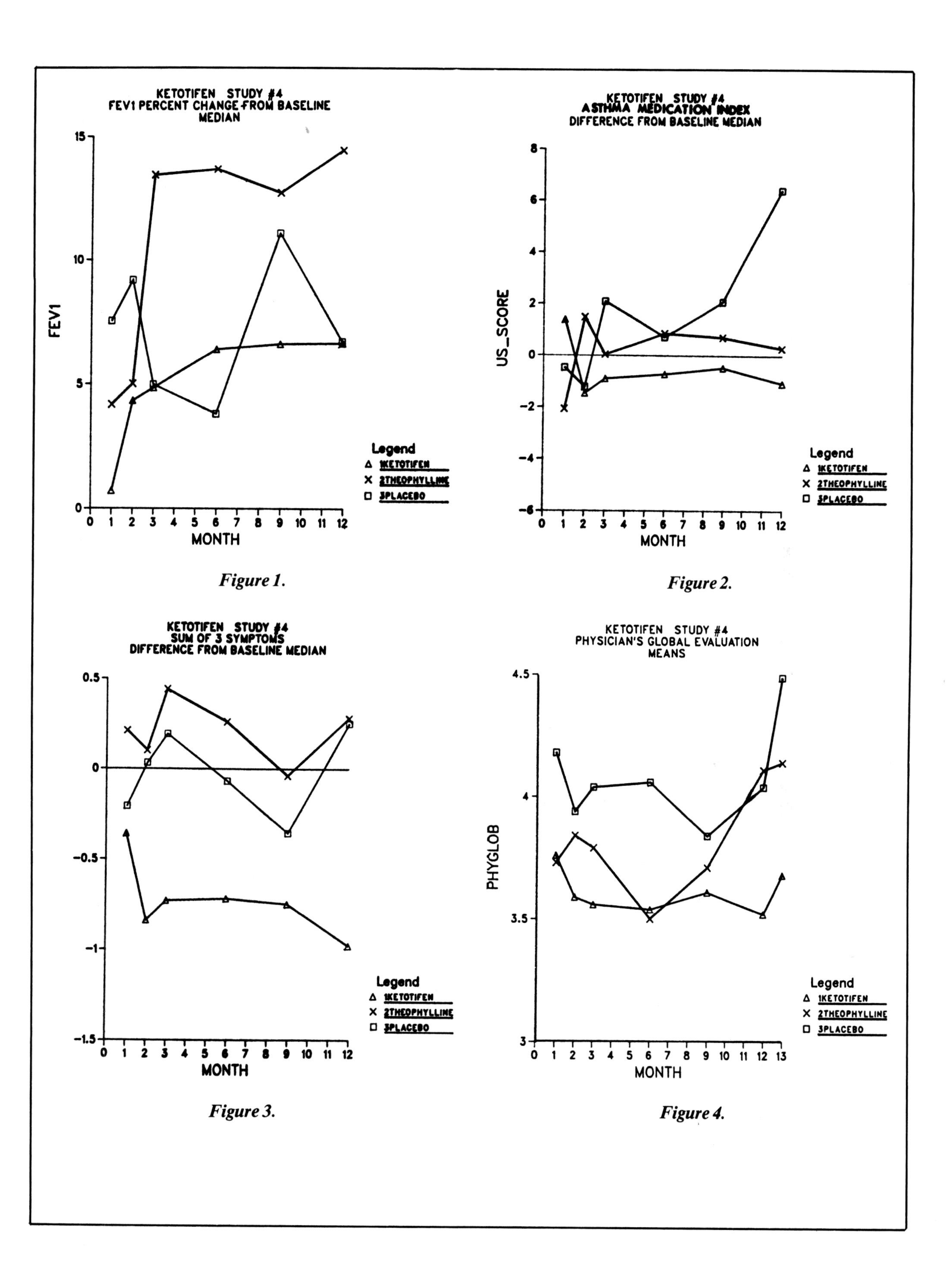

Figure 1.

Figure 2.

Figure 3.

Figure 4.

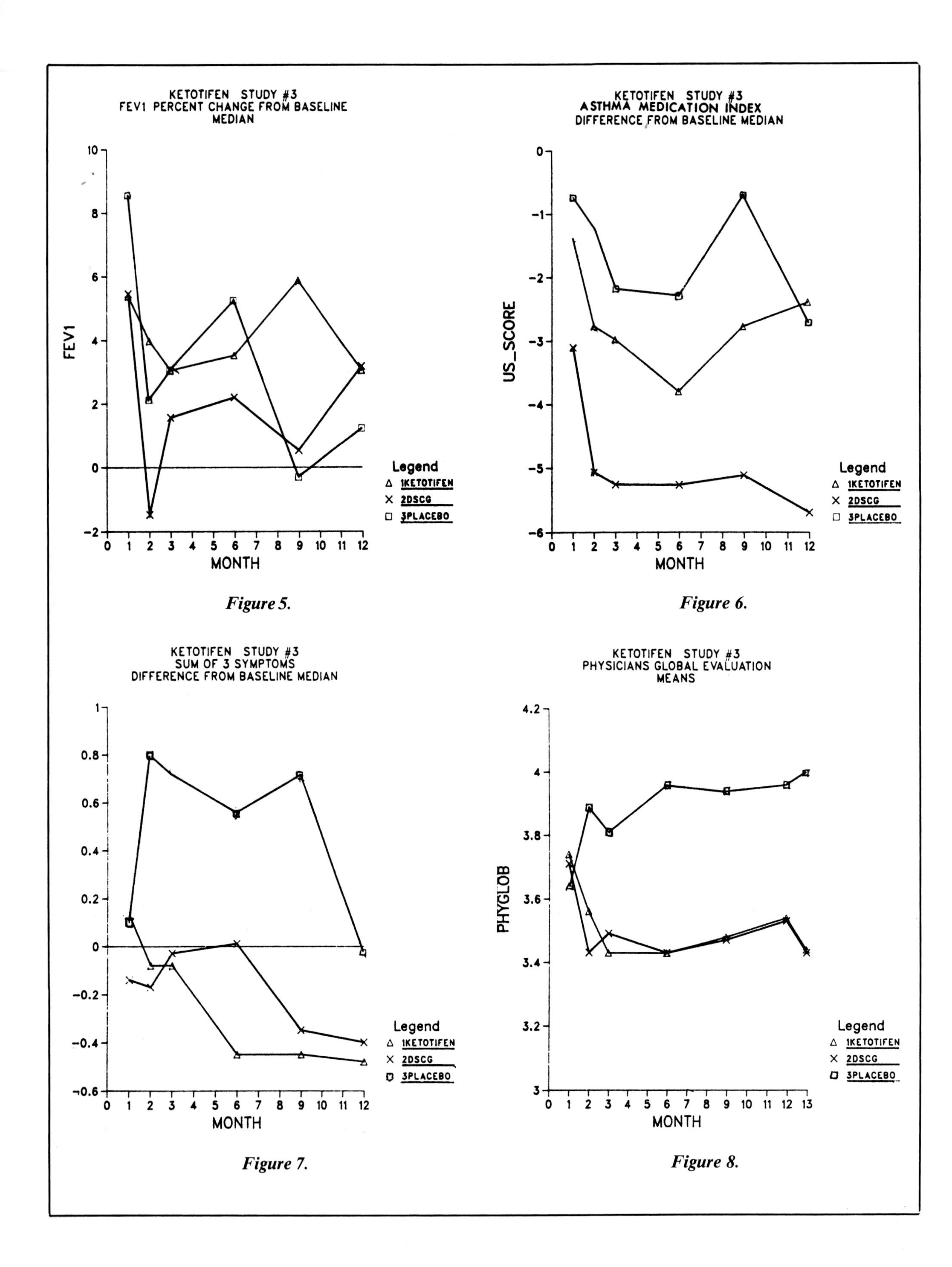

Figure 5.

Figure 6.

Figure 7.

Figure 8.

toms begin to increase. In this study, they followed the instructions so that there is a marked decrease in concomitant medication, but only a slight decrease in symptoms, while in the other study there was a larger decrease in symptoms and a smaller decrease in concomitant medication - or translated - the patients enjoyed feeling better and didn't decrease their medication in the other study.

As in the previous study, for the FEV_1's there is a slight increase for the majority except at one timepoint for DSCG, which is insignificant. For the Asthma Medication Index, the DSCG group had the greatest decrease in concomitant medication followed by the ketotifen and placebo groups. However, when one looks at the symptomatology, you can see that while the decrease in concomitant medication was not as great for the ketotifen group, the decrease in symptomatology was greater than that seen in the DSCG group, so that when these two are put together in the physician's global evaluation, both drugs are rated comparable.

This interpretation of the patient's overall condition by the investigator shows that they did take into account all the variables we have discussed, and it therefore allows a comparison of the different patient responses seen in the two studies. In the physician's global evaluation for the two studies, ketotifen was consistently producing a clinical effect which was obvious to the investigators. In the second study, the investigator also rated DSCG superior to placebo, which is in agreement with its clinical effects when used properly, thereby substantiating our rating system. The poor showing of theophylline would indicate that while it is effective in the acute situation, for the prophylactic situation a different mode of action is more appropriate.

Approximately a third of the patients in both studies dropped out before the full year for a variety of reasons. The between-group differences were in the treatment failure, uncooperative, and side effect areas. As would be expected, the placebo group has the higher percentage of the treatment failures (17%), followed by theophylline (14%), DSCG (11%) and the least with ketotifen (9%). A high percent of uncooperative patients in the DSCG group (14%) is difficult to explain; the most likely explanation would be problems with the use of the inhaler, but the other two groups in the study were also using a placebo inhaler, and their incidence was only 8%. An interesting aspect is the lack of side effect dropouts in the theophylline group compared to the 4% in the other groups.

The principal side effect seen with ketotifen was drowsiness, as would be expected from its pharmacological profile. The overall incidence of patients who reported any instance of drowsiness in both studies was approximately 19%, with the placebo groups and the positive controls being in the 3-4% range. The drowsiness with ketotifen, however, is relatively self-limiting and does not cause much of a problem after the first month. On a visit-by-visit basis, after two weeks and after an additional month on therapy, the incidence drops from 13% to 6% in one study and from 15% to 10% in the other, and thereafter drops markedly.

The next most prevalent side effects in these studies were headache, nausea and vomiting, which not too surprisingly were seen most commonly in the theophylline groups (16% for each), yet none of these patients dropped out, possibly because they were conditioned to expect and to tolerate these effects of theophylline.

In summary, these two studies show that in the long-term one-year clinical trials comparing ketotifen to the two most commonly-used prophylactic agents in asthma, DSCG and theophylline, Zaditen was shown to be an effective and safe therapeutic agent at a dose of lmg bid. While there was an initial incidence of drowsiness, this was transient and a tachyphylaxis developed to it. The physician consistently rated the Zaditen patients as improved over baseline. This combined with the case of administration of Zaditen compared to DSCG and the lack of gastrointestinal side effects compared to theophylline make this an ideal prophylactic agent. The clinical use of Zaditen may require some re-education of patients, since Zaditen is a truly prophylactic agent, and as such, has virtually no immediate effect which can be appreciated by the patients as an improvement in their condition. Patients must be instructed that the maximum effects of Zaditen may not be discerned for several weeks but that these effects will then allow them to decrease or completely eliminate their other asthma medications.

There are many other aspects of the therapeutic profile of Zaditen which are now under clinical investigation. As one would expect, we are extending our asthma prophylaxis studies into children. We will also be initiating studies in the urticaria/angioedema area, since early indications from Europe and New Zealand are that Zaditen will be a very effective agent in these indications. We are beginning pilot studies in food allergy and in urticaria secondary to other ideologies-e.g. mastocytosis. At this time the results are still preliminary, but hopefully will be proven in double-blind studies.

The NDA, based upon the studies I have presented, has been under review for a little over a year, and we are hoping for an approval.

REFERENCES

1. Craps, L. Ketotifen in the Prophylaxis of Bronchial Asthma. Clin. Ther. 5, 129-135, 1982.
2. Burns, R. B., et al. Factorial Rating System for Comparative Efficacy of Antiasthmatic Medication: A Multicentric Study Report. J. Asthma, Vol. 20, No. 2: 105-113, 1983. □

Chapter XXI

Icotidine,* An Antagonist of Histamine at Both H_1 and H_2 Receptors

C. R. Ganellin, R. C. Blakemore, T. H. Brown, D. G. Cooper, G. J. Durant, C. A. Harvey, R. J. Ife, D. A. A. Owen, M. E. Parsons, A. C. Rasmussen, G. S. Sach (England)

ABSTRACT

SK&F 93319 (icotidine), 2-[4-(3-methoxypyrid-2-yl)butylamino]-5-[(6-methylpyrid-3-yl)-methyl]-pyrimidin-4-one trihydrochloride, has been identified as a novel agent which combines into one molecule the ability to antagonize the actions of histamine at H_1 and H_2 receptors across a similar concentration or dose range. The degree of antagonism of vascular responses to histamine exceeds that possible with either an H_1- or H_2-receptor histamine antagonist alone. SK&F 93319 may have therapeutic utility in conditions requiring simultaneous antagonism of histamine at H_1 and H_2 receptors.

RATIONALE FOR COMBINING H_1- AND H_2-ANTAGONIST ACTIVITIES IN ONE MOLECULE

The actions of histamine on peripheral tissues have been characterized as being mediated mainly by two types of histamine receptors,[1,2] designated H_1 and H_2, based on the specific competitive reversible blockade by antagonist drugs. Thus, for example, specific antagonists such as pyrilamine, benadryl, or chlorpheniramine (well known 'antihistamines' now more specifically designated as H_1-receptor histamine antagonists) inhibit histamine-induced contraction of smooth muscle from the guinea-pig ileum and bronchus. H_2-receptor histamine antagonists, such as cimetidine and ranitidine, inhibit histamine-induced stimulation of gastric acid secretion and histamine stimulation of the rate of beating of the atrium.

Some effects of histamine, however, appear to be mediated by both receptors. As long ago as 1910, Dale and Laidlaw reported[3] that histamine caused dose-dependent depressor responses in the cat and dog. Following the discovery of the H_1-receptor antihistamines, Folkow, Haeger and Kahlson examined their effects on histamine-induced depressor responses and reported[4] in 1948 that the "maximal vasodilatation produced by low doses of histamine could be completely blocked by benadryl and related compounds but that the effect of larger doses of histamine, is not annulled or even diminished by any amount of antagonist drug." Indeed, they further suggested that "there are two types of receptors sensitive to histamine, only one of which can be blocked by benadryl and related compounds."

After our discovery (at SK&F, England) of the H_2-receptor histamine antagonist, burimamide,[2] preliminary experiments showed that the depressor responses to large doses of histamine, which are refractory to H_1-receptor antagonists could be abolished by burimamide.[2] Subsequent work by Black, Owen and Parsons[5] with the selective H_1-receptor antagonist pyrilamine (mepyramine) and the selective H_2-receptor antagonist

---

Smith Kline and French Research Limited, The Frythe, Welwyn, Hertfordshire, AL6 9AR, U.K.

Lecture delivered at the National Symposium on H_1 and H_2 Histamine Receptors, Brown University, Rhode Island Hospital, December 7th, 1983, by C. Robin Ganellin, Ph.D., Vice-President—Chemical Research, Honorary Professor of Medicinal Chemistry, University of Kent at Canterbury, England

* *An experimental drug currently being evaluated*

metiamide demonstrated that the depressor responses to histamine, in anesthetized cats and dogs, involved H_1 and H_2 receptors, both types producing a common response, i.e. a fall in blood pressure.

An extremely important message to emerge from the work of Black et al[5] is that simultaneous blockade of both H_1 and H_2 vascular receptors is required to fully inhibit histamine. They also showed that in the absence of an H_1-receptor antagonist, the H_2-receptor antagonism may be masked.

Further work with selective agonists and antagonists had demonstrated a number of complicating features, two of which are very pertinent to the present considerations:

(i) the relative sensitivities of the receptor responses to histamine varies considerably with the vascular bed and species,
(ii) there may be a temporal difference between the responses mediated by the two types of histamine receptor in the vasculature.

An indication of the importance of H_2 receptors in human peripheral vasodilation came from the studies of Wyllie et al (1972) with the first H_2-antagonist, burimamide.[6] Facial flushing is observed during infusion of histamine in man; this is not abolished by premedication with an H_1-antagonist, but subsequent infusion of burimamide completely abolished this response.

In human skin, histamine-induced wheal apparently involves both H_1 and H_2 receptors and responses to histamine are more effectively reduced by simultaneous use of both types of antagonist than by either singly (e.g. Marks and Greaves[7]).

Chipman and Glover (1976)[8] showed that pyrilamine (H_1-antagonist) reduced the immediate histamine-induced increase in forearm blood flow in man, although the response developed during the infusion. In contrast, metiamide (H_2-antagonist) had minimal effects on the immediate response but caused a quicker recovery after cessation of the infusion. A combination of pyrilamine and metiamide virtually abolished the vasodilator response to histamine throughout the histamine infusion.

The apparent importance of H_1 receptors in the immediate vasodilator response to histamine, changing to a more important role for H_2 receptors in the sustained response has also been demonstrated in various animal studies (see Levi, Owen, Trzeciakowski).[9] Thus, treatment with an H_1-receptor antagonist delays the vasodilator response to histamine, although a response develops with time during continuous exposure to histamine. In contrast, treatment with an H_2-receptor antagonist has little effect on the immediate vasodilator response to histamine, although the response to histamine fades substantially even when exposure to histamine continues. The response to histamine can be abolished only by simultaneous treatment with both types of antagonist.

These observations raise the question of whether there may be clinical circumstances involving vascular effects of histamine where it might be therapeutically advantageous to block simultaneously both H_1- and H_2-receptor mediated effects, e.g. conditions involving acute inflammation, urticaria, and vascular shock.

This analysis prompted us at SK&F to initiate clinical studies under the direction of Dr. W. L. Burland to investigate the use of cimetidine (as the H_2-antagonist) concomitantly with an H_1-receptor antagonist such as chlorpheniramine. Evidence has accrued to suggest that combined treatment with H_1- and H_2-antagonists is likely to be of benefit in pruritic, urticarial, and some other inflammatory skin diseases where histamine may be a major component in the initiation and/or maintenance of the skin's inflammatory vascular response (Burland and Mills, 1982).[10]

There is a difficulty, however, in using cimetidine and chlorpheniramine for concomittant drug treatment since these substances are very different in pharmacodynamic behaviour. Cimetidine is a weak base (pK_a 6.8 at 37°C so that 80% of molecules are unprotonated at pH 7.4),[11] very polar (octanol: water partition 2.5)[11] and has a short half-life for elimination of approximately 120 minutes. Chlorpheniramine, by contrast, is typical of H_1-antihistamines in being a much stronger base (pK_a of approximately 8.8 at 37°C; so that 96% of molecules are protonated at pH 7.4)[12] and lipophilic (octanol:water partition 5600).[12] Such differing physicochemical properties lead to different distribution and elimination characteristics within the body and it is unlikely that concentrations of each drug are maintained in balance for adequate simultaneous blockade of both H_1 and H_2 receptors.

To simplify the pharmacokinetic problem it seemed to us worthwhile to combine in one molecule the two actions of H_1 and H_2 receptor blockade. This approach does, however, introduce a new problem since *a priori* there is no indication of what relative potencies H_1:H_2 are required for such a combination to provide effective antagonism of histamine. As a starting point, it seemed reasonable to aim at a compound having comparable potency to antagonize histamine at both H_1 and H_2 receptors. It was anticipated that the pharmacological studies might indicate a requirement for a different balance and, if so, there would thus be a clear basis from which to project a more desirable ratio of activities.

MEDICINAL CHEMISTRY

Several chemical approaches were investigated in attempts to combine activities in one molecule; the

Table I

Chemical Structures Indicating Some of the Steps Taken for the Discovery of SK&F 93319

		pA_2
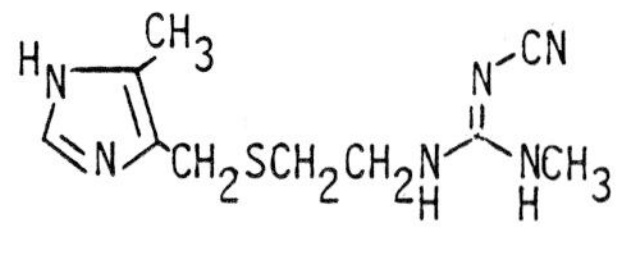 cimetidine	H_2	6.1
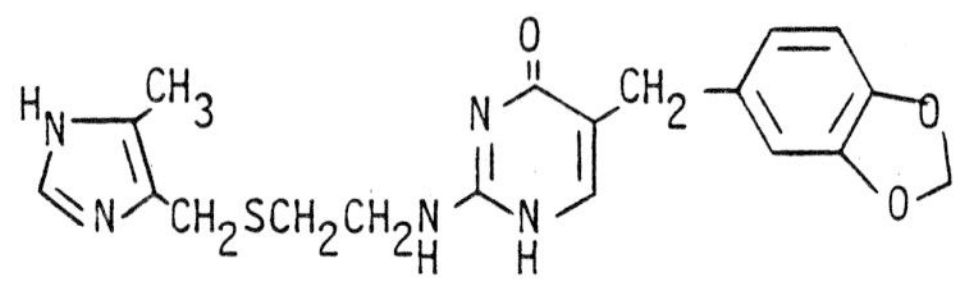 oxmetidine (SK&F 92994), H_2-antagonist, also possesses weak H_1-antagonist activity		
	H_2	*ca* 6.9
	H_1	5.4
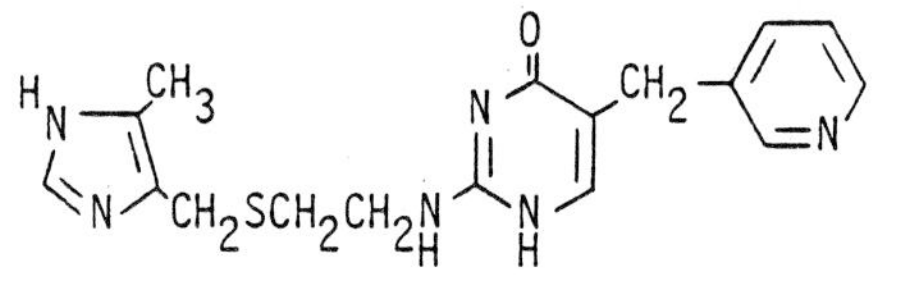 3-picolyl* in place of methylenedioxybenzyl in the isocytosine 5-position, e.g. SK&F 93018		
	H_2	7.0
	H_1	5.2
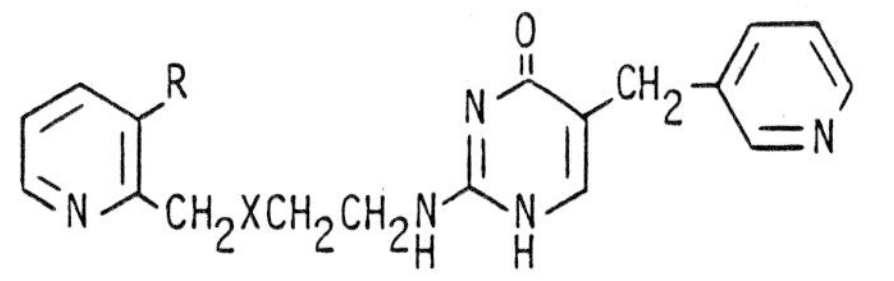 SERIES I (X = S) substituted pyridine in place of imidazole enhances H_1		
SERIES II (X = CH_2) $-CH_2$ in place of $-S-$ enhances H_1		
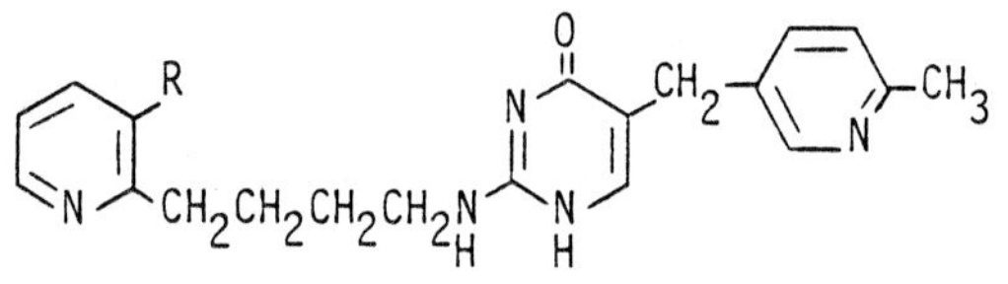 SERIES III 6-methyl-3-picolyl in the isocytosine ring; H_1 and H_2 antagonist potencies (in vitro) in balance when R = OCH_3 i.e. SK&F 93319		

* *picolyl = pyridylmethyl*

most successful approach was based on the observation that H_2-receptor histamine antagonists possessing a 5-substituted isocytosine moiety also had some (albeit weak) H_1-antagonist activity. For example, the H_2-antagonist oxmetidine SK&F 92994 and the corresponding picolyl analogue SK&F 93018 (Table 1) had pA_2 values 5.2–5.4 as H_1-antagonists on the isolated guinea-pig ileum.[13] Oxmetidine, like cimetidine, is an imidazole derivative and it was demonstrated that replacement of the imidazole ring by a pyridine ring retained H_2-antagonist activity and enhanced H_1-antagonist activity. Additionally, it was shown that replacing the thioether linkage ($-S-$) in the side chain by a methylene linkage ($-CH_2-$) further enhanced H_1 antagonist activity.

In the above structures it was found that activity was sensitive to the substituent in the pyridine ring at the position adjacent to the side chain. Various descriptions of the substituents were examined to correlate structure with activity and it appeared that activity was relatable to substituent size. Figure 1 shows linear correlations of H_1-receptor antagonist activity (determined in vitro on the guinea-pig ileum) for two series of substituted pyridines, I and II, where X = S and X = CH_2 respectively, using one of the steric parameters for the substituents as defined by Verloop et al.[14] This particular parameter represents the van der Waals radius of the substituent in the plane of the pyridine ring measured towards the CH_2 of the side chain. There is a consistent increase in potency of at least one pA_2 unit between the two series for any given substituent.

Figure 2 shows a correlation for the closely related series III, X = CH_2, in which a 6-methyl group is present

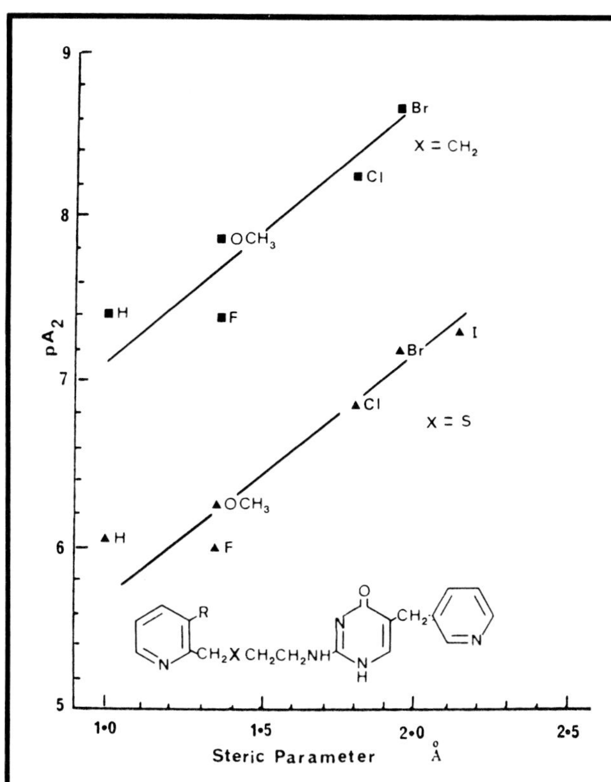

Figure 1. *Correlation between H_1-receptor histamine antagonism (in vitro against histamine-induced contractions of the guinea-pig ileum, represented as the pA_2 value on the ordinate axis) for two series of substituted pyridine derivatives, series I, X = CH_2 (upper line), series II, X = S (lower line), and a steric parameter (Verloop et al)[14] for the respective substituents (abscissa, Å). Antagonists were introduced into contact with the tissue for 8 minutes prior to histamine assay, except for compounds X = CH_2, R = F; X = S, R = F, OCH_3, Br, which had only 2 minutes contact.*

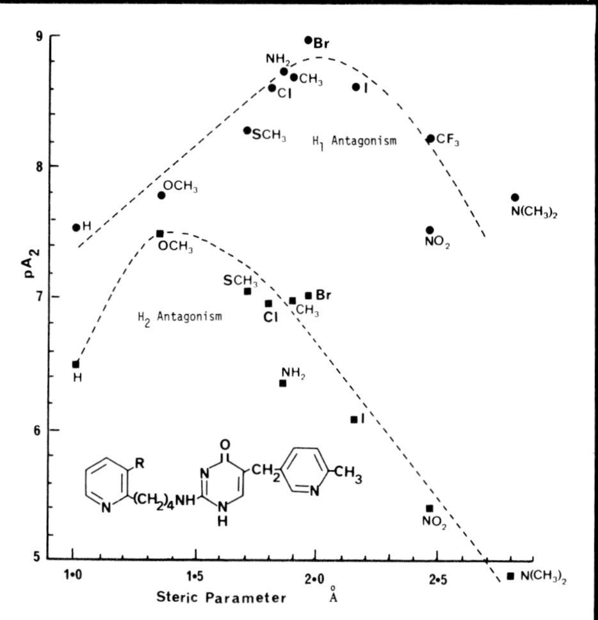

Figure 2. *Relationship between H_1-receptor histamine antagonism (upper curve, in vitro against histamine-induced contractions of the guinea-pig ileum) and H_2-receptor histamine antagonism (lower curve, in vitro against histamine stimulation of the rate of beating of the guinea-pig right atrium), represented as the pA_2 values on the ordinate axis, and a steric parameter (Verloop et al)[14] for the respective substituents (abscissa, Å) in substituted pyridylbutylisocytosines (series III). SK&F 93319 has R = OCH_3. H_1 antagonism was assayed after 8 minutes contact between the tissue and the antagonist; H_2 antagonism was assayed after 60 minutes contact, except for the compounds R = H and Cl which had 8 minutes.*

in the isocytosine 5-picolyl substituent, using the same set of Verloop parameters for an extended range of substituents. Both H_1 (ileum) and H_2 (atrium) antagonist potencies are plotted and it can be seen that in this series, for each compound, H_1 potency is greater than H_2, and the two activities appear to have different optima with respect to substituent size. The two activities are almost in balance when R = OCH_3, viz. for SK&F 93319, for which we propose the name "icotidine" (accepted by the USAN Council as a non-proprietary name).

Some useful chemical properties of SK&F 93319 are recorded in Table 2. SK&F 93319 has three weakly basic centres in the molecule and forms a stable trihydrochloride solid salt which is water soluble. The pK_a values are respectively 3.15, 5.5, and 5.9 so that at physiological pH the compound is mainly unionized. This is in contrast to conventional (H_1) antihistamines which are mainly in the cationic form at pH 7.4. SK&F 93319 has an octanol:water partition coefficient of 435:1 which is much higher than is usual for H_2-receptor antagonists (e.g. cimetidine partition coefficient = 2.5) but is less than that of most H_1-receptor antihistamines.

PHARMACOLOGY OF SK&F 93319

SK&F 93319 inhibited H_1-receptor histamine-induced contractions of the isolated guinea-pig ileum in a concentration dependent manner. Antagonism rapidly reached equilibrium with pA_2 values after 2 and 8 minute incubations 7.67 (7.20–8.50) and 7.77 (6.85–8.39)

Table II

Some Chemical Properties of SK&F 93319

Structure:	[chemical structure] OCH_3; $CH_2CH_2CH_2CH_2N$ H; N, N H, O; CH_2; N; CH_3; 3HCl
Name:	2-[4-(3-Methoxypyrid-2-yl)butylamino]-5-[(6-methyl-pyrid-3-yl)-methyl]-pyrimidin-4-one trihydrochloride
Formula:	$C_{21}H_{25}N_5O_2.3HCl$
Molecular Weight:	488.87 (Base weight 379.47)
Solubility:	The trihydrochloride is freely soluble in water.
Stock Solution:	A solution is prepared by dissolving 3.22g of SK&F 93319 .3HCl in 0.9% w/v saline made up to 100 ml; this is equivalent to 2.5% w/v of SK&F 93319 base, or 6.58×10^{-2} molar.
Stability:	A 3.22 w/v solution of the trihydrochloride salt (natural pH 2.3) did not show any evidence of decomposition on storing at room temperature for 26 weeks protected from light. The pH can be raised to a maximum of 4.2 by the addition of sodium hydroxide solution, but precipitation of the base occurs at pH 7.4. A solution of 18.04 mg of SK&F 93319 .3HCl (equivalent to 14 mg of SK&F 93319 base) in 3.0 ml of water made up to 15 ml with 0.9% w/v sodium chloride solution (natural pH 3.2) showed no evidence of decomposition after four weeks at room temperature.
Basicity:	The molecule has three basic centres with pK_a's at 37°C of 3.15 (measured) and 5.5, 5.9 (estimated) due to protonation of the pyrimidone, methoxypyridine and methylpyridine groups respectively.
Acidity:	The 2-aminopyrimid-4-one (isocytosine) group has an acidic pK_a at 37°C of 9.78 (measured) and SK&F 93319 is freely soluble in strong aqueous base.
Partition Coefficient:	P (octanol/water) at 37.5°C = 435 at pH 7.5 (log P = 2.64).

respectively; slopes of the Schild plots were not significantly different from unity suggesting competitive antagonism. SK&F 93319 antagonized the response to carbachol on the ileum at high concentrations giving an approximate pA_2 value of 4.8, i.e. a thousand fold separation between activities on histamine H_1 and muscarinic receptors.[15]

On the isolated guinea-pig atrium (H_2) SK&F 93319 antagonized the positive chronotropic action of histamine. After 8 minutes incubation of the tissue the pA_2 value was 6.66 (6.48–6.88) with a slope of 0.89 ± 0.33 but full development of antagonism was slow and after 60 minutes incubation the pA_2 value was 7.49 (7.00–8.50) with a Schild plot slope of 0.95 ± 0.17 (mean ±95% confidence limits). Concentrations up to 160μM did not cause parallel displacement of the isoprenaline dose-response curve but did depress the maximal response indicating a very big separation between activities at histamine H_2 and β-adrenergic receptors.[15]

To assess the relative potencies as an antagonist at H_1 and H_2 receptors *in vivo*, SK&F 93319 was examined in anesthetized guinea-pigs prepared to allow measurement of airways resistance and heart rate. Intravenous injection of histamine caused simultaneous and dose-dependent bronchoconstriction, an H_1-receptor action, and tachycardia, an H_2-receptor action (Figure 3).

Intravenous administration of SK&F 93319, 0.01 and 0.1 μmol/kg/min caused displacement to the right of the histamine dose-response curves for both bronchoconstriction and tachycardia indicating antagonist activity of SK&F 93319 at both H_1 and H_2 receptors over the same dose range (Figure 4). In contrast, pyrilamine caused major displacements to the right of the bronchoconstriction dose-response curve with little or no displacement of the tachycardia responses; cimetidine displaced the tachycardia dose-response curve to histamine but had no effect on the bronchoconstriction (Figure 4).

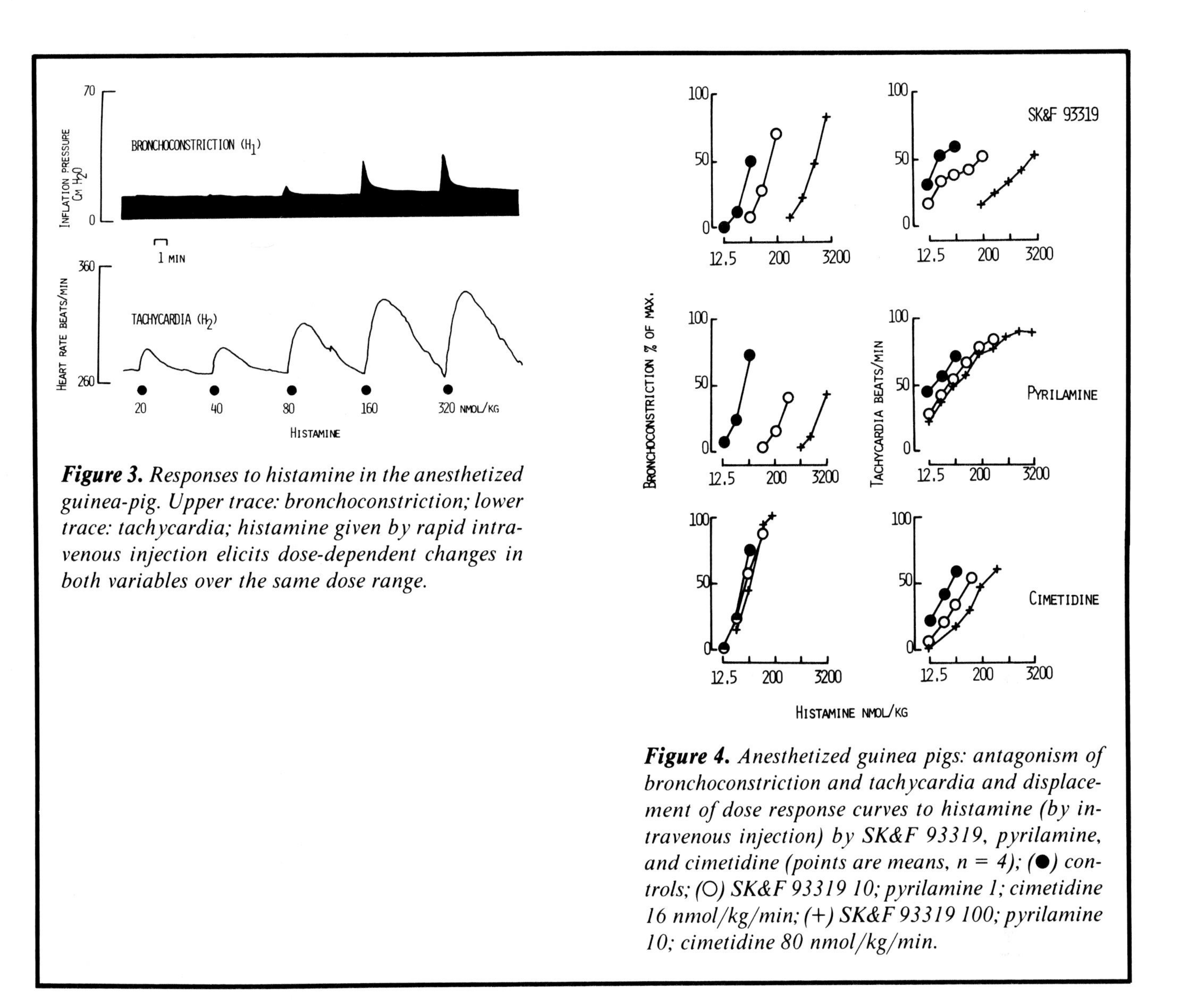

Figure 3. *Responses to histamine in the anesthetized guinea-pig. Upper trace: bronchoconstriction; lower trace: tachycardia; histamine given by rapid intravenous injection elicits dose-dependent changes in both variables over the same dose range.*

Figure 4. *Anesthetized guinea pigs: antagonism of bronchoconstriction and tachycardia and displacement of dose response curves to histamine (by intravenous injection) by SK&F 93319, pyrilamine, and cimetidine (points are means, n = 4); (●) controls; (O) SK&F 93319 10; pyrilamine 1; cimetidine 16 nmol/kg/min; (+) SK&F 93319 100; pyrilamine 10; cimetidine 80 nmol/kg/min.*

H_2-Receptor antagonism by SK&F 93319 *in vivo* was also demonstrated[15] by inhibition of histamine-stimulated gastric acid secretion in the rat and dog. In the perfused stomach preparation of the anesthetized rat, 50% peak inhibition was obtained at an intravenous dose of 0.21 μmol/kg (cf. 1.37 μmol/kg for cimetidine). In the conscious Heidenhain pouch dog, following the establishment of a steady acid secretory response stimulated by an infusion of histamine at a rate of 20 μmol/hour, doses of SK&F 93319 of 0.5 and 1.0 μmol/kg intravenously (by bolus injection) gave mean peak inhibitions of 42% and 86% respectively (cf. cimetidine 70% inhibition at 4 μmol/kg, in the same group of animals; n = 5). The activity of SK&F 93319 was also determined in the dog by the oral route (given in capsules), a dose of 2.5 μmol/kg (i.e. 1.2 mg/kg of the trihydrochloride salt of SK&F 93319) gave a mean peak inhibition of approximately 70% within 1.5 hours (cf. cimetidine 82% inhibition at 20 μmol/kg per os in the same group of animals; n = 5). This is shown in Figure 5.

Combined antagonism of SK&F 93319 at H_1 and H_2 receptors was demonstrated by inhibition of vascular responses to histamine and selective histamine-receptor agonists.[16] Experiments were made in cats, anesthetized with sodium pentobarbitone, 60 mg/kg i.p. Antagonism of depressor responses to intravenous injections of histamine, 2-(2-aminoethyl)pyridine (an H_1-receptor agonist), dimaprit and impromidine (H_2-receptor agonists) by SK&F 93319 were assessed by measurement of displacement of dose-response curves to each agonist. Similarly, the antagonism of vasodilator responses to intra-arterial injections of histamine and histamine receptor agonists were made in the acutely denervated femoral and gastric vasculature.[16]

Infusion of SK&F 93319 at 0.08 and 0.4 μmol/kg/

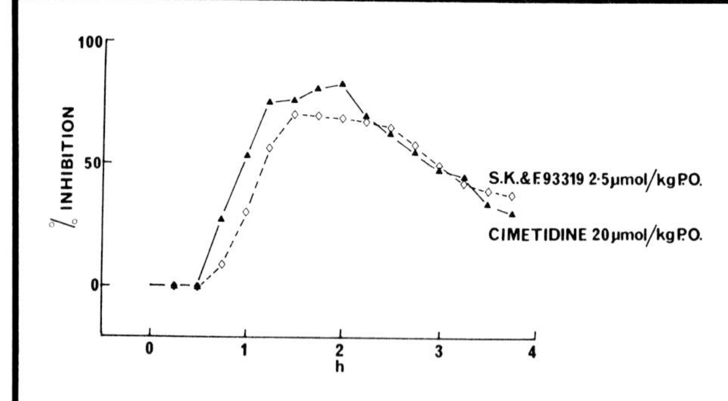

Figure 5. *Inhibition of maximal histamine-stimulated gastric acid secretion in the conscious Heidenhain pouch dog by orally administered SK&F 93319 and cimetidine respectively. Secretion stimulated by a continuous intravenous infusion of histamine at a rate of 20 μmol/hour. Ordinate axis: percentage inhibition of acid output. Abscissa: time in hours. Drugs given at time 0 when plateau secretion established (n = 5).*

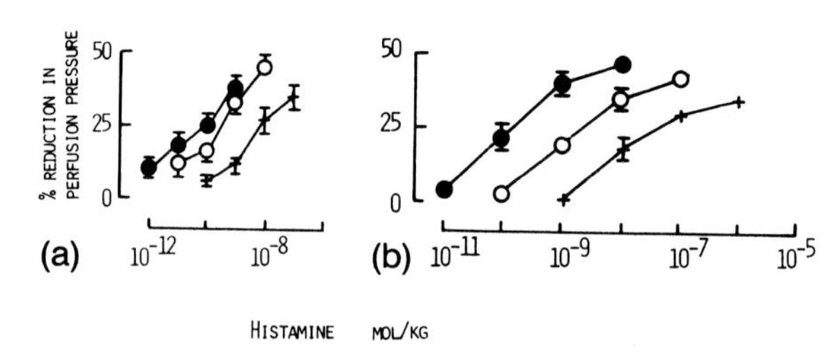

Figure 6. *Antagonism of vasodilator responses to histamine by SK&F 93319. (a) Femoral vasculature: control dose-response curve (●); histamine during infusion of SK&F 93319, 0.08 μmol/kg/min (○); histamine during infusion of SK&F 93319, 0.4 μmol/kg/min. (+); Values are mean of n = 4; s.e. indicated by vertical lines. (b) Gastric vasculature: control dose-response curve (●); histamine during the infusion of SK&F 93319, 0.08 μmol/kg/min (○); histamine during the infusion of SK&F 93319, 0.1 μmol/kg/min. (+); values are mean of n = 4; s.e. indicated by vertical lines.*

min caused parallel displacement to the right of the histamine and 2-(2-aminoethyl)pyridine dose-response curves for both depressor and vasodilator responses with similar dose-ratios for both agonists.[16] Antagonism of the responses to the H_2-receptor agonist dimaprit occurred additionally at 0.016 μmol/kg/min and greater dose-ratios were obtained for dimaprit than for histamine or 2-(2-aminoethyl)pyridine at any given dose of SK&F 93319. In a study comparing antagonism of depressor responses to histamine, dimaprit and impromidine, SK&F 93319 at 0.016 μmol/kg/min had no significant effect on the histamine dose-response curves but caused parallel displacement to the right for both the dimaprit and impromidine dose-response curves with similar dose-ratios for both agonists.[16]

The inhibition by SK&F 93319 of vasodilator responses to histamine in both the femoral and gastric vasculature is illustrated in Figure 6. The considerable displacement seen for the histamine dose-response curve in the gastric vasculature is of interest because it raises the possibility that combined blockade of histamine receptors may be of importance for treatment of gastric hemorrhage. The role of local blood vessel function in the genesis or healing of gastric ulcers has not been clearly established, nevertheless, gastric mucosal damage has been associated with histamine release and inhibition of the consequent vascular response requires use of both H_1- and H_2-receptor antagonists.[17]

It is apparent from these results that SK&F 93319 antagonized peripheral vascular responses to histamine *in vivo* at both H_1 and H_2 receptors. The displacement of the histamine dose-response curve achieved at the higher infusion rates of SK&F 93319 exceeded the maximum displacement possible with either an H_1- or H_2-receptor antagonist alone.

SK&F 93319 also antagonized the reduction in total peripheral resistance caused by intravenous infusion of histamine. The pharmacology of the vasodilator response to histamine infusions has been shown to have a time-base with a predominant role for H_1 receptors in the immediate peak response, within one minute of the start of the intravenous infusion, which changes to a predominant role for H_2 receptors in the sustained response when infusions exceed 2 or 3 minutes. This time base was first observed by Chipman and Glover[8] in human forearm and has now been found in a variety of vascular beds in different species including the peripheral vasculature in anesthetized cats (Harvey and Owen[16]; Owen et al.,[18]). SK&F 93319 was an effective antagonist of both the early and sustained vasodilator responses to histamine in the peripheral circulation, indicative of its antagonist activity at both H_1 and H_2 receptors on peripheral resistance vessels.

SPECIFICITY

Even when administered, to the anesthetized cat, at the high infusion rate of 2 μmol/kg/min, which essentially abolished the responses to the large doses of exogenous histamine used, there were no measurable changes in resting hemodynamic variables. No changes in resting hemodynamics were seen with i.v. bolus injections of 20 μmol/kg. Neither was any effect seen on autonomic function.

There was no effect detected on renal function[19] or pulmonary function[20] in the dog at doses of up to 20 μmol/kg.

Many H_1-receptor histamine antagonists (antihistamines) are known to cause sedation or drowsiness and it was therefore important to examine SK&F 93319 for such effects. In doses of up to 200 μmol/kg subcutaneously SK&F 93319 did not appear to affect locomotor or exploratory activity in mice.[21]

SK&F 93319, like other H_2-receptor antagonists is a very polar H-bonding molecule and, H_2-antagonists generally appear to have difficulty in penetrating the blood brain barrier. However, in view of the apparent lipophilicity of SK&F 93319 which has an octanol:water partition ratio of 435:1 (at 37.5°C and pH 7.5)[22] it seemed essential to provide a further check. Tests were therefore performed with ^{14}C labelled SK&F 93319 in rats, and it was verified that there was negligible penetration into the brain.[23]

STUDIES IN MAN

Studies in man by Johnson et al[24] (healthy volunteers) suggest that SK&F 93319 is well absorbed when given orally and has good bioavailability (range 47–65%), peak blood concentrations occurred within 60 minutes after oral admnistration. It has a high degree of serum protein binding (99.8%) and a mean plasma elimination half-life of 8.6 ± 1.6 hours.

In summary, SK&F 93319 has been identified as a novel agent which antagonizes the actions of histamine at H_1 and H_2 receptors across a similar concentration or dose range. The degree of antagonism of vascular responses to histamine by SK&F 93319 exceeds that possible with either an H_1- or H_2-receptor antagonist alone and can only be achieved by combined use of both types of antagonist.

SK&F 93319 is thus likely to be a useful tool in the study of histamine and its pharmacology and may have therapeutic usefulness in conditions requiring simultaneous antagonism of histamine at H_1 and H_2 receptors e.g. some inflammatory skin diseases such as the urticarias and mastocytosis, and in some cases of circulatory shock as may occur following anaphylactoid reactions to drugs or anesthetics.[25]

REFERENCES

1. Ash ASF, Schild HO. Receptors mediating some actions of histamine. Brit J Pharmacol 27:427–439, 1966.
2. Black JW, Duncan WA, Durant GJ, Ganellin CR, Parsons ME. Definition and antagonism of histamine H_2-receptors. Nature (London) 236:385–390, 1972.
3. Dale HH, Laidlaw PP. The physiological action of β-iminazolylethylamine. J Physiol 41:318–344, 1910.
4. Folkow B, Haeger K, Kahlson G. Observations on reactive hyperaemia as related to histamine, on drugs antagonizing vasodilatation induced by histamine and on vasodilator properties of andenosinetriphosphate. Acta Physiol Scand 15:264–278, 1948.
5. Black JW, Owen DA, Parsons ME. An analysis of the depressor responses to histamine in the cat and dog: involvement of both H_1- and H_2-receptors. Br J Pharmacol 54:319–324, 1975.
6. Wyllie JH, Hesselbo T, Black JW. Effects in man of histamine H_2-receptor blockade by burimamide. Lancet ii:1117–1120, 1972.
7. Marks R, Greaves MW. Vascular reactions to histamine and compound 48/80 in human skin: suppression by a histamine H_2-receptor blocking agent. Br J Clin Pharmacol 4:367–369, 1977.
8. Chipman P, Glover WE. Histamine H_2-receptors in the human peripheral circulation. Br J Pharmacol 56:494–496, 1976.
9. Levi R, Owen DAA, Trzeciakowski J. Action of histamine on the heart and vasculature. Ch 6. In: Pharmacology of Histamine Receptors. Ganellin CR, Parsons ME (Eds) Wright PSG, Bristol, London, Boston, 1982, pp. 236–297.
10. Burland WL, Mills JG. The pathophysiological role of histamine and potential therapeutic uses of H_1 and H_2 antihistamines. Ch 11. In: Pharmacology of Histamine Receptors. Ganellin CR, Parsons ME (Eds) Wright PSG, Bristol, London, Boston, 1982, pp. 436–481.
11. Brimblecombe RW, Duncan WA, Durant GJ, Emmett JC, Ganellin CR, Parsons ME. Cimetidine: a non-thiourea H_2-receptor antagonist. J Int Med Res 3:86–92, 1975.
12. Testa B, Murset-Rossetti L. The partition coefficient of protonated antihistamines. Its calculation and interpretation in terms of hydrophobic fragmental constants. Helv Chim Acta 61:2530–2537, 1978.
13. Blakemore RC, Brown TH, Durant GJ, Emmett JC, Ganellin CR, Parsons ME, Rasmussen AC. SK&F 92994: a new histamine H_2-receptor antagonist. Br J Pharmacol 70:105P, 1980.
14. Verloop A, Hoogenstraaten W, Tipker J. Development and application of new steric substituent parameters in drug design. Ch 4. In: Drug Design. Vol 7. Ariens EJ (Ed) Academic Press, New York, 1976, pp. 165–207.
15. Blakemore RC, Brown TH, Cooper DG, Durant GJ, Ganellin CR, Ife RJ, Parsons ME, Rasmussen AC, Sach GS. SK&F 93319: a specific antagonist of histamine at H_1- and H_2-receptors. Br J Pharmacol 80:437P, 1983.
16. Harvey CA, Owen DAA. Inhibition of vascular responses to histamine by SK&F 93319, a histamine antagonist at H_1- and H_2-receptors. Br J Pharmacol 80:438P, 1983. Cardiovascular studies with SK&F 93319, an antagonist of histamine at both H_1- and H_2-receptors. Br J Pharmacol 83:427–432, 1984.
17. Owen DAA, Harvey CA, Parsons ME, Pipkin G, Price CA. Histamine H_1- and H_2-receptor antagonists. Effects on gastric blood flow and experimental gastric hemorrhage in the rat. In: Microcirculation of the Alimentary Tract. Koo A, Lam SK, Smaje LH (Eds) World Scientific Publ Singapore, 1983, pp. 317–326.
18. Owen DA, Harvey CA, Boyce MJ. Effects of histamine on the circulatory system. Klin Wochenschr 60:972–977, 1982.
19. Dr V Weibelhaus, R&D Division, Smith Kline and French Laboratories, Philadelphia, PA.
20. Dr RD Krell, R&D Division, Smith Kline and French Laboratories, Philadelphia, PA.
21. Dr CR Calcutt, Smith Kline and French Research Limited, Welwyn, Hertfordshire, England.
22. Dr RC Mitchell, Smith Kline and French Research Limited, Welwyn, Hertfordshire, England.
23. Dr R Griffiths, Smith Kline and French Research Limited, Welwyn, Hertfordshire, England.
24. Johnson P, Griffiths R, Lee RM, McDowall RD, Doyle E, Taylor DC, Burland WL. The pharmacokinetics in man of SK&F 93319—a new antagonist at histamine H_1 and H_2 receptors. Xenobiotica 14:589–593, 1984.
25. Ahnefeld FW, Doenicke A, Lorenz W (Eds). Histamine and Antihistamines in Anesthesia and Surgery. Klin. Wochenschrift 60:871–1062, 1982.
26. Lorenz W, Doenicke A. H_1 and H_2 blockade: A prophylactic principle in anaesthesia and surgery against histamine-release responses of any degree of severity. NER Allergy Proc 6:37–57, 174–194, 1985. □

Chapter XXII

Loratadine: A Potent, Nonsedating, and Long-Acting H_1 Antagonist

Harold M. Friedman, M.D.

ABSTRACT

Loratadine, a nonclassical selective, peripheral H_1-receptor antagonist has undergone extensive preclinical studies and clinical trials in over 6,000 patients. In the treatment of allergic rhinitis, loratadine has efficacy equivalent to clemastine, terfenadine, astemizole, and mequitazine. Its duration of action is 18–24 hours making once daily dosing practical. Loratadine is virtually devoid of sedating or other CNS effects.

The classical H_1 antagonists may cause excessive sedation and anticholinergic effects, limiting their clinical usefulness.[1] It is likely that these unwanted effects occur because these drugs enter the central nervous system and interact with neuroreceptors.

In recent years, newer antihistamines have been developed that do not readily concentrate in the brain, producing fewer undesirable side effects. However, currently available nonsedating antihistamines either require frequent dosing or several days of administration for a full response.

A more ideal antihistamine would be nonsedating, possess a rapid onset of action, and provide 24-hour relief of histamine-mediated symptoms with a single dose. Its H_1-receptor-binding affinity should be high, but not so strong as to preclude performing skin tests for several weeks once the drug is discontinued. Loratadine meets these requirements.

PHARMACOLOGY

Loratadine is a piperidine compound related to azatadine. It is relatively specific in blocking peripheral H_1-receptors with very little H_2-receptor antagonism.[2] Even at large multiples of the dose needed to inhibit histamine-induced bronchospasm, loratadine has insignificant effects on platelet-activating factors or methacholine bronchial challenges.

Loratadine, like several other antihistamines, does stabilize mast cell membranes. *In vitro*, loratadine inhibited the release of histamine and leukotrienes from human lung fragments, cloned murine mast cells, and rat peritoneal mast cells.[2]

Guinea pigs were protected from the lethal effects of intravenous histamine for 18–24 hours when pretreated with loratadine. In equipotent doses, terfenadine protection lasted for 6 hours and astemizole protection for 12 hours.[3]

In mice and rats, loratadine had no effects in tests of motor activity, tone, and mydriasis in doses as high as 300 mg/kg, while terfenadine and diphenhydramine had pronounced effects in similar dose ranges. Behavioral changes in monkeys and dogs were much less influenced by loratadine than with diphenhydramine, chlorpheniramine, promenthazine, and terfenadine.

The fatal effects of physostigmine in mice could be blocked by classical antihistamines while loratadine was not capable of altering the death rate, consistent with its lack of anticholinergic actions.

The paucity of central nervous system side effects caused by loratadine may be due to both its inability to penetrate the blood-brain barrier and its lack of affinity for the brain receptors associated with sedation.

Distribution of ^{14}C-labeled loratadine was determined 3 hours to 3 days after its administration to rats. Extremely low levels of radioactivity were present in the brains of these animals at all times. At 3 hours after dosing, the concentration of ^{14}C was 40-fold higher in lung tissue than in the brain (Fig. 1).

Associate Professor of Clinical Medicine, Dartmouth Medical School, Hanover, NH

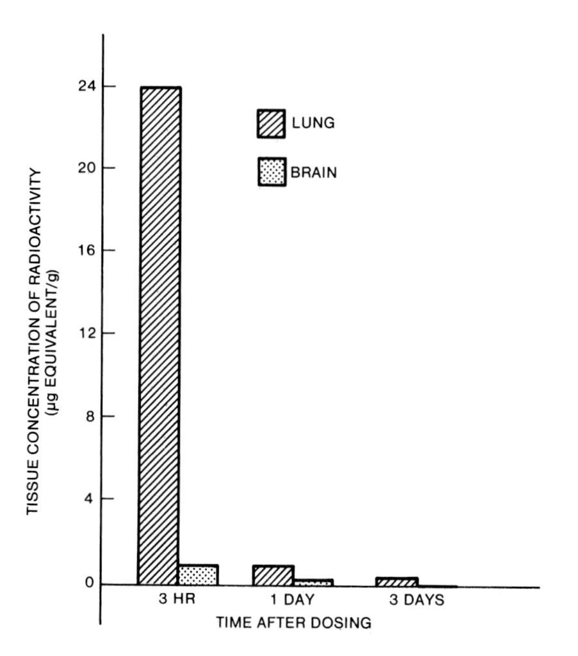

Figure 1. *Relative concentration of loratadine in lung and brain.*

Classical antihistamines cross the blood-brain barrier and produce sedation largely by occupying H_1-receptors in the brain. In contrast to the results found with competitive binding studies using older antihistamines, loratadine, at twice its peripheral antihistamine dose, could not inhibit the binding of ^{3}H-mepyramine to mouse cerebral cortex. In addition, radioligand binding studies confirmed that the loratadine indeed exhibited greater affinity for peripheral rather than central H_1-receptors. Identical studies with terfenadine, astemizole, mequitazine, and chlorpheniramine indicated no such selective peripheral binding.[4]

CLINICAL PHARMACOLOGY

Oral loratadine is well absorbed and extensively metabolized.[5] In man, loratadine is present in measurable levels in plasma within 15 minutes and reaches peak levels within 1 hour after a single oral dose. The elimination half-life of loratadine and its active metabolite is 18 hours, permitting once a day dosing.

The suppression of histamine-induced skin wheals is regarded as a standard model for demonstrating the activity of H_1-receptor antagonists in man. Using this model, loratadine, in single and multiple doses, was significantly more effective ($p = 0.001$) than placebo in suppressing the formation of histamine-induced skin wheals.[6–8] The suppression of wheal formation was noted within 2 hours after the first dose of loratadine. Tachyphylaxis did not occur over a 28-day study (Fig. 2).

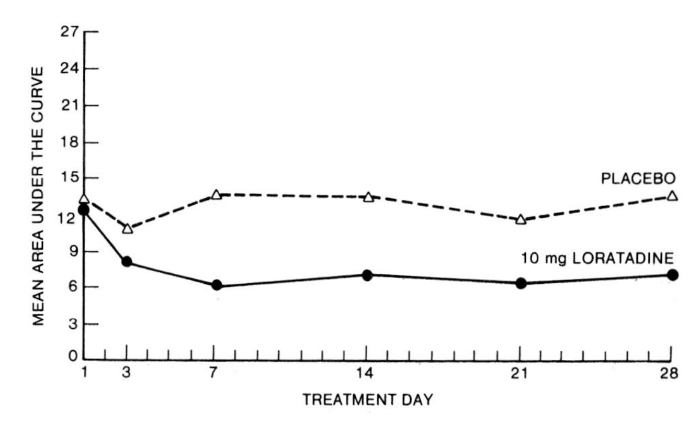

Figure 2. *Mean area under the curve (0–12 hours) for mean daily adjusted wheal area.*

CLINICAL EFFICACY

Seasonal Allergic Rhinitis

The effects of loratadine in relieving the symptoms of seasonal allergic rhinitis have been evaluated worldwide in 34 clinical studies in 113 centers.

In all studies, a standard protocol was used to measure changes from baseline scores for symptoms that included nasal discharge, stuffiness, itching and sneezing, as well as itching, burning, tearing, and redness of the eyes, and itching of the ears and palate.

The percent change in symptom scores in the multiple studies is shown in Figure 3. Improvement in mean total symptom scores in patients taking loratadine was statistically better than a placebo ($p < 0.05$) and was similar to that observed for the nonsedating antihistamines, terfenadine and astemizole, and the sedating antihistamine, clemastine.[9]

In one spring study conducted in the United States, 108 patients in each treatment group received either loratadine, 10 mg daily, clemastine, 1 mg b.i.d., or placebo.[10] The percent improvement was 46% on day 3 for loratadine-treated patients compared with 41%

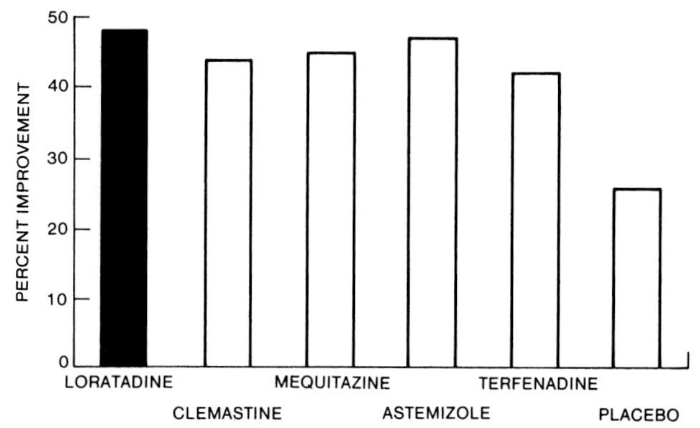

Figure 3. *Loratadine in seasonal allergic rhinitis: percent improvement in mean total symptom score.*

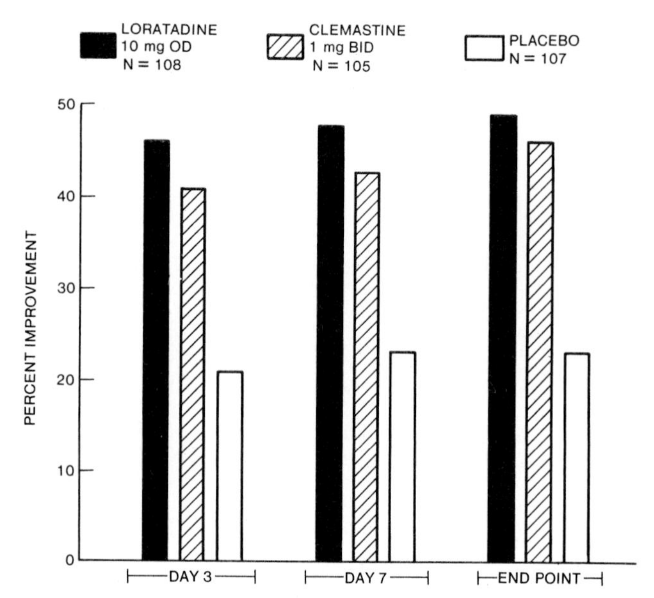

Figure 4. *Percent improvement in mean total symptom scores in spring study.*

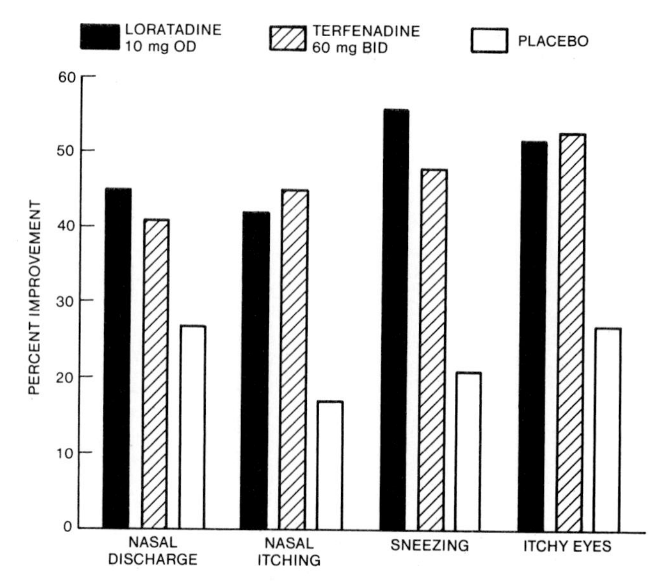

Figure 5. *Percent improvement in mean individual symptom scores at first (day 3) evaluation.*

for those treated with clemastine and 21% in the placebo group (Fig. 4). The symptom improvement remained constant throughout the duration of the study.

Essentially identical results were found in a springtime Canadian study with terfenadine, 60 mg b.i.d., as the control antihistamine.[11] There was a 48% improvement in symptoms for patients treated with 10 mg of loratadine daily, with 46% improvement present at the conclusion of the study.

Loratadine was shown to be especially effective in relieving sneezing, nasal discharge, nasal itching, and the conjunctival symptoms of ocular itching and burning (Fig. 5). The onset of symptom relief was often within 30 minutes of ingestion of the loratadine. The combination of loratadine and pseudoephedrine sulfate has been shown to further increase the relief of symptoms and enhance the relief of nasal congestion.

Perennial Allergic Rhinitis

Loratadine, 10 mg daily, has been shown to be useful in the treatment of perennial allergic rhinitis. The symptoms of nasal discharge, stuffiness, postnasal drainage, nasal itching, sneezing, and itchy and watery eyes were evaluated in several double-blind studies. These trials compared loratadine, 10 mg daily, with terfenadine, 60 mg b.i.d., clemastine, 1 mg b.i.d., and a placebo. The patients were treated and followed for up to 6 months.

Loratadine was comparable to other antihistamines in lowering symptom scores. Throughout the duration of the study there was a 45–50% decline in the complaints of nasal stuffiness, postnasal drainage, and nasal discharge (Fig. 6).

Chronic Urticaria

Patients with chronic urticaria were studied in several randomized, double-blind, 28-day trials.[12] The efficacy of loratadine, 10 mg o.d., was compared with terfenadine, 60 mg b.i.d. and placebo in alleviating the symptoms of itching, erythema, and wheal number and size. Loratadine was more effective than a placebo ($p < 0.05$) and equal to terfenadine in providing symptomatic relief (Fig. 7).

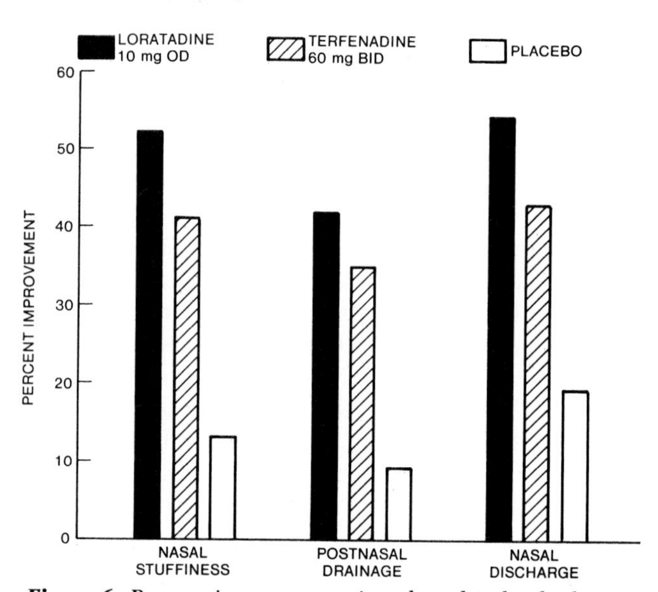

Figure 6. *Percent improvement in selected individual symptoms in patients with perennial allergic rhinitis.*

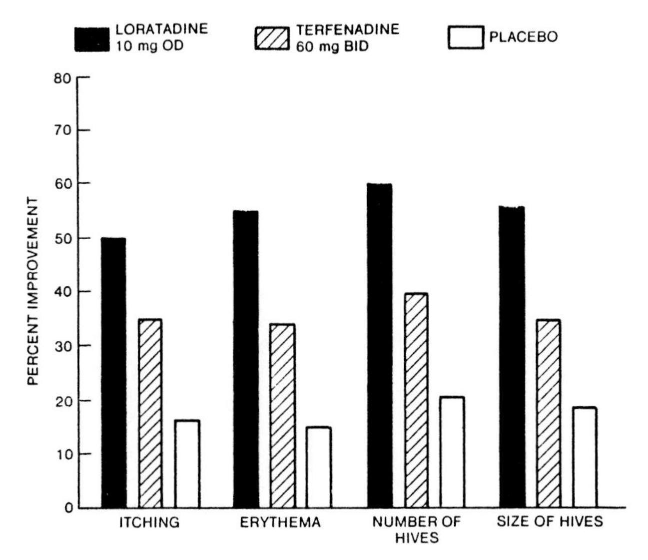

Figure 7. Percent improvement in individual symptoms in patients with chronic urticaria.

CLINICAL SAFETY

Over 2,500 patients treated with loratadine were evaluated for safety. These included over 1,000 patients with perennial allergic rhinitis or allergic skin disorders treated with loratadine for up to 6 months. The results confirm that loratadine is nonsedating, safe, and well tolerated.[9–12]

Sedation occurred in 8% of the patients treated with loratadine, 8% with terfenadine, and 6% with a placebo (Fig. 8). The highest incidence of sedation was reported in those patients receiving clemastine (21%). The incidence of sedation in patients receiving loratadine was statistically less than in those treated with clemastine and no different than in those receiving terfenadine or a placebo. A dry mouth was reported in 3% of patients treated with loratadine as compared with 2% in the placebo group. The incidence and profile of adverse experiences did not change as the studies were extended from 2 weeks to 6 months.

To further investigate the central nervous system effects of loratadine, several special studies were conducted in volunteers. Assessment of objective performance demonstrated no declines in psychomotor function or the appearance of sedation while patients were receiving loratadine.[13] In contrast, diphenhydramine significantly ($p < 0.05$) reduced psychomotor performance and increased daytime sleepiness.[14]

The comparative anticholinergic effects of single oral doses of loratadine, 10 mg, were evaluated by measuring salivary flow, sedation, heart rate, and blood pressure in a randomized, double-blind trial.[9] Loratadine did not cause reduction in salivary flow or any changes in heart rate or blood pressure. Promethazine significantly ($p < 0.05$) reduced salivary flow.

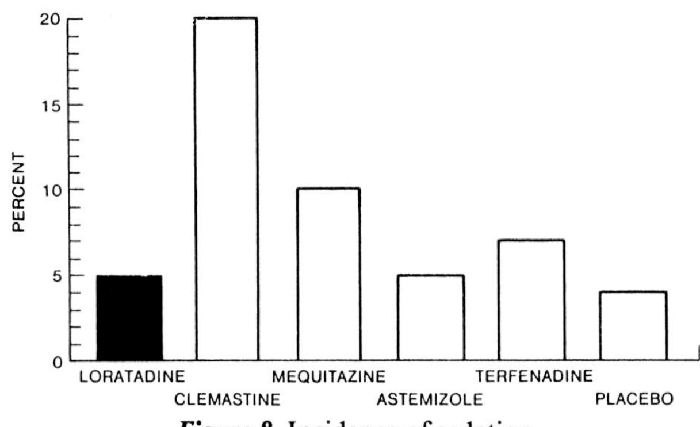

Figure 8. Incidence of sedation.

SUMMARY

Loratadine has been shown to be a safe and effective nonsedating antihistamine for the treatment of seasonal and perennial allergic rhinitis, conjunctivitis, and chronic urticaria. Loratadine is comparable in efficacy to terfenadine,[11] astemizole,[15,16] and clemastine.[10,17] Its clinical advantages of prompt onset of action and long duration of effect permit once daily dosing, yet elimination is rapid enough for accurate skin testing within 72 hours after the drug is discontinued.

REFERENCES

1. Drouin MA. H_1 histamines: perspective on the use of the conventional and new agents. Ann Allergy 55:747–752, 1985.
2. Kreutner W, Chapman RW, Gulbenkian A, Siegel MI. Antiallergic activity of loratadine, a non-sedating antihistamine. Allergy 42:57–63, 1987.
3. Barnett A, Iorio LC, Kreutner W, Tozzi S, Ahn HS, Gulbenkian A. Evaluation of the CNS properties of SCH 29851, a potential non-sedating antihistamine. Agents Actions 14:590–597, 1984.
4. Ahn HS, Barnett A. Selective displacement of ^{3}H-mepyramine from peripheral vs central nervous system receptors by loratadine, a non-sedating antihistamine. Eur J Pharmacol 127:153–155, 1986.
5. Katchen B, Cramer J, Chung M, et al. Disposition of ^{14}C-SCH 29851 in humans. Ann Allergy 55:293, 1985.
6. Batenhorst RL, Batenhorst AS, Graves DA, Foster TS, Kung M, Gural RP, Amkraut HJ. Pharmacologic evaluation of loratadine (SCH 29851), chlorpheniramine, and placebo. Eur J Clin Pharmacol 31:247–250, 1986.
7. Kassem N, Roman I, Gural R, Dyer G, Robillard N. Effects of loratadine (SCH 29851) in suppression of histamine-induced skin wheals. Ann Allergy, in press, 1986.
8. Roman IJ, Kassem N, Gural RP, Herron J. Suppression of histamine-induced wheal response by loratadine (SCH 29851) over 28 days in man. Ann Allergy 57:253–356, 1986.

9. Roman IR. Loratadine—clinical profile (Abstract). Presented at European Academy of Allergology and Clinical Immunology, Budapest, May 1986.
10. Dockhorn RJ, Bergner A, Connell JT, Falliers CJ, Grabiec SV, Weiler JM, Shellenberger MK. Safety and efficacy of loratadine (SCH 29851), a new non-sedating antihistamine in seasonal allergic rhinitis. Ann Allergy, in press, 1987.
11. Gutkowski A, Shulz JI, Herbert J, Turenne Y, Prevost M, Del Carpio J, Nedilski MM, Bedard P. Efficacy of loratadine 10 mg OD vs terfenadine 60 mg BID and placebo in patients with seasonal allergic rhinitis (Abstract). Presented at European Academy of Allergology and Clinical Immunology, Budapest, May 1986.
12. Pedrali P, Bruttmann G. Efficacy of loratadine in the management of idiopathic chronic urticaria (Abstract). Presented at European Academy of Allergology and Clinical Immunology, Budapest, May 1986.
13. Bradley CM, Nicholson AN. Studies on the central effects of the H_1-antagonist, loratadine. Eur J Clin Pharmacol, in press, 1987.
14. Roth T, Roehrs T, Zorick F. Central effects of H_1 antihistamines (Abstract). Presented at European Academy of Allergology and Clinical Immunology, Budapest, May 1986.
15. Oei HD, Verheij E, Schwab D, Lherminier M, Bruynzeel PLB. A comparative study of the efficacy of loratadine and astemizole (Abstract 263). Presented at American Academy of Allergy and Immunology, Washington, DC, Feb 1987 J Allergy Clin Immunol, 79:190, 1987.
16. Kaminszczik I, Soto-Roman L, Kutwak A, Rodriguez L, Cataldo J, Ronaj H, Fantuzzi Alliende H. Loratadine vs astemizole: onset of allergy symptoms relief (Abstract). Presented at European Academy of Allergology and Clinical Immunology, Budapest, May 1986.
17. Kemp JP, Meltzer EO, Orgel HA, Welch MJ, Bahna SL, Chervinsky P, Rachelefsky GS, Seltzer JM, Vande Stouwe RA, Valero RN. A comparison of loratadine, clemastine and placebo in patients with seasonal rhinitis (Abstract 264). Presented at American Academy of Allergy and Immunology, Washington, DC, Feb 1987 J Allergy Clin Immunol 79:190, 1987. □

Chapter XXIII

Cetirizine, a Novel Antihistamine

Sheldon L. Spector, M.D.,* Robert Altman, M.D.**

ABSTRACT

Cetirizine, an oxidative metabolite of hydroxyzine, is a cyclizine class H_1-receptor antagonist with diminished CNS activity currently under investigation. It has a novel pharmacokinetic profile with a 9-hour half-life, lower volume of distribution and total body clearance, minimal metabolism and essentially renal excretion. Minimal binding to CNS receptors has been demonstrated in animal models. In contrast to its parent compound and diphenhydramine, cetirizine has an effect comparable to placebo on psychomotor function and multiple sleep latency tests. Inhibition of histamine-induced bronchospasm and mild bronchodilation has also been demonstrated. U.S. and European clinical trials have affirmed its safety and efficacy in histamine-associated disorders.

A new class of H_1 antihistamines with reduced CNS soporific side effects but effective in blocking respiratory and cutaneous effects of histamine has been developed. Cetirizine, a human metabolite of hydroxyzine, is a potent and effective example of this class of drug, which is currently under investigation.

Cetirizine is a H_1-receptor antagonist of the cyclizine class. It is an oxidative metabolite of hydroxyzine in which the terminal primary alcohol of the side chain has been converted to a carboxylic acid (Fig. 1). The polarity thus created theoretically diminishes blood-brain penetration, which in addition to histamine receptor specificity, accounts for its improved side effect profile.

* *Clinical Professor of Medicine, UCLA School of Medicine, Los Angeles, CA*

** *Senior Associate Medical Director, Pfizer Pharmaceuticals, New York, NY*

PHARMACOKINETICS

The half-lives of H_1-receptor antagonists vary greatly ranging from a few hours for terfenadine and triprolidine[1,2]; to about 9 hours for cetirizine, azatadine, and loratadine; to approximately 20–25 hours for hydroxyzine, chlorpheniramine, and brompheniramine[1]; to 5–14 days for astemizole.[2] Most of these antihistamines including cetirizine have shorter elimination half-life values in children than in adults.

Simons and co-workers[1-3] have reported that regardless of the age of patients, apparent volume of distribution and total body clearance appear to be large, i.e., 3.4–18.5 liters/kg and 4.4–32.1 ml/min/kg for most of the H_1-receptor antagonists except for cetirizine for which values are 0.8 liter/kg and 0.5 ml/min/kg respectively.[4] Urinary excretion of unchanged antihistamine is higher after cetirizine (60% of dose) than after any other H_1 blocker.[4] After multiple doses (10 mg daily) of cetirizine, steady state is attained by the third dose with no apparent accumulation in plasma drug concentrations.[4]

Wood and Chasseaud[4,5] have reported on the metabolism and pharmacokinetics of ^{14}C-cetirizine in man. Six healthy male volunteers received a 10-mg oral dose of radiolabeled cetirizine. The drug was rapidly absorbed with peak mean concentrations of radioactivity

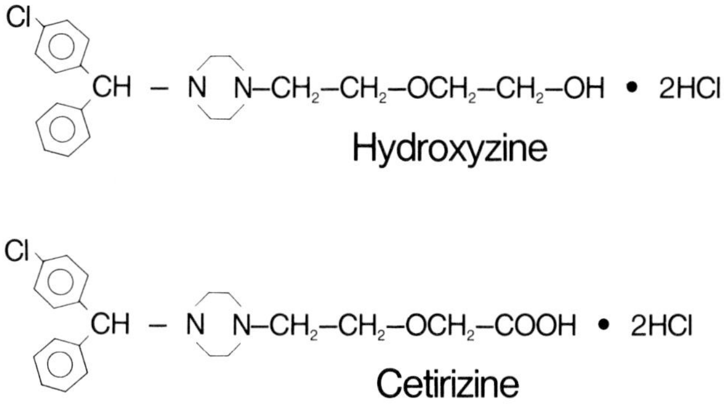

Cl
CH – N N–CH_2–CH_2–OCH_2–CH_2–OH • 2HCl
Hydroxyzine

Cl
CH – N N–CH_2–CH_2–OCH_2–COOH • 2HCl
Cetirizine

Figure 1.

(374 ng equivalents/ml) of unchanged drug achieved within 1 hour. Concentrations of radioactivity initially declined with a half-life of about 9 hours, but the terminal half-life was longer. The former corresponds to the known half-life of cetirizine. Radioactivity was initially excreted quite rapidly during the first day (61% of dose in urine and 1% in feces) and then more slowly (10% in urine, 9% in feces) during the next 4 days.

Examination of the thin-layer chromatographic profiles of radioactive compounds excreted in urine and present in plasma has indicated that there is little metabolism of cetirizine in man. Essentially, only one minor metabolite, which formed by oxidative *O*-dealkylation of the cetirizine side chain, was observed in plasma and urine.

Matzke and co-workers[4,5] reported on the pharmacokinetics of cetirizine in the elderly and in patients with renal insufficiency. In 16 geriatric patients the elimination half-life, apparent total body clearance, and area under the serum concentration time curve were significantly different from those in adult normal subjects, but the apparent volume of distribution was not. The pharmacokinetic parameters correlated with both age and renal function. The effect of renal function was more important than age, suggesting that the age effect may actually result from decreased renal function in the geriatric patients.

PHARMACOLOGIC ATTRIBUTES

In preclinical studies, cetirizine was shown to be capable of antagonizing the actions of histamine in a variety of animal and human models, including survival from anaphylactic hypotension, while being devoid of CNS effects. Because the drug does not prevent histamine release at physiologic concentrations in most model systems, it is thought to act exclusively on the H_1-receptor.

Snyder and Snowman[5] demonstrated that cetirizine, hydroxyzine, and terfenadine had similar binding affinity for guinea pig brain and lung histamine receptors. They concluded that the diminished sedative effects of cetirizine were probably not attributable to lesser affinity for brain versus peripheral receptors. In comparison with terfenadine and hydroxyzine, cetirizine was most selective for histamine H_1-receptors, while at clinically effective doses, terfenadine and hydroxyzine occupied serotonin, dopamine, α-adrenergic, and calcium channel receptors to a similar extent as the histamine receptor. In a comparison experiment of peripherally administered antihistamines in rats, d-chlorpheniramine and hydroxyzine occupied a majority of histamine H_1-receptors while neither cetirizine nor terfenadine significantly occupied histamine H_1-receptors in the brain. Thus, it may be concluded that terfenadine and cetirizine entered the brain to occupy histamine receptors less than other antihistamines.

CLINICAL PHARMACODYNAMICS

Using single doses of medication in healthy controls, Gengo et al.[6] assessed the CNS effects of cetirizine with psychomotor function tests. CNS effects were measured in 12 subjects using critical flicker fusion frequency Stroop word testing and perceived feelings of drowsiness using visual analog scales. In a second study of 15 subjects cetirizine, doses of 5, 10, and 20 mg were compared with diphenhydramine, 50 mg, and placebo. The CNS effects were measured using digit-symbol substitution, maze tracking, and a driving performance analyzer that evaluated choice reaction time and vigilance. Skin wheal response to dermal histamine was also assessed. The results suggested that cetirizine, in contrast to hydroxyzine or diphenhydramine, produced significant antihistamine effects without CNS changes.

Dement et al.[4,5] also found no difference between 5, 10, or 20 mg of cetirizine and placebo with regard to a direct EEG measure of sleepiness: sleep latency tests involving 20-minute opportunities to try to fall asleep in bed while EEG and eye movements were recorded. Interestingly, although hydroxyzine significantly reduced sleep latency, subjects who received it were apparently unaware of their sleepiness or impaired performance.

Tashkin and co-workers[7] studied the effectiveness of 5, 10, and 20 mg of cetirizine and 25 mg of hydroxyzine versus placebo in 10 asthmatics with a mean age of 27.7 ± 9.4 and FEV_1 70% of predicted value. Production of bronchodilatation and protection against bronchoconstriction induced by histamine inhalation (0.03–20 μg/ml) were measured. For all 10 subjects, the provocative concentration of histamine causing a 20% decline in FEV_1 from the postdiluent control value (PC_{20}) was more than 4-fold greater after each active drug than placebo. Cetirizine provided significantly greater protection against histamine-induced bronchospasm than placebo ($p < 0.001$); moreover, a dose-dependent protective effect was noted with cetirizine. Significant bronchodilation was also found at 60 min: FEV_1 increased significantly after all active antihistamines compared with placebo and after cetirizine, 20 mg, compared with hydroxyzine ($p < 0.05$).

EUROPEAN CLINICAL TRIALS[1]

Clinical efficacy has been shown in numerous European studies.[5] In seasonal allergic rhinitis, a total of 228 patients were treated in double-blind, placebo-controlled studies with 10 mg of cetirizine once a day for 3 weeks. Another 40 patients were treated with 10 mg of cetirizine q.d. or terfenadine, 60 mg, b.i.d. for 3 weeks. In every instance, cetirizine was better than placebo and/or had a therapeutic index comparable with terfenadine.

In perennial allergic rhinitis, a total of 252 patients

were treated with cetirizine, 10 mg once a day, in double-blind, crossover studies with terfenadine and placebo control periods. Another 40 were treated in a crossover design against placebo alone, and another 40 in parallel against terfenadine. In six studies cetirizine was superior to terfenadine; in six it was equal to terfenadine. No significant side effects were observed in any study.

In chronic idiopathic urticaria, a total of 147 patients were studied with cetirizine, 10 mg q.d., in double-blind, crossover studies with a placebo control period. Treatment periods ranged from 7–14 days. Another 30 patients were treated with cetirizine, 5 mg b.i.d., in a double-blind, crossover study versus placebo, with treatment periods of 21 days each. Cetirizine was superior to placebo in all these studies.

In other urticaria trials cetirizine, 10 mg q.d., terfenadine 60 mg b.i.d., and placebo were compared in double-blind, crossover manner, with treatment periods of 14 days. In addition, 30 patients were similarly studied but with a 20-mg cetirizine q.d. dose. The advantage of cetirizine over terfenadine was statistically significant in selected parameters of some studies. No significant side effects were observed in these studies.

Long-term open tolerance studies (26 patients for 6 months, 65 patients for 12 months) revealed no significant adverse effects and indicated persistent effectiveness throughout the study period.

U.S. CLINICAL TRIALS

Cetirizine has also been administered to more than 1500 patients in the United States in Phase I, II, and III studies for periods up to 6 months.[5]

Cetirizine, at doses of 5, 10, and 20 mg q.a.m. was compared with placebo in a parallel study of 1 week's duration in 419 patients at nine sites during the typical ragweed season. Cetirizine was significantly more effective than placebo at all doses in reducing typical rhinitis symptoms. A dose-response relationship was demonstrated as the 20-mg dose of cetirizine was significantly more effective than 5 mg.

In a perennial rhinitis trial cetirizine doses of 10 and 20 mg q.a.m. was compared with placebo in a 4-week parallel study of 220 patients at six study sites. Both cetirizine doses were effective in reducing rhinitis symptoms and maintained their superiority to placebo over the course of the study.

The effect of cetirizine on chronic idiopathic urticaria was studied in 144 patients at six study sites. Cetirizine doses of 10 and 20 mg q.h.s. were compared with placebo in a parallel design over a four-week study period. Urticaria lesion scores and pruritus were evaluated by patients and physicians and indicated superiority of both cetirizine doses to placebo.

The incidence of sedation with doses of cetirizine greater than 5 mg in these trials was higher than with placebo. Nevertheless, this side effect was generally mild and self-limiting and rarely required a change in the therapeutic regimen.

In conclusion, cetirizine was shown to be safe and effective treatment for symptoms of seasonal and perennial allergic rhinitis and idiopathic urticaria. The slight sedation shown at the higher doses might limit its appeal.

REFERENCES

1. Simons FER, Simons KJ. H_1 receptor antagonists: clinical pharmacology and use in allergic disease. Pediatr Clin North Am 30:899–914, 1983.
2. Simons FER, Simons KJ, LG Reid. Comparison of the suppressive effect of astemizole, terfenadine and hydroxyzine on histamine induced wheals and flares in humans. J Allergy Clin Immunol 77:355, 1968.
3. Simons FER, Simons KJ, Frith EM. The pharmacokinetics and antihistaminic effects of the H_1-receptor antagonist hydroxyzine. J Allergy Clin Immunol 73:69, 1984.
4. Data on file, Department of Clinical and Scientific Affairs, Pfizer Pharmaceuticals, New York.
5. Proceedings of Investigators' Symposium, "Cetirizine: A Recent Advance in Selective Antihistamine Therapy." Ann Allergy 59 (no. 6): 1–68, 1987.
6. Gengo FM, Dabronzo J, Yurchak A, Love S, Miller K. The relative antihistaminic and psychomotor effects of hydroxyzine and cetirizine. Clin Pharmacol Ther 42:265–272, 1987.
7. Brik A, Tashkin DP, Gong H Jr., Dauphinec B, Lee E. Effect of cetirizine, a new histamine H_1-antagonist on airway dynamics and responsiveness to inhaled histamine in mild asthma. J Allergy Clin Immunol 80:51–56, 1987. □

Chapter XXIV

Epilogue: New H_1-Receptor Antagonists

F. Estelle R. Simons, M.D., Keith J. Simons, Ph.D.** (Canada)

ABSTRACT

The new H_1-receptor antagonists such as astemizole, cetirizine, loratadine, levocabastine, ketotifen, and azelastine have diverse pharmacokinetics, pharmacodynamics, and potency. Astemizole, for example, is the most long-acting of the new drugs and is not suitable for sporadic use. Cetirizine, the carboxylic acid metabolite of hydroxyzine, unlike other H_1-receptor antagonists, is minimally metabolized in the body and is primarily excreted in unchanged form in the urine. Levocabastine is the most potent of the new drugs and can be applied topically to the conjunctivae or to the nasal mucosa for relief of allergic rhinoconjunctivitis. Ketotifen and azelastine have well-described antiallergic effects in addition of their antihistaminic effects. None of the new H_1-receptor antagonists is any more effective in relieving nasal congestion than the first-generation H_1-receptor antagonists are. Most, but not all, of the new H_1-receptor antagonists lack anticholinergic effects and are relatively nonsedating.

The perfect H_1-receptor antagonist would be highly potent and would produce clinical benefits within an hour after ingestion. It would have a duration of action of at least 24 hours. It would be completely devoid of undesirable effects. No first-generation H_1-receptor antagonist fulfils all these criteria, but some of the new, interesting H_1-receptor antagonists currently undergoing clinical trials may meet these expectations.

* *Faculty of Medicine, Section of Allergy & Clinical Immunology, Department of Pediatrics and Child Health, University of Manitoba, Winnipeg, Manitoba, Canada R3A 1S1*

** *Faculty of Pharmacy, University of Manitoba, Winnipeg, Manitoba, Canada R3T 2N2*

PHARMACOKINETICS AND PHARMACODYNAMICS

Like their predecessors,[1-9] the new H_1-receptor antagonists have variable pharmacokinetics (Table I). Some of the new drugs are unique. *Astemizole*, for example, has a half-life of approximately 5 days (parent compound), but its metabolites have a half-life of approximately 18 days. It takes weeks to reach steady-state serum concentrations with this drug and to achieve peak effects.[10-16] This disadvantage can be partially overcome if a loading dose is given during the first week of treatment.[17] Studies of astemizole pharmacodynamics suggest that it is unsuitable for sporadic use or for *rapid* relief of allergic rhinitis or urticaria symptoms.

Cetirizine is a carboxylic acid metabolite of the piperazine, hydroxyzine. Unlike other H_1-receptor antagonists, it does not undergo transformation in the liver. Its pharmacokinetic characteristics differ considerably from those of other H_1-receptor antagonists. Even when cetirizine is administered in tablet or capsule formulations, peak serum cetirizine concentrations occur within 1 hour. Plasma protein binding is high. Cetirizine is eliminated primarily by renal clearance, with 70% of the drug being excreted in unchanged form in the urine within 24 hours after ingestion of a dose. Cetirizine has a half-life of 8–9 hours in adults. In elderly patients with renal impairment, the half-life may increase to 11 or 12 hours. Significant wheal and flare suppression lasts for 24 hours after one 10-mg dose.[18-20]

Loratadine in the usual dose of 10 mg gives peak serum concentrations within a few hours. The half-life is approximately 12 hours, but the suppressive effect on the histamine-induced wheal and flare lasts for 12–24 hours.[21-24]

Levocabastine, at least in animal studies, is 15,000 times as potent as chlorpheniramine, 1,500 times as

Table I

Some New Histamine H_1-Receptor Antagonists

Drug	Molecular Structure	Dose	Serum Elimination Half-Life (hr)	Duration of Action After a Single Dose	Efficacy Compared to Chlorpheniramine*
Astemizole†	Tricyclic	10 mg once daily	120	Weeks	>
Cetirizine	Tricyclic	10 mg once daily	8.5	24 hr	=
Loratadine	Tricyclic	10 mg once daily	12	12–24 hr	=
Levocabastine	Cyclohexylpiperidine	0.2 mg of 0.5% solution topically twice daily	35	Up to 72 hr	>
Ketotifen	Tricyclic (thiophene)	1 mg twice daily	20.4	12 hr	=
Azelastine	Phthalazinone	2 mg twice daily		12 hr	=

* *Direct double-blind comparison in humans not available yet for all drugs.*
† *Loading dose should be given.*

potent as terfenadine, and 65 times as potent as astemizole. It is water-soluble and effective when applied topically to the nasal mucous membrane and the conjunctivae. A single topical application of levocabastine blocks the nasal and conjunctival response to histamine or antigen challenge for 24–72 hours.[25–28] Some systemic absorption occurs from the mucosa, the serum concentrations being about 1/30 of the steady-state level achieved after giving 0.5 mg of levocabastine by mouth.

Ketotifen has multiple effects in addition to its antihistaminic effect. Among other things, it prevents mediator release from human mast cells, basophils, and chopped lung, inhibits calcium transport across cell membranes, has a weak anti-serotonin effect and reduces human neutrophil activation induced by PAF-acether. Ketotifen has a serum elimination phase half-life value of 20.4 hours and a duration of action of at least 12 hours. It is maximally effective after 6–12 weeks of treatment, at least in asthma.[29–31]

Azelastine is a phthalazinone and, it, too, has antiallergic effects as well as antihistaminic effects. In addition, it has been reported as having anti-leukotriene effects, at least in the guinea pig. The exact mechanism of action of the antiallergic effect of this drug is unknown, but antagonism of Ca^{2+}-dependent steps in the process of mediator secretion has been postulated. Azelastine has a serum elimination half-life of approximately 12 hours and twice daily dosage is required.[32,33]

For all H_1-receptor antagonists studied to date[34–37] in children, clearance rates are more rapid and half-life values are shorter than in adults (Table II).

ADVERSE EFFECTS

Most of the new H_1-receptor antagonists are not very lipid-soluble and do not cross the blood-brain barrier to any extent. They are, therefore, relatively nonsedating, meaning that in clinical trials, they cause the same incidence of sedation as placebo. This property is not universal. Azelastine occasionally causes marked drowsiness. Ketotifen has sedative effects in about 15% of adults, when given in the usual dose of 1 mg twice daily; this tends to be worse in the first week of treatment and ameliorates over time. The absence of sedation from the new H_1-receptor antagonists is not necessarily a welcome feature for all patients, especially those with itchy skin secondary to urticaria or atopic dermatitis who may actually miss the sedative effect of the first-generation drugs.[38,39]

The new H_1-receptor antagonists do not have clinically significant anticholinergic effects. Some of them, such as ketotifen and astemizole, may cause excessive weight gain, possibly due to their anti-serotonin effects. Azelastine causes a dose-related, dry, metallic taste in the mouth.

The safety of the new drugs in pregnancy has not been determined at this time. H_1-receptor antagonists as a class are consumed ubiquitously worldwide with and without prescription, and no major problems with teratogenicity have been observed. However, in rats, norcyclizine, a metabolite of some of the piperazine antihistamines, is a teratogen. Although it is somewhat reassuring that none of the new H_1-receptor antagonists with a tricyclic structure, including cetirizine, is metabolized to norcyclizine, the use of any of these new drugs should be avoided by women in the first trimester of pregnancy, until further studies have been performed.

EFFICACY

While some of the new H_1-receptor antagonists will no doubt be used in a traditional role for control

Table II

Pharmacokinetics of H_1-Receptor Antagonists

	$T_{1/2}$ (hr)	
	Children	**Adults**
Chlorpheniramine	11.0	24.4
Hydroxyzine	7.1	20.0
Terfenadine*	2.0	4.5
Cetirizine	6.2	8.3

* *Terfenadine metabolite I.*

of itching, sneezing, and rhinorrhea in patients with allergic rhinitis and for control of itching in patients with urticaria and atopic dermatitis, one can envisage expanded and different roles for many of the new drugs. For example, levocabastine as a topical agent will be extremely useful in the management of allergic conjunctivitis, as well as in the management of allergic rhinitis. Ketotifen and azelastine will probably find their chief applications in the treatment of asthma and will be especially useful in patients with mild asthma who also have some other allergic disorder such as allergic rhinoconjunctivitis or urticaria.

The relative potency of the new H_1-receptor antagonists is not perfectly understood at this time, as direct comparative studies in humans are not yet available for most of the new drugs. Astemizole[10–17] and levocabastine[25–28] are more potent than chlorpheniramine and terfenadine. Astemizole rivals hydroxyzine for potency as long as loading doses of astemizole are given in the first week of treatment.[17] Apart from these two exceptions, the new H_1-receptor antagonists are no more potent than the H_1-receptor antagonists presently in use. Loratadine and cetirizine seem to have potency comparable to that of chlorpheniramine and terfenadine.

It is unrealistic to expect any of the new drugs to be more effective than the old drugs in relieving nasal congestion, a symptom notoriously not well relieved by H_1-receptor antagonists.

CLINICAL INVESTIGATION FACILITATED BY THE NEW, NONSEDATING H_1-RECEPTOR ANTAGONISTS

The new H_1-receptor antagonists have been particularly useful in providing insights into the class of drugs as a whole. For example, they have facilitated studies of subsensitivity to H_1-receptor antagonist activity. Their relative lack of sedation leads to improved compliance in dosing regimens over weeks and months of treatment, in contrast to the noncompliance due to sedation that may occur when antihistamines such as hydroxyzine or chlorpheniramine are given over long periods of time.[40,41] Some of the apparent "subsensitivity" to the first-generation drugs may have been due to noncompliance, as subsensitivity does not appear to develop readily to nonsedating drugs such as terfenadine and loratadine.[22,42] Also, there is little evidence that autoinduction of enzymes metabolizing the H_1-receptor antagonists contributes to subsensitivity.[43]

The new, nonsedating H_1-receptor antagonists can be tested in a truly double-blind fashion in chronic or induced asthma. Their efficacy in prevention or relief of bronchospasm has led to the definite conclusion that H_1-receptor antagonists individually and as a class are not, per se, harmful to patients with asthma who happen to require these drugs for an allergic disorder such as rhinitis.[29–33,44–48]

In vitro studies comparing ketotifen with first-generation H_1-receptor antagonists such as chlorpheniramine have led to our understanding that many of the first-generation drugs have antiallergic effects in addition to their antihistaminic effects.[49]

Investigation of drugs such as levocabastine has shown that an H_1-receptor antagonist applied topically to mucous membranes does not necessarily result in sensitization of the patient to the drugs.[25–28]

SUMMARY

H_1- receptor antagonist research has entered a phase of unprecedented activity. Information about individual new H_1-receptor antagonists is exciting, but, best of all, this information is contributing to our increased understanding of these drugs as a class and is helping investigators to shed light on many of the old, intriguing questions about these most useful pharmacologic compounds.

REFERENCES

1. Simons FER, Simons KJ. H_1-receptor antagonists: clinical pharmacology and use in allergic disease. Pediatr Clin North Am 30:899–914, 1983.
2. Vallner JJ, Needham TE, Chan W, Viswanathan CT. Intravenous administration of chlorpheniramine to seven subjects. Curr Ther Res 26:449–453, 1979.
3. Yacobi A, Stoll RG, Chao GC, Carter JE, Baaske DM, Kamath BL, Amann AH, Lai CM. Evaluation of sustained-action chlorpheniramine-pseudoephedrine dosage forms in humans. J Pharm Sci 69:1077–1081, 1980.
4. Huang S-M, Athanikar NK, Sridhar K, Huang YC, Chiou WL. Pharmacokinetics of chlorpheniramine after intravenous and oral administration in normal adults. Eur J Clin Pharmacol 22:359–365, 1982.
5. Kotzan JA, Vallner JJ, Stewart JT, Brown WJ, Viswanathan CT, Needham TE, Dighe SV, Malinowski R. Bioavailability of regular and controlled-release chlorpheniramine products. J Pharm Sci 71:919–923, 1982.
6. Simons FER, Frith EM, Simons KJ. The pharmacokinetics and antihistaminic effects of brompheniramine. J Allergy Clin Immunol 70:458–464, 1982.
7. Findlay JWA, Butz RF, Coker GG, DeAngelis RL, Welch

RM. Triprolidine radioimmunoassay: disposition in animals and humans. J Pharm Sci 73:1339–1344, 1984.
8. Simons KJ, Singh M, Gillespie CA, Simons FER. An investigation of the H_1-receptor antagonist triprolidine: pharmacokinetics and antihistaminic effects. J Allergy Clin Immunol 77:326–330, 1986.
9. Simons FER, Simons KJ, Frith EM. The pharmacokinetics and antihistaminic effects of the H_1-receptor antagonist hydroxyzine. J Allergy Clin Immunol 73:69–75, 1984.
10. Richards DM, Brogden RN, Heel RC, Speight TM, Avery GS. Astemizole: a review of its pharmacodynamic properties and therapeutic efficacy. Drugs 28:38–61, 1984.
11. Callier J, Engelen RF, Ianniello I, Olzem R, Zeisner M, Amery WK. Astemizole (R 43 512) in the treatment of hay fever. An international double-blind study comparing a weekly treatment (10 mg and 25 mg) with a placebo. Curr Ther Res 29:24–35, 1981.
12. Howarth PH, Emanuel MB, Holgate ST. Astemizole, a potent histamine H_1-receptor antagonist: effect in allergic rhinoconjunctivitis, on antigen and histamine-induced skin wheal responses and relationship to serum levels. Br J Clin Pharmacol 18:1–8, 1984.
13. Howarth PH, Holgate ST. Comparative trial of two non-sedative H_1 antihistamines, terfenadine and astemizole, for hay fever. Thorax 39:668–672, 1984.
14. Malmberg H, Holopainen E, Grahne B, Binder E, Savolainen S, Sundberg S. Astemizole in the treatment of hay fever. Allergy 38:227–231, 1983.
15. Bernstein IL, Bernstein DI: Efficacy and safety of astemizole, a long-acting and non-sedating H_1-antagonist for the treatment of chronic idiopathic urticaria. J Allergy Clin Immunol 77:37–42, 1986.
16. Fox RW, Lockey RF, Bukantz SC, Serbousek D. The treatment of mild to severe chronic idiopathic urticaria with astemizole: double-blind and open trials. J Allergy Clin Immunol 78:1159–1166, 1986.
17. Gendreau-Reid L, Simons KJ, Simons FER. Comparison of the suppressive effect of astemizole, terfenadine, and hydroxyzine on histamine-induced wheals and flares in humans. J Allergy Clin Immunol 77:335–40, 1986.
18. Simons FER, Simons KJ, Yeh J, Chung DM. The comparative pharmacokinetics of H_1-receptor antagonists. Ann Allergy In press.
19. Wood S, Chasseaud LF. The metabolism and pharmacokinetics of ^{14}C-cetirizine in man. Ann Allergy In press.
20. Gengo FM, Dabronzo J, Yurchak A, Love S, Miller JK. The relative antihistaminic and psychomotor effects of hydroxyzine and cetirizine. Clin Pharm 42:265–272, 1987.
21. Batenhorst RL, Batenhorst AS, Graves DA, Foster TS, Kung M, Gural RP, Amkraut HJ. Pharmacologic evaluation of loratadine (SCH 29851), chlorpheniramine and placebo. Eur J Clin Pharmacol 31:247–250, 1986
22. Barnett A, Iorio LC, Kreutner W, Tozzi S, Ahn HS, Gulbenkian A. Evaluation of the CNS properties of SCH 29851, a potential non-sedating antihistamine. Agents Actions 14:590–597, 1984.
23. Roman IJ, Kassem N, Gural RP, Herron J. Suppression of histamine-induced wheal response by loratadine (SCH29851) over 28 days in man. Ann Allergy 57:253–256, 1986.
24. Bruttmann G, Pedrali P. Loratadine (SCH29851) 40 mg once daily versus terfenadine 60 mg twice daily in the treatment of seasonal allergic rhinitis. J Int Med Res 15:63–70, 1987.
25. Feinberg G, Stokes TC. Application of histamine-induced conjunctivitis to the assessment of a topical antihistamine, levocabastine. Int Arch Allergy Appl Immunol 82:537–538, 1987.
26. Pecoud A, Zuber P, Kolly M. Effect of a new selective H_1-receptor antagonist (levocabastine) in a nasal and conjunctival provocation test. Int Arch Allergy Appl Immunol 82:541–543, 1987.
27. Pipkorn U, Bende M, Hedner J, Hedner T. A double-blind evaluation of topical levocabastine, a new specific H_1 antagonist in patients with allergic conjunctivitis. Allergy 40:491–496, 1985.
28. Kolly M, Pecoud A. Comparison of levocabastine, a new selective H_1-receptor antagonist, and disodium cromoglycate, in a nasal provocation test with allergen. Br J Clin Pharmacol 22:389–394, 1986.
29. Simons FER, Luciuk GH, Becker AB, Gillespie CA. Ketotifen: a new drug for prophylaxis of asthma in children. Ann Allergy 48:145–150, 1982.
30. Craps LP. Immunologic and therapeutic aspects of ketotifen. J Allergy Clin Immunol 76:389–393, 1985.
31. Tinkelman DG, Moss BA, Bukantz SC, Sheffer AL, Dobken JH, Chodosh S, Cohen BM, Rosenthal RR, Rappaport I, Buckley CE, Chusid EL, Deutsch AJ, Settipane GA, Burns RBP. A multicentre trial of the prophylactic effect of ketotifen, theophylline, and placebo in atopic asthma. J Allergy Clin Immunol 76:487–497, 1985.
32. Diamantis W, Harrison JE, Melton J, Perhach JL, Sofia RD. In vivo and in vitro H_1 antagonist properties of azelastine. Pharmacologist 23:149, 1981.
33. Zechel H-J, Brock N, Lenke D, Achterrath-Tuckermann U. Pharmacological and toxicological properties of azelastine: a novel antiallergic agent. Arnzeim-Forsch/Drug Res 31:1184–1193, 1981.
34. Simons FER, Luciuk GH, Simons KJ. Pharmacokinetics and efficacy of chlorpheniramine in children. J Allergy Clin Immunol 69:376–381, 1982.
35. Simons FER, Simons KJ, Becker AB, Haydey RP. Pharmacokinetics and antipruritic effects of hydroxyzine in children with atopic dermatitis. J Pediatr 104:123–127, 1984.
36. Uden D. Clinical pharmacokinetics of cetirizine 5 mg po in pediatric patients with allergic rhinitis. Cetirizine Investigators Manual New York: Pfizer, 1986.
37. Simons FER, Watson WTA, Simons KJ. The pharmacokinetics and pharmacodynamics of terfenadine in children. J Allergy Clin Immunol In Press.
38. Krause LB, Shuster S. The effect of terfenadine on dermographic wealing. Br J Dermatol 110:73–79, 1984.
39. Krause LB, Shuster S. Mechanism of action of antipruritic drugs. Br Med J 287:1199–1200, 1983.
40. Taylor RJ, Long WF, Nelson HS. The development of subsensitivity to chlorpheniramine. J Allergy Clin Immunol 76:103–107, 1985.
41. Long WF, Taylor RJ, Leavengood DC, Nelson HS. Skin test suppression by antihistamines and the development of subsensitivity. J Allergy Clin Immunol 76:113–117, 1985.
42. Simons FER, Gillespie CA, Simons KJ. Does sub-sensitivity to terfenadine develop during chronic dosing? Clin Invest Med 10:49, 1987.
43. Simons KJ, Simons FER. The effect of chronic administration of hydroxyzine on hydroxyzine pharmacokinetics in dogs. J Allergy Clin Immunol 79:928–932, 1987.
44. Clee MD, Ingram CG, Reid PC, Robertson AS. The effect of astemizole on exercise-induced asthma. Br J Dis Chest 78:180–183, 1984.
45. Holgate ST, Emanuel MB, Howarth PH. Astemizole and other H_1-antihistaminic drug treatment of asthma. J Allergy Clin Immunol 76:375–380, 1985.
46. Brik A, Tashkin DP, Gong H, Dauphinee B, Lee E. Effect of

cetirizine, a new histamine H_1 antagonist, on airway dynamics and responsiveness to inhaled histamine in mild asthma. J Allergy Clin Immunol 80:51–56, 1987.

47. Ollier S, Gould CAL, Davies RJ. The effect of single and multiple dose therapy with azelastine on the immediate asthmatic response to allergen provocation testing. J Allergy Clin Immunol 78:358–364, 1986.

48. Kemp JP, Meltzer EO, Orgel HA, Welch MJ, Bucholtz GA, Middleton E, Spector SL, Newton JJ, Perhach JL. A dose-response study of the bronchodilator action of azelastine in asthma. J Allergy Clin Immunol 79:893–899, 1987.

49. Church MK, Gradidge CF. Inhibition of histamine release from human lung in vitro by antihistamines and related drugs. Br J Pharmacol 69:663–667, 1980. □

Chapter XXV

Summary of H_1 and H_2 Histamine Receptors

Guy A. Settipane, M.D.

Histamine, a B-imidazolylethylamine, is predominantly found in tissue mast cells and circulating basophils. The tissue content of histamine corresponds to the number of those cells in the tissue or fluids studied. The release of histamine from mast cells and circulating basophils predominantly occur in response to an antigen-IgE antibody interaction or by nonspecific stimulus that degranulate these cells. Some of the nonspecific causes are certain drugs such as opiate derivatives and intravenous or intraarterial radiopaque contrast media used in diagnostic studies. Other nonspecific stimuli may be trauma or other physical agents. In chapter I, Beaven and WoldeMussie state that histamine is found in blister fluid produced by trauma (skin suction and heat, cold, solar radiation or pressure). The average tissue histamine levels in adults are 5–10 $\mu g/g$. Histamine levels in plasma are 1% of that in blood and less than 0.01% of that in tissue. Cerebral spinal fluid has high concentrations of histamine with levels slightly lower than that found in blood. Histamine levels in tears and gastric juice and saliva are higher than that found in plasma. The turnover rate of histamine is about 1% per day of the total body pool of histamine and represents a combination of degranulation of basophils and mast cells.

Rapid inactivation of histamine mainly occurs in the vascular endothelial cells with the involvement of two enzymes: histamine-N-methyltransferase and diamine oxidase. Less than 3% of injected histamine appears unchanged in the urine. To produce generalized symptoms, usually the plasma histamine level should be above 1 ng/ml. Since there are potentially lethal quantities of histamine present in our tissues, efficient mechanisms for histamine clearance and inactivation are necessary for survival. A large intravenous injection of histamine is usually cleared from the plasma in five minutes.

In pathological conditions, changes in histamine levels are usually well correlated with changes in pathophysiological parameters. Examples of such correlations are diseases associated with abnormal numbers of mast cells (mastocytosis) and basophils (chronic myelogenous leukemia, polycythemia vera) or reactions associated with mast cell degranulation (asthmatic attacks, physically-induced urticarias, anaphylactic or drug reactions). Procedures developed by Beaven and WoldeMussie as well as other laboratories and the precautions that should be observed in the measurement of histamine in body fluids are critically reviewed in Chapter I.

Classically there are two different types of histamine receptors: H1 receptors and H2 receptors. The H2 receptors which regulate gastric acid secretion were formally identified in 1972 with the discovery of a newly synthesized compound, burimamide, which blocked the H2 receptor. Later two different types of histamine analogues, which selectively stimulate the H1 and H2 receptors were discovered. The upper respiratory tract is predominantly effected by the H1 receptors and the gastrointestinal tract is predominately effected by the H2 receptors. A summary of the major histamine responses by receptor subtypes are listed in Chapter II by Casale. He states that the mediation of histamine's actions occurs as a consequence of the generation of either cyclic GMP or cyclic AMP subsequent to the stimulation of specific H1 or H2 receptors, respectively. The development of specific histamine receptor agonists and antagonists and radioligand binding techniques have proved useful in the elucidation of the precise sequence of events following histamine receptor interactions. In addition, knowledge of histamine receptor subtypes and histamine-induced post-receptor events has proven beneficial in the development of treatment modalities for diseases such as anaphylaxis and the Zollinger-Ellison syndrome.

In Chapter III, Beer discusses the abnormalities in the histamine-induced suppressor cell network in atopic subjects. He states that antibody responses of the IgE isotype, like other immunoglobulin classes, are regulated by a finely-tuned network of complex positive and negative regulatory factors. In atopic subjects, there is a reduction in the generation of histamine-induced suppressor cell activity which positively correlates with decreased phenotypic expression of histamine-type 2 receptors on T lymphocytes. Nonatopic control subjects with systemic mastocytosis have normal functional and phenotypic data, suggesting that chronic in vivo activation by histamine of T cells from atopics does not explain the abnormal histamine-induced suppressor response. Proper functioning of the histamine-induced suppressor cell system involves obligatory interactions between lymphocytes and monocytes. Monocytes from atopic subjects produced significantly less prostaglandin E2 in response to exogenous histamine-induced suppressor factor. A new immunostimulatory drug, Fanetizole mesylate, partially corrects the abnormal histamine-induced suppressor response. Clinical application of this information may lead to new treatments of the atopic diathesis.

In chapter IV Kaliner describes the role of histamine receptors in anaphylaxis, which is an acute medical emergency caused by systemic mast cell degranulation in response to diverse stimuli. The etiology of anaphylaxis ranges from IgE-mediated allergic reactions to anaphylactoid responses caused by infusions of radiocontrast media. The common thread in the spectrum of causes is mast cell degranulation with systemic release of mediators, particularly histamine. As histamine is one of the predominant causes of the clinical changes occurring in anaphylaxis, treatment of anaphylaxis requires both H1 and H2 histamine receptor antagonists in addition to epinephrine.

The most frequent causes of human anaphylaxis include penicillin reactions, insect stings, and radiocontrast dye reactions. The primary organs involved are cutaneous, gastrointestinal, respiratory, and cardiovascular systems, all of which contain the richest sources of mast cells. The usual progression of symptoms begins within minutes of exposure to the inciting agent, peaks within 15–30 minutes and is complete within hours. Symptoms of anaphylaxis can be attributed primarily to the local actions of the many mast cell mediators and the circulating effect of histamine. The majority of the changes occurring in anaphylaxis can be attributed to histamine (acting through H1 and H2 receptors), prostaglandins, and leukotrienes.

The diagnosis most easily confused with anaphylaxis is a vasovagal reaction which is associated with pallor, extreme diaphoresis and bradycardia with the absence of flushing, urticaria, angioedema, pruritus and asthma. Bradycardia may be the most important differential point since anaphylaxis is associated with marked tachycardia or shock.

Kaliner emphasizes that a recent complexity in the treatment of anaphylaxis has developed with the increased use of β-adrenergic blocking agents in many subjects (e.g., headaches, hypertension, heart failure, glaucoma). It appears that β-adrenergic receptor antagonists potentiate allergic reactions, possibly by reducing the normal homeostatic influences induced by circulating catecholamines. Treatment of anaphylaxis in the presence of β-adrenergic blockade should be essentially unchanged, recognizing the fact that agents such as epinephrine that ordinarily stimulate both α- and β-adrenergic receptors will act predominately upon α-receptors under these circumstances. Asthma developing as part of the spectrum of anaphylaxis should not be treated solely with β-adrenergic agonists as they are likely to be ineffective. When searching for underlying causes of unexplained anaphylaxis, attention should be directed at topical β-adrenergic antagonists used in the treatment of glaucoma.

The next chapter deals with neural-chemical receptors found in the nose and upper respiratory tract. There are six neural-chemical receptors identified in the nose. Five of these are highly functional and play important roles in the physiology of the nose. These nasal receptors are the α-adrenoceptor, β2 adrenoceptor, cholinoceptor, H1 histamine receptor, H2 histamine receptor (essentially nonfunctional), and the irritant receptor.

The H1 histamine receptor is stimulated by histamine, which causes a direct and indirect increase in nasal airway resistance. If histamine is placed in one nasal canal, both canals will have an increased nasal resistance to airflow, but the side without histamine will be congested only about 60% as much as the side with histamine. Therefore, it is postulated that about 60% of the nasal congestion is indirectly produced by histamine through neural reflex action. Repeated application of histamine to the nasal mucosa will produce tachyphylaxis of this neural reflex but will not inhibit the direct action of histamine on the mucosa. H1 antihistamines block the H1 receptors, greatly diminishing the effect of histamine. H1 antihistamines do not improve nasal airway resistance, but they do suppress sneezing, itching and hypersecretion.

The H2 histamine receptor is essentially nonfunctioning in the nose. The anatomic location, description, function, and physiology of this receptor are described in detail in sections of this book. Essentially, it is stimulated by histamine and is blocked by cimetidine and other newer types of H2 antihistamines. H1 antihistamines have no effect on the H2 histamine receptors. The alpha adrenoceptor is stimulated by neosynepherine and norepinephrine-like drugs causing a decreased nasal airway resistance. Most topical nasal medications are directed toward the alpha adrenoceptor. Reserpine and reserpine-like drugs deplete natural occurring norepinephrine from neural junctions, causing an increased nasal airway resistance.

Unlike its effect on the lung, stimulation of the $\beta 2$-adrenoceptor increases airway resistance in the nose. Isoproterenol application to the nose causes an increased airway resistance, which is blocked by propranolol. One hypothesis for this opposite action on the nose compared to the lung is that $\beta 2$ adrenoceptor agonists cause relaxation of smooth muscles. In the lung, this action results in bronchial dilation. The only smooth muscle present in the nose is associated with the blood capillary walls, and relaxation of these muscles result in dilation of the capillaries, engorgement of blood vessels, and extravasation of fluid. The end result is nasal congestion.

The cholinoceptor is part of the parasympathetic system and is stimulated by methacholine which causes profuse rhinorrhea. The cholinoceptor is blocked by atropine. Antihistamines have no effect on this receptor.

The irritant receptor is an extremely important receptor, whose significance has been appreciated only recently. This receptor is stimulated by nonspecific chemicals such as dust, histamines, NH3 and SO2. Most of the action of this receptor is through neural reflex action and is inhibited by atropine. Local anesthetics to the nose, such as lidocaine, will also inhibit this reflex. Antihistamines, both H1 and H2 do not inhibit actions initiated by the irritant receptor.

The irritant receptor plays an important role in the rhinobronchial reflex. Stimulation of neural receptors in the nose, pharyngeal and sinus areas can produce bronchospasm through neural reflexes. The receptors involved are the histamine (H1) and irritant receptors which send afferent neural impulses through the Trigeminal, Facial and Glossopharyngeal nerve to the medulla oblongata where the vagal nucleus is stimulated. The efferent arm of this reflex is the vagal nerve with its ramifications sending neural impulses to the bronchial tree causing bronchospasm.

There are other important neural reflexes involving the nose. The most common is the sneezing reflex. An extremely important reflex is the submersion reflex, which results in apnea, bradycardia, and increased blood pressure. This reflex is related to that of aquatic mammals and is responsible for saving the lives of many children who otherwise would have drowned.

The next two chapters discuss lower airway receptors. Barnes states that there appears to be two major cellular systems that initiate responses and both are activated by receptors on the cell surface. Receptors are activated by specific agonists which lead to the response either by changing intracellular cAMP or by increasing intracellular calcium. Receptors which involve cAMP activate or inhibit adenylate cyclase involve a linking protein, nucleotide regulatory protein which either stimulates or inhibits the enzyme. Other receptors which result in increases in intracellular CA^{2+} cause hydrolysis of phosphatidyl inositol in the membrane. In the lungs, the autonomic neural receptors are β-adrenoceptors, α-adrenoceptors, cholinergic receptors and possibly the nonadrenergic noncholinergic receptors (the peptides, VIP and substance P). The mediator receptors in the lungs are H1 and H2 histamine receptors, leukotriene receptors (B4, C4, D4, E4); prostaglandin receptors (prostacyclin, PGD2, PGF2, PGE2 and thromboxane A2), adenosine receptors, platelet activating factor (PAF), and bradykinin receptors.

The receptors whose action causes bronchial constriction are as follows: α-adrenoceptors, cholinergic receptors, noncholinergic excitatory receptors (activated by substance P), H1 histamine receptors, leukotrienes (B4, C4, D4 and E4), prostaglandin receptors (PGD2, PGF2α, thromboxane A2), adenosine receptors, PAF receptors and bradykinin receptors.

Receptors whose action causes bronchial dilatation are as follows: β-adrenoceptors, nonadrenergic inhibitory receptors (activated by the peptide VIP), and prostaglandin E2 receptor.

The function of β-adrenoceptors have been further elaborated. Barnes states that relaxation by exogenous β-agonists is mediated by $\beta 2$-receptors, but relaxation by sympathetic nerve stimulation is mediated by $\beta 1$-receptors. These findings are consistent with the view that $\beta 1$ receptors are regulated by sympathetic nerves (neuronal β-receptors), whereas $\beta 2$-receptors are regulated by circulating epinephrine (hormonal β-receptors). In human airway smooth muscle which has no sympathetic innervation, no $\beta 1$-receptor mediated effects occurs. This has been confirmed in functional studies in vitro, in which relaxation of central and peripheral airways is mediated only by $\beta 2$-receptors. Autoradiographic studies of β-receptor subtypes in human lung have confirmed that β-receptors of human airway smooth muscle from bronchi to terminal bronchioles are entirely of the $\beta 2$-subtype.

In his chapter, Braman reviews evidence that the human lungs have both H1 and H2 histamine receptors, but H1-receptors, which mediate bronchoconstriction, predominate. H1 receptor antagonist can produce significant bronchodilatation in some asthmatics, block bronchoconstriction induced by antigen and histamine inhalation challenge, and have some protective effect against exercise and aspirin-induced bronchoconstriction. H2 receptors mediate bronchidilatation, but this effect is relatively weak in man. However, H2 receptors increase vascular permeability, bronchial mucous production and bronchial epithelial permeability. It is probable that several mechanisms of histamine-induced bronchial smooth muscle contraction are important. These include:

1) direct smooth muscle stimulation by the H1 receptor,

2) neural receptor mediated reflex cholinergic bronchoconstriction.

3) the release of secondary mediators (prostaglandins, thromboxanes, etc.) through activation of both H1 and H2 receptors.

The role of classic antihistamines (H1 receptor antagonists) in the treatment of asthma has not been established. Since factors that precipitate asthma are quite varied, these agents may provide benefit in selected patients.

The main objection to using antihistamine in asthma is sedation, and the dryness that is produced by their anticholinergic effect. Newer, nonsedating antihistamines especially those still under investigation are devoid of cholinergic effect (drying) and therefore, are more acceptable for use in asthmatic patients. Recently, we treated 10 patients with both asthma and rhinitis with 4 mg of chlorpheniramine or placebo on a double blind basis. No significant difference was found in pulmonary function tests three hours later, and no patient complained of sedation or dryness. We concluded that oral chlorpheniramine may have no ill effect on stable asthmatic patients and feel that FDA warning labels placed on antihistamines for use in asthma may be unnecessary.

Hirschowitz discusses histamine receptors and the gut. The gastric mucosa of all vertebrates is relatively rich in histamine which is a strong stimulus for secretion of gastric acid. Histamine stimulation of acid secretion is mediated via cAMP, and this effect is blocked by very small amounts of prostaglandins E2. With few exceptions, the H2 antagonists have been potent inhibitors of acid secretion in all animal species tested. H2 antagonists do not inhibit cholinergic muscarinic stimuli. Histamine stimulates the secretion of pepsin co-equally with gastric acid. This secretion is unaffected by H1-antagonists but is inhibited by H2 antagonists. H2 antagonists have no direct effect on serum gastrin.

As a rule, muscular contraction of the gut including the stomach, pylorus and intestine occurs with stimulation of H1 histamine receptors. H2 receptor agonists relax the smooth muscle of the stomach and the gallbladder.

A practical clinical application of the H2 antagonist is the suppression of gastric acid secretion. Since its release eight years ago, cimetidine has been used in perhaps 30 million patients and is the largest selling drug in the world. In the last few years, ranitidine another more potent H2 antagonist, with a nitrofuran configuration, has also come into general use for the treatment of duodenal ulcer and hypersecretory states.

Worldwide endoscopically-controlled double-blind trials of cimetidine and ranitidine tested against each other or against placebo have demonstrated in duodenal ulcers a healing rate of 76% at 4 weeks and 87% at 6 weeks with both drugs, compared to 40% and 45% respectively for placebo. Upon withdrawal of H2 antagonist treatment after healing, there is a recurrence rate of 50–90% in one year. H2 antagonists also have been found to be clinically effective in gastric ulcers, Zollinger-Ellison Syndrome, control of acid secretion in systemic mastocytosis and basophil leukemia, and in erosive gastritis.

Histamine receptors in the heart are discussed by Levi and his colleagues. They state that cardiac manifestations of systemic anaphylaxis range from transient electrocardiographic changes to ventricular fibrillation with complete circulatory collapse. Many of these cardiovascular events are attributable to the stimulation of cardiac H1 and H2 receptors by histamine released during anaphylaxis. Indeed, the heart itself has been shown to contain high concentrations of histamine, which can be released not only by IgE-mediated hypersensitivity reactions, but by various drugs and chemicals as well. Release of cardiac histamine is accompanied by changes in rate, rhythm, contractility, and electrical conduction which can be reproduced by the administration of exogenous histamine. H2-receptors have been shown to mediate histamine-induced increases in sinus rate, myocardial contractility, and electrical automaticity, while decreases in contractility and atrioventricular conduction velocity are H1-mediated.

Histamine receptors in the brain are discussed by Garbarg and Schwartz. They state that in mammalian brain, neuronal histamine is likely to act as a neurotransmitter and is recognized by the two classes of histamine receptors (H1 and H2) previously characterized in peripheral organs. Cerebral H1 receptors can be selectively labeled by a tritiated antagonist mepyramine, in particulate fractions or in the living animal. Cerebral H1 receptors mediate the glycogen hydrolysis and the breakdown of inositol phospholipids elicited by the amine. They are indirectly involved in the histamine-mediated accumulation of cyclic AMP. All these biochemical responses mediated by H1 receptors are calcium-dependent. H2 receptors are coupled to an adenylate cyclase. In addition, a novel class of histamine receptors (H3) are presynaptic autoreceptors that modulate the release of neuronal histamine. The biochemical events mediated by these receptors, in agreement with anatomical and electrophysiological knowledge, suggest for histaminergic neurons a role in the regulation of general levels of activity, of energy reserves, and of vascular controls in large areas of the brain.

There are H1 and H2 histamine receptors associated with skin blood vessels. Frequently an H1 antihistamine is sufficient in treating urticaria but in certain resistant cases of chronic urticaria a combination of H1 and H2 antihistamine has been more successful in treatment than an H1 antihistamine alone. Histamine content of the skin from patients with chronic urticaria is higher than that found in normal skin. Patients with severe cold-induced urticaria appear to develop the highest levels of plasma histamine.

The next chapter deals with histamine release in anesthesia and surgery. Moss states that histamine release can occur in response to anaphylactic or chemically mediated anaphylactoid reactions during general anesthesia. Narcotics and muscle relaxants have been demonstrated both *in vitro* and *in vivo* to cause significant histamine release. This histamine release appears to be directly related to changes in the cardiovascular system that are often seen during anesthesia. The use of combined H1 and H2 antagonists to attenuate the effects of anaphylactoid reactions in humans has been shown in several controlled trials. In addition, recent experience with chymopapain administration suggests that the use of H1 and H2 antagonists may be useful in the prophylaxis of immunologically mediated reactions. The muscle relaxants, especially succinylcholine are most often implicated as the cause of immunologic reactions to anesthetic agents. Cardiovascular collapse followed by bronchospasm are important components of true immunologically-mediated reactions to anesthetic drugs.

The last series of chapters in this book is devoted to specific antihistamines both those presently commercially available and those still under investigation. The lead chapter in this series is on methods of studying antihistamines. Connell states that there are four general methods for studying efficacy of antihistamines. They are the outpatient methods, field trials, challenge trials, and skin test wheal studies. In the outpatient method, subjects are given the treatments to take at home while exposed to the antigen in their usual environment. In the field trial, all subjects are observed at the same time for limited periods while in the same location. The challenge techniques utilize quantitated or semiquantitated amounts of antigen administered to the shock tissue. In the skin test method, antigen is injected into the skin and the reaction observed and measured. Each method has its own advantages and defects. Regardless of the techniques used, it is desirable to use a positive control (known active drug) and a placebo control. Needless to say, it is imperative that the treatments be double-blinded since all of the assays are subjective. These controls help to determine the accuracy of the results and assess the proficiency of each laboratory where the study is conducted. Lastly, a proper informed consent is a prerequisite for any clinical study. Food and Drug Administration (FDA) guidelines are available for these informed consent forms as well as guidelines for institutional review of the protocol for human testing.

The classical H1 antihistamines are discussed by Dr. Cooper. He states that these antihistamines appear to be well absorbed orally and have protein binding that varies from 72% with chlorpheniramine to 98% with diphenhydramine. Metabolism appears to be primarily hepatic with little renal effect. The elimination half-life is reported to be from five hours with triprolidine up to 15–25 hours with chlor- and brompheniramine. Newer agents have even longer half-lives ranging from 16–23 hours with terfenadine, 38 hours with mequitazine and 104 hours with astemizole. In terms of pharmacodynamic distribution of the antihistamines, the highest concentrations appear to be found in the lungs and lower concentrations in spleen, kidneys, brain, muscle and skin. Small amounts of the drug appear to be distributed into breast milk. Onset of action varies from 15–60 minutes by the oral route, parenterally from 15 to 30 minutes, and rectally from 30–45 minutes. Peak effect is usually seen within three to 12 hours with non-sustained release formulations and in eight to 24 hours with prolonged release dosage forms. In this chapter, he lists the various classes of H1 antihistamines together with their pharmacologic actions. Important side effects of these drugs are sedation, mouth drying, irritability, and mood changes. In addition, tachyphylaxis (loss of effectiveness) can occur after a few weeks of using the same antihistamines. Changing from one class of antihistamine to another class will relieve tachyphylaxis.

In the next chapter, Feldman discusses H2 receptor antagonists. He states that the advent of H2 receptor antagonists has dramatically advanced the understanding and treatment of peptic ulcer disease. Ranitidine and cimetidine have been shown to be safe and effective in healing duodenal and gastric ulcers and in prevention of duodenal ulcer relapse. Due to differences in chemical structure, ranitidine is more potent and has a longer duration of action and fewer side effects than cimetidine. The current trend in therapy is toward less frequent dosing patterns with more attention toward controlling nocturnal acid secretion.

Newer antihistamines and histamine-release inhibitors are discussed by Dr. Johnson who states that traditional H1 receptor antagonists are a mainstay of drug therapy for the allergic state, but cause numerous discomforting side effects which often hinder compliance. Newer H1 antagonists, including astemizole and terfenadine, appear remarkably free of central side effects and may provide a therapeutic breakthrough for clinicians. H2 antagonists have revolutionized drug therapy for hypersecretory states. Ranitidine appears to have fewer side effects than cimetidine at this stage in its utilization history, but has not been used as extensively. Other antisecretory agents of promise include some tricyclic antidepressants, prostaglandin derivatives, and potassium-hydrogen ATPase inhibitors. The standard drug for suppression of mediator release from mast cells is cromolyn sodium (disodium cromoglycate). DSCG also is reported to block exercise-induced bronchospasm and late phase reactions as well as sulfur dioxide-induced bronchoconstriction, where mediator release may not be implicated. A major limitation to DSCG therapy has been that the only effective route of administration is insufflation, which some patients find uncomfortable. More recently developed drugs show therapeutic promise. Newer histamine-release inhibitors (ketotifen, oxatimide) are effective orally and offer better patient compliance.

Terfenadine is a novel piperidine-type antihistamine. The structural basis for terfenadine's lack of side effects may reside in the tertiary butyl group and hydroxyl group proximate to the phenyl ring. The tertiary butyl group may retard the ability of terfenadine to pass the blood brain barrier. Terfenadine is discussed by Buckley and colleagues. In their study the effectiveness of 60 mg b.i.d. of terfenadine was compared with an active control, 4 mg t.i.d. of chlorpheniramine, and placebo in many patients with seasonal allergic rhinitis. In contrast to the gradual decrease in seasonal symptoms observed over a 7 day period of study in placebo-treated patients, both antihistamines produced a prompt significant decrease in sneezing and rhinorrhea, and a gradual decrease in nasopharyngeal pruritis. Terfenadine-related sedation did not differ from that produced by the placebo and was less than the sedation produced by the active control.

An extremely promising drug still under development is azelastine (Wallace Laboratories) which is a novel, orally effective and long-acting drug with histamine (H1)-receptor blocking properties. It also exerts receptor blocking activities towards leukotrienes, serotonin, acetylcholine and bradykinin but at concentrations greater than that required to block H1-receptors. In addition azelastine is a potent inhibitor of the allergic and nonallergic chemical mediator release. An exciting finding is that azelastine was found to produce clinically significant bronchodilation of long duration in moderate to severe reversible lower airway disease.

The development of the new antihistamine astemizole (Janssen Pharmaceutical) is discussed by Ray. Astemizole's chemical structure is unrelated to that of histamine and the classic antihistamines. It is an extremely potent and specific H1 antagonist. It does not produce sedation and has an extraordinarily long duration of action lasting over several days. In addition, astemizole lacks anticholinergic activity.

Ketotifen (Sandoz Inc.) is another drug still in the development stage. It initially was studied in asthmatic patients. It is a benzocycloheptathiophene derivative which is orally active. Structurally the compound resembles cyproheptadine and azadatine. The three compounds are all tricyclic with the similar side chain; however, in ketotifen the typical benzene ring has been replaced by a 5-membered sulphur-containing thiophene ring. The compound with this modification retains its antihistaminic effect, but acquires: the ability to stabilize mast cells and inhibit the release of histamine and SRS-A; the ability to effect beta-receptor mediator responses in a manner similar to corticosteroids; the ability to prevent anaphylactic reactions in animals rendered tachyphylactic to DSCG or isoprenoline; and the ability to inhibit calcium transport across mast cell and smooth muscle membranes. The activity of ketotifen in the prophylaxis of asthma is probably due to a combination of these effects. Presently it is being studied in urticarial/angioedema where it appears to be very effective. It is used as an oral preparation.

Ganellin and his colleagues discuss the exciting new drug still under investigation, Icotidine (Smith, Kline & French Laboratories). Icotidine, 2-[4-(3-methoxy-pyrid-2-yl)butylamino]-5-[6-methylpyrid-3-yl)-methyl]-pyrimidine-4-one trihydrochloride, has been identified as a novel agent which combines into one molecule the ability to antagonize the actions of histamine at H1 and H2 receptors across a similar concentration or dose range. The degree of antagonism of vascular responses to histamine exceeds that possible with either an H1- or H2-receptor histamine antagonist alone. Icotidine may have therapeutic utility in conditions requiring simultaneous antagonism of histamine at H1 and H2 receptors.

Another new H_1 antihistamine that is undergoing investigative clinical trials is Loratadine (Schering). It is an tricyclic compound with a half life of 8.5 days and a duration of action of 24 hours. Its efficacy is equivalent to chlortrimeton and virtually is devoid of sedation and has no anticholinergic action. Clinical trials appear promising.

The chapter on cetirizine (Pfizer Pharmaceuticals) by Spector and Altman outlines another exciting H_1 receptor antagonist that is still under investigation in the United States. Cetirizine, a metabolite of hydroxyzine, is in the cyclizine class of H_1 antihistamines and appears to have diminished central nervous system activity. It has a half-life of nine hours. Inhibition of histamine induced bronchospasm with mild bronchodilation has been demonstrated. Thus far clinical trials have affirmed its safety and efficacy.

An epilogue of the new H_1-receptor antagonists by Estelle and Keith Simons concludes the section on new H_1 antihistamines. They point out that H_1 receptor antagonist research has entered a phase of unprecedented activity. They state that the perfect H_1 receptor antihistamine would be highly potent with beneficial effects within one hour and a duration of action of at least 24 hours. Also, it must be devoid of any undesirable effects. Although this perfect antihistamine has not been discovered yet, the newer antihistamines appear to be approaching these expectations. The Simons' compare the molecular structure, dose, half-life, duration of action, and efficacy (compared to chlortrimeton) of astemizole, cetirizine, loratadine, temelastine, levocabastine, ketotifen, and azelastine. Astemizole, levocabastine, and ketotifen have a serum half life of over 20 hours. Most of these new antihistamines have a duration of action over 24 hours except for ketotifen and azelastine which have a duration of action of about 12 hours. Astemizole and levocabastine have a greater efficacy then chlortrimeton. Details of side effects are still under investigation, but the drugs with less sedation appear to have a definite advantage.

In summary, the very important actions of histamine and its receptors have been fully reviewed with emphasis placed on tissue concentration, release mechanism, target organ effect and treatment with H1 and H2 antihistamines. The rapid development of these antihistamines is having a profound effect on patient care and the practice of medicine. It is hoped that the information from this book will culminate in another long step in the evolution of modern medicine. □

INDEX

Note: Page numbers in *italics* refer to figures. Page numbers followed by t refer to tables.